# Pain in Horses: Physiology, Pathophysiology and Therapeutic Implications

*Guest Editor*

WILLIAM W. MUIR, DVM, PhD

# VETERINARY CLINICS OF NORTH AMERICA: EQUINE PRACTICE

www.vetequine.theclinics.com

*Consulting Editor*
A. SIMON TURNER, BVSc, MS

December 2010 • Volume 26 • Number 3

SAUNDERS an imprint of ELSEVIER, Inc.

**W.B. SAUNDERS COMPANY**
*A Division of Elsevier Inc.*

1600 John F. Kennedy Boulevard ● Suite 1800 ● Philadelphia, Pennsylvania 19103

http://www.vetequine.theclinics.com

**VETERINARY CLINICS OF NORTH AMERICA: EQUINE PRACTICE Volume 26, Number 3**

December 2010 ISSN 0749-0739, ISBN-13: 978-1-4377-2502-5

Editor: John Vassallo; j.vassallo@elsevier.com
Developmental Editor: Jessica Demetriou

*Veterinary Clinics of North America: Equine Practice* (ISSN 0749-0739) is published in April, August, and December by Elsevier Inc., 360 Park Avenue South, New York, NY 10010-1710. Business and Editorial Offices: 1600 John F. Kennedy Blvd., Suite 1800, Philadelphia, PA 19103-2899. Subscription prices are $238.00 per year (domestic individuals), $373.00 per year (domestic institutions), $117.00 per year (domestic students/residents), $277.00 per year (Canadian individuals), $466.00 per year (Canadian institutions), $320.00 per year (international individuals), $466.00 per year (international institutions), and $159.00 per year (international and Canadian students/residents). To receive student/resident rate, orders must be accompanied by name of affiliated institution, date of term, and the signature of program/residency coordinator on institution letterhead. Orders will be billed at individual rate until proof of status is received. Foreign air speed delivery is included in all *Clinics* subscription prices. All prices are subject to change without notice. **POSTMASTER:** Send address changes to *Veterinary Clinics of North America: Equine Practice*, 3251 Riverport Lane, Maryland Heights, MO 63043. Customer Service (orders, claims, online, change of address): Elsevier Health Sciences Division, Subscription Customer Service, 3251 Riverport Lane, Maryland Heights, MO 63043. Tel: 1-800-654-2452 (U.S. and Canada); 314-447-8871 (outside U.S. and Canada). Fax: 314-447-8029. E-mail: journalscustomer service-usa@elsevier.com (for print support); E-mail: journalsonlinesupport-usa@elsevier (for online support).

*Reprints*. For copies of 100 or more of articles in this publication, please contact the Commercial Reprints Department, Elsevier Inc., 360 Park Avenue South, New York, NY 10010-1710. Tel.: 212-633-3812; Fax: 212-462-1935; E-mail: reprints@elsevier.com.

*Veterinary Clinics of North America: Equine Practice* is covered in *MEDLINE/PubMed (Index Medicus)*, *Excerpta Medica, Current Contents/Agriculture, Biology and Environmental Sciences*, and *ISI*.

Printed and bound by CPI Group (UK) Ltd, Croydon, CR0 4YY

Transferred to Digital Print 2011

# Contributors

## CONSULTING EDITOR

**A. SIMON TURNER, BVSc, MS**
Diplomate, American College of Veterinary Surgeons; Professor, Department of Clinical
Sciences, College of Veterinary Medicine and Biomedical Sciences, Colorado State
University, Fort Collins, Colorado

## GUEST EDITOR

**WILLIAM W. MUIR, DVM, PhD**
Diplomate, American College of Veterinary Anesthesiologists; Diplomate, American
College of Veterinary Emergency and Critical Care; Equine Anesthesia and Analgesia
Consulting Services, Columbus, Ohio

## AUTHORS

**SIMON N. COLLINS, PhD**
School of Veterinary Science, The University of Queensland, Gatton, Queensland,
Australia; Orthopaedic Research Group, Centre for Equine Studies; Neuromuscular
Research Group, Animal Health Trust, Lanwades Park, Kentford, Newmarket, Suffolk,
United Kingdom

**R. EDDIE CLUTTON, BVSc, MRCVS, DVA, MRCA**
Diplomate, European College of Veterinary Anaesthesia and Analgesia; Professor of
Veterinary Anaesthesiology, Easter Bush Veterinary Centre, University of Edinburgh,
Easter Bush, Roslin, Midlothian, Scotland, United Kingdom

**JANNY C. DE GRAUW, DVM**
Junior Research Fellow, Department of Equine Sciences, Faculty of Veterinary Medicine,
Utrecht University, Yalelaan, Utrecht, The Netherlands

**THOMAS J. DOHERTY, MVB, MSc**
Diplomate, American College of Veterinary Anesthesiologists; Professor, Department
of Large Animal Clinical Sciences, College of Veterinary Medicine, The University
of Tennessee, Knoxville, Tennessee

**KEVIN K. HAUSSLER, DVM, DC, PhD**
Diplomate, American College of Veterinary Sports Medicine and Rehabilitation; Assistant
Professor, Gail Holmes Equine Orthopaedic Research Center, Department of Clinical
Sciences, College of Veterinary Medicine and Biomedical Sciences, Colorado State
University, Fort Collins, Colorado

**KASPAR MATIASEK, DVM, DrMedVet, DrMedVetHabil, FTA-Neuropath, MRCVS**
Neuromuscular Research Group; Neuropathology Laboratory, Animal Health Trust,
Kentford, Newmarket, Suffolk, United Kingdom

**WILLIAM W. MUIR, DVM, PhD**
Diplomate, American College of Veterinary Anesthesiologists; Diplomate, American College of Veterinary Emergency and Critical Care; Equine Anesthesia and Analgesia Consulting Services, Columbus, Ohio

**CLAUDIO C. NATALINI, DVM, MS, PhD**
Professor, Departamento de Farmacologia, Instituto de Ciências Básicas da Saúde, Universidade Federal do Rio Grande do Sul, Porto Alegre RS, Brazil

**CHRISTOPHER POLLITT, BVSc, PhD**
School of Veterinary Science, The University of Queensland, Gatton, Queensland, Australia

**SHEILAH A. ROBERTSON, BVMS, PhD, MRCVS**
Diplomate, American College of Veterinary Anesthesiologists; Diplomate, European College of Veterinary Anaethesia and Analgesia; Professor of Anesthesiology, Section of Anesthesia and Pain Management, Department of Large Animal Clinical Sciences, College of Veterinary Medicine, University of Florida, Gainesville, Florida

**L. CHRIS SANCHEZ, DVM, PhD**
Diplomate, American College of Veterinary Internal Medicine; Associate Professor of Medicine, Department of Large Animal Clinical Sciences, College of Veterinary Medicine, University of Florida, Gainesville, Florida

**M. REZA SEDDIGHI, DVM, PhD**
Assistant Professor, Department of Large Animal Clinical Sciences, College of Veterinary Medicine, The University of Tennessee, Knoxville, Tennessee

**ALEXANDER VALVERDE, DVM, DVSc**
Diplomate, American College of Veterinary Anesthesiologists; Associate Professor, Department of Clinical Studies, Ontario Veterinary College, University of Guelph, Guelph, Ontario, Canada

**P. RENÉ VAN WEEREN, DVM, PhD**
Diplomate, European College of Veterinary Surgeons; Professor of Equine Musculoskeletal Biology, Department of Equine Sciences, Faculty of Veterinary Medicine, Utrecht University, Yalelaan, Utrecht, The Netherlands

**ANN E. WAGNER, DVM, MS**
Diplomate, American College of Veterinary Pathologists; Diplomate, American College of Veterinary Anesthesiologists; Professor, Department of Clinical Sciences, College of Veterinary Medicine and Biomedical Sciences, Colorado State University, Fort Collins, Colorado

**CLAIRE E. WYLIE, BVM&S, MRCVS, MSc**
Epidemiology Research Group, Centre for Preventive Medicine, Animal Health Trust, Kentford, Newmarket, Suffolk, United Kingdom

# Contents

Pain is a multidimensional sensory phenomenon that has evolved as a protective method for maintaining homeostasis and facilitating tissue repair. Both excitatory and inhibitory physiologic and pathologic mechanisms are involved in its generation and maintenance. Untreated pain and nervous system changes (plasticity) that occur during chronic pain make pain much more difficult or impossible to effectively treat. Therapies directed toward the treatment of pain should be mechanism based and preventative whenever possible. Prospective, randomized clinical trials conducted in horses that suffer from naturally occurring pain will help to determine the current best approaches to effective pain therapy.

The stress response represents an animal's attempt to reestablish the body's homeostasis after injury, intense physical activity, or psychological strain. Two different neuroendocrine pathways may be activated in stressful situations: the hypothalamic-pituitary-adrenocortical axis, leading to increased cortisol levels, and the sympathoadrenomedullar system, leading to increased catecholamine levels. By applying some of the evaluation methods described in this article in the appropriate clinical situations, equine veterinarians can almost certainly improve their ability to recognize and manage pain in horses.

Opioid analgesics have been the foundation of human pain management for centuries, and their value in animals has increased since it was proposed that it is the veterinarian's duty to alleviate pain whenever it may occur. Compared with other domesticated species, the horse has benefitted less from the increased understanding of opioid pharmacology in animals, because early literature was overlooked and later work, which examined adverse side effects rather than analgesia, concluded that analgesic and excitatory doses were irreconcilably close. More recent studies have indicated a widening role for opioid analgesics in equine pain management, and radioligand studies have revealed a basis for the equine response pattern to opioid analgesics.

Alpha-2 agonists, such as xylazine, clonidine, romifidine, detomidine, medetomidine, and dexmedetomidine, are potent analgesic drugs that also induce physiologic and behavioral changes, such as hypertension, bradycardia, atrioventricular block, excessive sedation and ataxia, all of which can potentially limit their systemic use as analgesics in some clinical cases. The use of medetomidine and dexmetomidine has been introduced for equine anesthesia/analgesia, and although not approved in this species, their increased specificity for alpha-2 receptors may offer some potential advantages over the traditional alpha-2 agonists. Similarly, other routes of administration and benefits of alpha-2 agonists are recognized in the human and laboratory animal literature, which may prove useful in the equine patient if validated in the near future. This review presents this relevant information.

This article describes the rationale behind the use of systemically administered lidocaine as an analgesic. The analgesic efficacy of intravenously administered lidocaine is well documented by studies in human patients and laboratory animals. The mechanism by which systemically administered lidocaine produces analgesia is uncertain but is thought to include action at sodium, calcium, and potassium channels and the N-methyl-D-aspartate acid receptor. In addition, the anti-inflammatory actions of lidocaine are important in producing analgesia because inflammatory mediators augment neuronal excitability. The available studies of systemically administered lidocaine in horses provide evidence for the analgesic and anesthetic effects of intravenous lidocaine in this species.

In the past 10 years, there have been many recent advances in spinal techniques in horses, both epidural and subarachnoid, to identify drugs or drug combinations that have sensory effects without motor nerve paralysis, thus providing pain control without these horses becoming recumbent. Opioids, alpha-2 agonists, dissociative drugs, and others have been investigated. Many of these drugs, which have serious side effects when injected systemically in horses, have been shown to have useful analgesic effects when injected spinally. Morphine-like opioids have the greatest potential for spinal use as they produce long-lasting analgesia without motor effects. Often the doses used spinally are significantly lower than those needed for systemic effects.

N-Methyl-D-aspartate (NMDA) is a synthetic chemical binding molecule (ligand) that selectively binds to the "slow response" glutamate NMDA receptor (NMDAR). NMDARs are important for normal brain function and play a central role in learning, memory, and the development of central nervous system hyperactive states. Diverse chemicals belonging to various drug families have demonstrated NMDAR antagonistic effects. Ketamine has been shown to produce antihyperalgesic effects produced by incision and tissue or nerve damage, and has become popular in equine practice as an anesthetic and more recently as an analgesic for standing surgical procedures and the treatment of laminitis. This review focuses on the development of ketamine as an anesthetic and analgesic in horses.

Manual therapy includes a diverse array of techniques, such as touch therapies, massage, physical therapy, osteopathy, and chiropractic, that were originally developed for use in humans and have been gradually applied to horses. All forms of manual therapy have variable reported levels of effectiveness for treating musculoskeletal issues in humans, but mostly only anecdotal evidence exists in horses. This article explores the scientific literature for evidence of efficacy, safety, and common mechanisms of action of the different forms of manual therapies for potential use in managing acute or chronic pain syndromes in horses. Currently, there is limited evidence supporting the effectiveness of spinal mobilization and manipulation in reducing pain and muscle hypertonicity. Further research is needed to assess the efficacy of specific manual therapy techniques and their contribution to multimodal protocols for managing specific somatic pain conditions in horses.

Identification and alleviation of visceral pain is a frequent concern for the equine owner and veterinarian. This article discusses sources, methods for identification and quantitation, and options for treatment of visceral pain in horses.

This article focuses on pain associated with osteoarthritis (OA). It first describes the basic biology of articular cartilage and other joint structures and the defining features of the osteoarthritic disease process. Subsequently, the possible origins of pain in OA are discussed before embarking on how to manage this clinical entity. The emphasis is on the pharmacologic management of joint pain, and attention is paid to systemic therapeutic strategies as well as to local (intra-articular) treatment modalities. Nonmedical ways of modulating joint pain are briefly mentioned, but not extensively discussed, as these are outside the scope of this article.

Laminitis poses a threat to all horses, and is widely considered as being one of the most important diseases of horses and a global equine welfare problem. The effects of laminitis lead to debilitation, development of pronounced digital pain, and great suffering in the afflicted animal. The precise pathophysiological processes that result in laminitic pain are poorly defined, and hence the delivery of effective palliative care is clinically challenging. Knowledge and understanding of pain states in other animal species may further aid the elucidation of equine laminitic pain mechanisms, guide the search for treatable causes of this multifactorial problem, and thereby help achieve enhanced therapeutic and palliative care. However, parallels drawn from pain states in other animals must consider species differences in both anatomy and physiology, and the specific nature of the laminitic disease process.

## FORTHCOMING ISSUES

*April 2011*
**Endocrine Diseases**
Ramiro E. Toribio, DVM, PhD,
*Guest Editor*

*August 2011*
**Regenerative Medicine**
Matthew C. Stewart, BVSc, PhD,
and Allison A. Stewart, DVM, MS,
*Guest Editors*

*December 2011*
**Clinical Neurology**
Thomas J. Divers, DVM,
and Amy L. Johnson, DVM,
*Guest Editors*

## RECENT ISSUES

*August 2010*
**Advances in Laminitis, Part II**
Christopher C. Pollitt, BVSc, PhD,
*Guest Editor*

*April 2010*
**Advances in Laminitis, Part I**
Christopher C. Pollitt, BVSc, PhD,
*Guest Editor*

*December 2009*
**Practice Management**
Reynolds Cowles, DVM
*Guest Editor*

---

**RELATED INTEREST**

*Veterinary Clinics of North America: Small Animal Practice*
November 2008 (Vol. 38, No. 6)
**Update on Management of Pain**
Karol A. Mathews, DVM, DVSc, *Guest Editor*

---

## THE CLINICS ARE NOW AVAILABLE ONLINE!

Access your subscription at:
**www.theclinics.com**

# Preface

# Pain in Horses: Physiology, Pathophysiology, and Therapeutic Implications

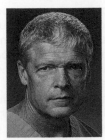

William W. Muir, DVM, PhD
*Guest Editor*

The study of pain mechanisms, processes, and therapies remains multidimensional and complex not only because of the consequences of pain's physical, physiological, and emotional (psychological) components but, and as importantly, because of our inability to develop or provide succinct and precise methods for its evaluation and therapy. Many advances have been made and continue to emerge regarding our understanding of the neurobiological mechanisms responsible for pain but a huge chasm exists between integration of mechanisms into clinical practice, and more importantly, their relevance to therapeutic strategies.

Most of what has been learned is extrapolated from experimental studies conducted in mice and rats. Almost all, if not all, clinically relevant "evidence" is derived from studies conducted in humans. Most studies conducted in animals are insufficiently powered, inadequately assessed, confounded, or biased. Even more disturbing is that pain therapies reported to be effective in rats, dogs, or humans are assumed to be equally and sometimes more effective in horses.

Pain therapy in horses, however, is in its infancy. We are just beginning to generate the types of data (pharmacokinetic, pharmacodynamic, experimental, clinical) that permit a rational approach to pain therapy. This issue of the *Veterinary Clinics of North America: Equine Practice* was organized and designed to serve as a source of information regarding our current understanding of pain processes, pain diagnosis, and pain therapy in horses. By default, much of what is believed to be fundamentally responsible for the production of pain in horses has been derived from other mammalian species and serves as a reasonable starting point given that most advanced mammals share biologically similar peripheral and central nervous systems.

doi:10.1016/j.cveq.2010.08.003
0749-0739/10/$ – see front matter
**vetequine.theclinics.com**

The first article (Muir) provides a definition of pain in animals and describes the various universal mechanisms currently believed to be responsible for pain. Toward this end, the "language" of pain is defined in order to facilitate a clearer understanding of what it is we are talking about. Article 2 (Wagner) describes the physiological, immunological, and emotional consequences of pain and provides explanations for how these responses lead to the development of pain scales. The article describes current methods for diagnosing and categorizing clinical pain in horses.

Emphasis throughout this issue has been placed upon pharmacologic and chiropractic approaches for treating pain since these therapies have demonstrated the greatest evolution and successes in recent years. Discussion of specific pharmacologic therapies for the treatment of pain includes individual articles on opioids (Clutton), alpha-2 agonists (Valverde), local anesthetics (Doherty and Seddighi), spinal anesthetics and analgesics (Natalini), and, N-methyl-D-aspartate (NMDA) inhibitors (Muir). The clinical use of chiropractic techniques that can be used alone or in conjunction with pharmacologic approaches to pain therapy is described (Haussler).

The final three articles address various clinical conditions in horses that commonly produce pain. The differences between visceral and somatic pain are considered and various therapies are proposed (Robertson and Sanchez). The pathophysiology of osteoarthritic pain (inflammatory pain; van Weeren and de Grauw) and laminitic pain (neuropathic/inflammatory pain; Collins and coworkers) are described in conjunction with critical comments on the use of nonsteroidal and steroidal anti-inflammatory drugs.

Most if not all other therapeutic approaches other than cyrotherapy remain to be validated in horses. Hopefully pain therapy in horses will continue to be a focus of clinical investigation for both the welfare of horses and the enjoyment of their human companions.

William W. Muir, DVM, PhD
Equine Anesthesia and Analgesia Consulting Services
338 West 7th Avenue
Columbus, OH 43201, USA

E-mail address:
monos369@gmail.com

# Pain: Mechanisms and Management in Horses

William W. Muir, DVM, PhD

**KEYWORDS**

- Pain • Nociception • Sensitization • Disinhibition
- Therapeutics

Pain, what an enigma, is often physically limiting and frustrating to treat. Pain evolved as a homeostatic warning system associated with tissue or nerve injury.[1] Pain is an everyday, albeit often brief, occurrence for all animals but a few unlucky humans with congenital insensitivity to pain (not yet reported in animals).[2] For some, pain persists or recurs long after the pain-producing stimulus has been removed resulting in pain as disease with little or no known cause.[3] Most of what we have learned concerning the mechanisms responsible for pain and its consequences continues to be clarified with key advances being made in the past 25 years.[4] Most of these advances in knowledge in mammalian species have evolved from studies conducted in rats and mice. This knowledge, however, has resulted in an improved understanding of pain and its ubiquitous involvement with all aspects of mammalian physiology. Once thought, as proposed by Rene Descartes, to be a "hard-wired" system wherein information is transmitted by pain-specific nerve fibers, it is now appreciated that pain is a multidimensional sensory experience that is subserved by so-called "wide dynamic range" (WDR) neurons that respond to both low- and high-threshold cutaneous stimuli and frequently involves multiple sensing systems, nerve fiber types, and areas of the central nervous system (CNS; spinal cord, brain).[5] Furthermore, the generation and persistence of pain can be elicited by neural mechanisms that not only activate or exaggerate excitatory activity (hypersensitivity, sensitization) but also by mechanisms that decrease inhibitory activity (disinhibition). Persistent (chronic) pain, for example, is now appreciated for its ability to modify nervous system physiology and anatomy and has led to the conclusion that the nervous system is malleable or plastic and that chronic pain can become pain as disease, leading to distress.[6] As new information and knowledge of the mechanisms responsible for pain emerge, new therapies evolve and many therapies become recognized for their potential therapeutic value.[7,8]

All animals are entitled to 5 freedoms: freedom from hunger and thirst; freedom from discomfort; freedom to express normal behavior; freedom from fear and distress; and

Equine Anesthesia and Analgesia Consulting Services, 338 West 7th Avenue, Columbus, OH 43201, USA

*E-mail address:* bill.muir@amcny.org

Vet Clin Equine 26 (2010) 467–480
doi:10.1016/j.cveq.2010.07.008
0749-0739/10/$ – see front matter © 2010 Elsevier Inc. All rights reserved.

freedom from pain, injury, and disease. Pain has been defined as, "an unpleasant sensory and emotional experience associated with actual or potential tissue damage or described in terms of such damage" (**Table 1**). A more appropriate definition for pain in animals states: "Animal pain is an aversive sensory and emotional experience representing an awareness by the animal of damage or threat to the integrity of its tissues; it changes the animal's physiology and behavior to reduce or avoid damage, to reduce the likelihood of recurrence and to promote recovery; unnecessary pain occurs when the intensity or duration of the experience is inappropriate for the damage sustained or when the physiologic and behavioral responses to it are unsuccessful at alleviating it."[9] The emotional component of this definition is all too often created by unexpected events, strange environments, and proceedings that produce fear. Pain in horses is a valuable clinical sign (apprehension, anxiety, reluctance to interact, lameness, stomping, rolling) and is often the first and only sign of a current or impending problem.[10] When pain is severe or becomes chronic, behavioral signs are exaggerated and can result in a failure to thrive ("sickness syndrome").[11] Pain prevention (preventative therapy) and treatment (palliative therapy) are dependent upon knowledge of the anatomy, physiology, and pathologic processes responsible for sensory processing in health and disease. This knowledge precludes and is prerequisite to the development and application of rational pain therapies and appreciation of their consequences.

Consider, for example, a 12-year-old, 510 kg, retired Thoroughbred racehorse trained as a children's hunter-jumper that is presented with an acute history of a deep wire cut on its left front pastern. The horse is noticeably lame on the affected limb. Historically the horse was reported to have "sensitive" front feet that responded to phenylbutazone, local steroid (methyprednisolone acetate) injections, and sarapin administration. Two weeks before this traumatic event the horse was moved to a new stable at which time the farm farrier "balanced" the feet resulting in severe lameness and swelling of both front limb fetlocks, which persisted for approximately 5 to 7 days. The horse was reluctant to move, almost 3-legged lame, refusing to put weight on its left front limb, standing with most of its weight on its hind limbs. The horse walked with a "rocking-horse" type gate, was alert and anxious, hypersensitive to touch on the affected limb, and highly sensitive to palpation of the wound and the affected limb. The horse was administered 2.5 µg/kg detomidine intravenously (IV) and a low palmar (volar) nerve block was performed by injecting 2.5 mL of 2% lidocaine in the area of the medial and lateral plantar nerves just distal to the buttons of the splint bones. The horse became sedate and markedly less painful on the left front limb when moved but noticeably lame on the right front limb. The horse's presenting signs are suggestive of acute adaptive primary and secondary hypersensitivity of the affected limb resulting in hyperalgesia and allodynia. Primary hypersensitivity was likely related to the wound and the development of peripheral sensitization. The horse's response to initial therapy is suggestive of a chronic painful condition, likely involving both front limbs, resulting from central sensitization and maladaptive pain. The wound was cleaned and bandaged and a multimodal therapeutic pain program recommended and instituted to be administered during the next 7 to 10 days. The program incorporated both intermittent and rescue recommendations that used multiple pharmacologic therapies, complementary remedies, and rehabilitative recommendations.

## NOCICEPTION AND PAIN TERMINOLOGY

The case presented in the preceding paragraph emphasizes that a cogent discussion of pain and pain therapy cannot occur without consensus regarding the terms and phrases used to describe pain and its causes (**Tables 1** and **2**).[12] These terms and phrases constitute the language of pain and have evolved from the neurobiological, biochemical, and pathophysiologic processes responsible for its production and effects. Nociception is a term used to describe the neural processes for the transduction (detection), transmission, modulation, projection, and central processing of actual or potentially tissue-damaging stimuli (**Fig. 1**). Nociception can occur without pain (general anesthesia). Nociception is inclusive of all the sensory neural mechanisms used to detect and process noxious (harmful) or pain-producing stimuli. Nociception begins in the periphery and is dependent upon the sensitivity and activity of nociceptors, nociceptive neurons, and the prevailing status of the central nervous system (spinal cord and brain). Under normal circumstances, noxious stimuli (mechanical, thermal, chemical, electrical) activate a variety of comparatively high threshold uni- and polymodal nociceptors located throughout the body. Nociceptive neurons express transient receptor potential (TRP) channels that subserve a protective function and are highly implicated in the immediate detection of noxious stimuli such as heat or tissue damage.[13] The TRP vanilloid (TRPV1) receptor, is activated by capsaicin, the hot ingredient in chili peppers, and has been identified in the central and peripheral nervous systems of most mammals, including horses.[14] It is known to play a central role in the development and/or maintenance of persistent pain states, particularly those caused by inflammation.[12] Noxious stimuli are converted (transduced) to electrical impulses by pain receptors or nociceptors. The electrical signals (action potentials) are transmitted to the spinal cord by thinly myelinated (A$\delta$) and unmyelinated (C) primary (first-order) sensory nerve fibers. The A$\delta$ nerve fibers transmit electrical nerve impulses much faster than C fibers and are responsible for the rapid onset of the sharp or first pain that triggers aversion and withdrawal from the stimulus. Activation of C fibers results in a slower onset pain (second pain) that in humans is associated with a dull throbbing or burning sensation. It is worth noting that visceral pain is transmitted exclusively by C fibers that travel with nerves of the autonomic nervous system, which may help to explain the exaggerated physiologic responses (tachycardia, hyperpnea, hypertension, sweating) associated with visceral pain.[15] First-order nerve fibers terminate and connect (synapse) on second-order nerve fibers located in the dorsal horn of the spinal cord. Second-order neurons and interneurons feed into nociceptive pathways that terminate in the brain. Nociceptive pain, sometimes referred to as "physiologic" pain, is produced by noxious stimuli that activate high-threshold nociceptors and continues to occur so long as the noxious stimulus is maintained, thereby serving as a warning system that protects against tissue injury (see **Table 2**). If the noxious stimulus is intense enough to cause tissue injury and a subsequent inflammatory response, pain persists and the sensory nervous system undergoes graded adaptive or maladaptive changes dependent upon the cause and severity of the pain-producing stimulus.[3] Said another way, the sensory nervous system is plastic, initially adapting (adaptive pain) to minimize or prevent tissue injury and subsequently through mechanisms that protect and aid in the healing and repair of the injured body part. Chemical substances (prostaglandins, leukotrienes, bradykinin, nerve growth factors, histamine) produced by tissue damage and inflammation, for example, activate and sensitize (decrease threshold) nociceptors resulting in peripheral sensitization, an exaggerated and prolonged response to noxious stimuli (hyperalgesia) and the sensation of pain by normally innocuous stimuli (allodynia). Severe or prolonged (chronic) pain can result in central sensitization, which is often initiated by peripheral sensitization and is frequently characterized by hyperalgesia, allodynia, and secondary hypersensitivity (pain outside the injured area). Maladaptive pain is uncoupled from the noxious stimulus or healing, is spontaneous or

**Table 1**
**Definitions of pain and associated terms**

| Term | Definition |
| --- | --- |
| Pain | An unpleasant sensory and emotional experience associated with actual or potential tissue damage or described in terms of such damage.<br>Note: Stress (anxiety, fear) and distress exaggerate pain. |
| Animal pain | Animal pain is an aversive sensory and emotional experience representing an awareness by the animal of damage or threat to the integrity of its tissues; it changes the animal's physiology and behavior to reduce or avoid damage, to reduce the likelihood of recurrence, and to promote recovery; unnecessary pain occurs when the intensity or duration of the experience is inappropriate for the damage sustained or when the physiologic and behavioral responses to it are unsuccessful at alleviating it. |
| Stress response | Responses to acute injury or environmental change that leads to an increase in metabolic rate, blood clotting, water retention, and immune function; a "fight or flight" alarm reaction with autonomic activation.<br>Note: Chronic stress results in "sickness syndrome" or a so-called "poor doer." |
| Noxious stimulus | An actual or potentially tissue-damaging event.<br>Note: A painful mechanical, chemical, thermal, or electrical event. |
| Nociceptor | A sensory receptor capable of transducing and encoding noxious stimuli. |
| Nociception | Neural process of encoding and processing noxious stimuli.<br>Note: Inclusive of the neural processes responsible for stimulus transduction, transmission, modulation, projection, and perception. |
| Nociceptive pain | Pain arising from activation of nociceptors.<br>Note: Generally considered to be "Physiologic or Adaptive" and serving as an alarm mediated by high-threshold ($A\delta$, C) sensory neurons. |
| Inflammatory pain | Pain caused by peripheral tissue inflammation.<br>Note: Inflammation can be acute or chronic and produces hypersensitivity (peripheral sensitization) that can lead to central sensitization. |
| Neuropathic pain | Pain arising as a consequence of a lesion or disease affecting the somatosensory (central or peripheral) nervous system.<br>Note: Pain may occur in the absence of a stimulus. |
| Dysfunctional pain | Amplification of nociceptive signaling in the absence of inflammation or neural lesions. |
| Adaptive pain | Pain that contributes to survival by the initiation of responses and behaviors that protect the animal from injury and promote healing when injury has occurred. |
| Maladaptive pain | Pain as disease; pain that is uncoupled from the noxious stimulus; an expression of abnormal sensory processing.<br>Note: Pain that persists or is recurrent after the healing process has occurred. |

|  |  |
|---|---|
| First pain | The initial well-localized and brief pain produced by a noxious stimulus.<br>Note: Produced by high-threshold pain receptors. |
| Second pain | The delayed, diffuse, and protracted pain produced by polymodal pain receptors. Second pain persists after the termination of the noxious stimulus.<br>Note: Severe acute painful events, chronic pain, and visceral pain are predominantly of the "second pain" type. |
| Superficial somatic pain | Pain associated with ongoing activation of nociceptors in the skin, subcutaneous tissue, or mucous membranes. |
| Deep somatic pain | Pain associated with ongoing activation of nociceptors in muscles, tendons, joint capsules, fasciae, or bones. |
| Visceral pain | Pain arising from visceral organs (eg, heart, lungs, gastrointestinal tract, liver, kidneys, bladder). |
| Perioperative pain | Pain that is present in a surgical patient because of preexisting disease; the surgical procedure. |
| Breakthrough pain | Pain that overwhelms or "breaks through" any pain relief afforded by ongoing analgesics. |
| Intractable pain | Intense, usually chronic and unremitting, pain for which no accepted medical intervention has provided relief. |
| Sensitization | Increased responsiveness to neurons to normal input or recruitment of a response to normally subthreshold inputs. |
| Peripheral sensitization | Increased sensitivity of peripheral nociceptive neurons owing to a decrease in threshold and increase in excitability.<br>Note: Hypersensitivity is produced by a variety of inflammatory mediators ("sensitizing soup"), including prostaglandins, bradykinin, serotonin, histamine, and $H^+$. |
| Central sensitization | Increased excitability and responsiveness of central (spinal dorsal horn) nociceptive neurons to normal subthreshold afferent input from synaptic facilitation or a decrease in inhibition.<br>Note: Involves activation of NMDA receptors. |
| "Windup" | The temporal summation of repetitive nociceptive neuron activity resulting ("use" or activity-dependent) in prolonged discharge of dorsal horn neurons. |
| Disinhibition | Removal of normal CNS inhibitory pathways that modulate the spinal transmission of nociceptive inputs.<br>Note: Predominantly GABA-ergic in the spinal cord. |
| Primary hypersensitivity | Pain produced by peripheral sensory neurons inside the inflamed or tissue-damaged area. |
| Secondary hypersensitivity | Pain produced by normal peripheral sensory neurons outside the inflamed or tissue-damaged area. |
| Hyperesthesia | Increased sensitivity to normal stimulation. |
| Paresthesia/Dysesthesia | Abnormal unpleasant sensation that can be spontaneous or evoked. |
| Hyperalgesia | An increased response to a stimulus that is normally painful. |

(continued on next page)

**Table 1**
*(continued)*

| Term | Definition |
|------|-----------|
| Allodynia | Pain caused by a stimulus that normally does not provoke pain, such as the light touch of a hand or finger. |
| Hyperpathia | A syndrome characterized by an abnormally exaggerated reaction to a stimulus, especially a repetitive stimulus. |
| Pain behavior | Nonverbal actions understood by observers to indicate that the animal is experiencing pain. <br> Note: Includes abnormal activities, gait and postures; avoidance of interaction or activity; abnormal expressions and vocalization. |
| Pain management | The systematic study of clinical and basic science and its application for the reduction of pain and suffering. |
| Analgesia | Absence of pain in response to a normally painful stimulus, typically without loss of consciousness. |
| Adjuvant | A medication that is not primarily an analgesic but that has independent or additive pain-relieving effects. |
| Multimodal analgesia | "Balanced analgesia": more than one method or modality of controlling pain (eg, drugs from 2 or more classes, plus nondrug treatment). <br> Note: With the goal of producing additive or synergistic effects, reducing side effects, or both. |
| Preemptive (preventative) analgesia | Interventions, frequently involving drug therapy, performed before a noxious event (eg, surgery) intended to minimize or prevent the impact of a pain-producing stimulus. <br> Note: Preventing peripheral and/or central sensitization. |
| Rescue analgesia | The administration of analgesic therapy for the treatment of pain. |
| Tolerance | Adaptation to a single (acute) or repetitive exposure to therapy that results in a diminution of one or more of the therapy's effects. |

*Abbreviations:* CNS, central nervous system; GABA, gamma-amino-butyric-acid; NMDA, N-methyl-D aspartate.

| | | Functional | |
| | Stimulus | Category/Response | |
| Type of Pain | Dependency | Characteristics | Clinical Examples |
|---|---|---|---|
| **Table 2** | | | |
| **Types of pain** | | | |
| Nociceptive "Physiologic" | Evoked by high-intensity (noxious) stimuli | Adaptive and protective: brief, localized; signals potential tissue damage | Response to everyday noxious stimuli: needle prick, hoof testers |
| Inflammatory | Evoked by low- and high-intensity stimuli secondary to tissue injury | Adaptive and reversible: protection and promotion of healing by producing sensory amplification (hypersensitivity); duration of pain parallels active inflammation (eg, tissue trauma) | Laceration, joint inflammation, sprain, strain, surgery |
| Neuropathic | Evoked by low- and high-intensity stimuli; peripheral or CNS neuropathies | Maladaptive and persistent: Independent of lesion or disease; central sensory amplification maintained; spontaneous or stimulus dependent; marked immune response | Nerve trauma, neuroma, viral infections |
| Dysfunctional | Evoked by low- and high-intensity stimuli or in the absence of a stimulus | Maladaptive, potentially persistent but often intermittent; sensory amplification maintained; spontaneous or stimulus dependent | Cause unknown: intermittent but chronic GI pain may be an example |

*Abbreviations:* CNS, central nervous system; GI, gastrointestinal.

recurrent, and results from the abnormal operation of the nervous system: it is pain as disease.[16]

## SENSITIZATION AND DISINHIBITION

Sensitization, involving the peripheral or central nervous systems, can be produced by the production and dissemination of the by-products of damaged or infected tissues (lymphocytes, neutrophils, mast cells, macrophages). Tissue

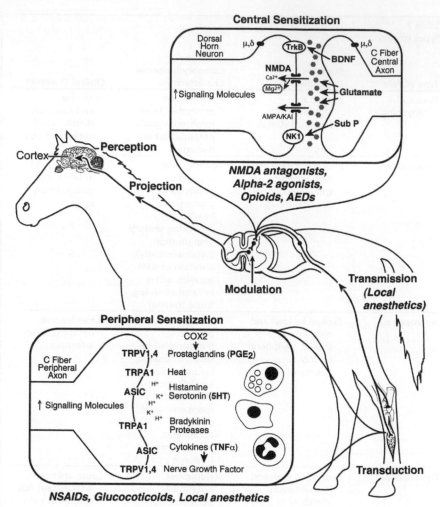

**Fig. 1.** Nociception includes the transduction, transmission, modulation, projection, and perception of noxious stimuli. Peripheral and central sensitization exaggerate and amplify the noxious stimulus. NSIADs, glucocorticoids, local anesthetics, opioids, alpha-2 agonists, NMDA antagonists and antiepileptic drugs (AEDs) are effective in modifying these responses.

trauma releases prostaglandins, bradykinin, and neurotrophic growth factors (NGFs) and ions (H⁺ K⁺) into the injured area and is responsible for peripheral sensitization and the development of primary hyperalgesia and allodynia. Activation of immune cells increases the production of cytokines (interleukin [IL]-1, IL-6, tumor necrosis factor [TNF]-α) that lower the threshold and activate central sensory neurons, amplifying the pain response.[4] Repetitive stimulation of peripheral sensory nerves can temporally summate to produce prolonged and exaggerated responses in dorsal horn sensory neurons resulting in central sensitization.[6,17] Central sensitization can last for hours to days, is largely caused by the removal of the magnesium blockade and activation of N-methyl-D-aspartate (NMDA) receptors by glutamate, and is believed to be responsible for pain outside the area of tissue injury (secondary hyperalgesia).[6] Central sensitization enables low-intensity stimuli to produce pain owing to changes in sensory processing in the spinal cord. Finally, descending pathways originating in the brain (amygdala, hypothalamus) and relayed via the brain stem and rostral ventral medulla to the spinal cord release inhibitory neurotransmitters (5-hydroxy tryptamine; norepinephrine; endogenous opioids) that provide tonic and phasic inhibitory control of nociceptive input.[18] Noradrenergic inhibition normally occurs because of activation of central alpha-2 receptors and the release of the inhibitory neurotransmitters, gamma-amino-butyric-acid (GABA) and lysine. Peripheral nerve injury caused by severe trauma or conditions that produce neuropathic pain (laminitis; neurodegenerative disease) contribute to hypersensitivity. Peripheral sensitization, central sensitization, and disinhibition represent a continuum of the pain process. Pain produces stress, which is short-lived in most horses because of the short duration of exposure to the stressor. Surgery and anesthesia are common sources of relatively short periods of pain and stress, respectively, in horses but osteoarthritis and laminitis can produce pain that persists for months or years and can lead to suffering.[19–21] Suffering occurs when horses are forced to endure the imposition of untreated or chronic painful conditions, is maladaptive, and initiates neural and endocrine responses that negatively affect homeostatic functions critical to the animal's well-being.[22]

## TREATING PAIN IN HORSES

Most studies examining the analgesic effects of drugs in horses lack controls, are inadequately powered, not objectively evaluated, or reflect the biases of the investigators.[23] Furthermore, most investigations have been conducted in experimental pain models (balloon colic, heat lamp, endotoxin administration, hoof nail) using otherwise normal horses. Few studies of therapeutic efficacy have been conducted in horses with naturally occurring disease, making it difficult to determine their clinical efficacy. Regardless, what has been learned suggests that horses respond to pain similar to other mammals and the data from alternate species are likely to be relevant in the horse. Pharmacologic approaches to the treatment of pain in horses should be mechanism based and selected for specific purposes (inflammation, nerve injury), for specific reasons (peripheral vs central sensitization), scaled to the severity and type of pain (somatic vs visceral; mild vs severe), and formulated to produce the greatest success (multimodal therapy; preventative; rescue).[16] Most drugs used for the treatment of pain in horses fall into 1 of 4 broad categories: steroidal and nonsteroidal anti-inflammatory drugs (NSAIDs), opioids, alpha2 agonists, and local anesthetics (Table 3). Similarly, complementary and alternative therapies that include acupuncture, chiropractic, and neutriceutical approaches to pain relief have only begun to be objectively evaluated in horses.[24] The terms complementary and alternative therapies are often used interchangeably but are distinct. Complementary therapies are used together with traditional therapies to produce the desired effect. For example, opioids may be combined with NSAIDs to manage breakthrough pain and are therefore complementary. Alternative therapies are frequently used in conjunction with conventional approaches.

## LOCAL ANESTHETICS

Local anesthetics (lidocaine, mepivicaine, bupivicaine, ropivicaine) are applied topically or injected at a specific site (local; perineurally [regional]) to produce a loss of sensation.[25] Analgesia is produced by the blockade of sodium ion channels,

**Table 3**
**Classes of analgesic drugs**

| Analgesic Drugs | | |
|---|---|---|
| **Drug Class Representative** | **Mechanism of Action** | **Evidence for Clinical Efficacy** |
| Opioids<br>　Morphine<br>　Meperidine<br>　Methadone<br>　Hydromorphone<br>　Fentanyl<br>　Butorphanol<br>　Buprenorpine | Primarily mu ($\mu$) opioid agonists;<br>　kappa ($\kappa$) opioid agonistic activity<br>　may be important for butorphanol | Good |
| Alpha-2 agonists<br>　Xylazine<br>　Detomidine<br>　Medetomidine<br>　Romifidine | Primarily alpha-2A receptor<br>　stimulants; possible imidazoline ($I_1$)<br>　receptor agonist | Good |
| NSAIDs<br>　Aspirin<br>　Phenylbutazone<br>　Flunixin<br>　Ketoprofen<br>　Firocoxib<br>　Diclofenac | Inhibition of cyclooxygenase<br>　and ↓ in prostaglandins:<br>　$PGE_2$, $PGI_2$, $TXA_2$ | Strong |
| Local anesthetics<br>　Lidocaine<br>　Mepivacaine<br>　Bupivacaine<br>　Ropivacaine | Block voltage–gated sodium channels<br>　($Na^+$ channels) – impair nerve<br>　conduction | Strong |
| Corticosteroids<br>　Triamcinolone acetonide<br>　Methylprednisolone acetate<br>　Dexamethasone | Inhibition of phospholipase A2 | Good |
| Others<br>　Ketamine, tiletamine<br>　Gabapentin<br>　Tramadol<br>　Capsaicin<br>　Sarapin | NMDA antagonist<br>Calcium channel $\alpha2$-$\delta$ blocker<br>Mu ($\mu$) opioid receptor agonist<br>Desensitization of C-fibers by<br>　overactivation of TRPV1 channel<br>Irritant | Good<br>Poor<br>Poor<br>Unknown (Fair)<br>Fair to Poor |

*Abbreviations:* NMDA, N-methyl-D aspartate; NSAID, nonsteroidal anti-inflammatory drug; TRPV1, transient receptor potential vanilloid.

thereby preventing the initiation and conduction of electrical impulses in small-diameter (C, A$\delta$) sensory nerve fibers. Larger (clinical) dosages of local anesthetics can produce a loss of motor function and temporary motor paralysis. Most local anesthetic drugs administered systemically produce mild CNS depression, are anesthetic sparing, and have antiarrhythmic, antishock, and gastrointestinal pro-motility effects. Large IV dosages, however, can produce hypotension, anxiety, seizures, and apnea. These effects are more common in stressed or sick horses.

## ANTI-INFLAMMATORY DRUGS

Nonsteroidal anti-inflammatory drugs (NSAIDs: phenylbutazone, flunixin meglumine, firocoxib) produce anti-inflammatory and analgesic effects by inhibiting cyclooxygenase (COX), the enzyme that metabolizes arachidonic acid to prostaglandins.[26] Prostaglandins and leukotrienes are key factors in the production of peripheral sensitization and likely are important in augmenting central sensitization. NSAIDs are effective analgesics for the treatment of mild to moderate inflammatory pain, emphasizing the importance of prostaglandin production in the initiation and maintenance of pain. Prostaglandins (PGE2, TXA$_2$) activate prostaglandin (EP) receptors throughout the body, producing pain, inflammation, and fever. They are also responsible for the production of a protective gastric barrier to intralumenal acidity, sustaining normal gastric secretory activity, and maintaining normal gut motility. Prostaglandins also regulate renal blood flow and maintain normal renal tubular function. There are 2 types of COX: COX-1 and COX-2. COX-1 is constitutive and helps to maintain normal cell homeostasis. COX-2 is also constitutive in the CNS, kidney, eye, and reproductive organs but becomes markedly upregulated during inflammation and infection. COX-1 inhibition can produce altered gastrointestinal motility and gastrointestinal ulceration, renal or liver toxicity, and has the potential to delay clotting. Both COX-1 or COX-2 inhibition can cause renal failure, which is more common in very young, old, or dehydrated horses. Glucocorticoids (triamcinolone, methyprednisolone acetate) act one step earlier in the metabolic cascade, producing anti-inflammatory effects by inhibiting phospholipase-A2, the enzyme that facilitates the break down of membrane phospholipids to arachadonic acid, subsequently leading to prostaglandin and leukotriene production.[27,28]

## OPIOIDS

Opioids (morphine, meperidine, methadone, hydromorphone, fentanyl, butorphanol, buprenorphine) are generally considered to be effective analgesics in horses, although their range of potential therapeutic effects likely overlaps with the development of side effects and toxicity. Furthermore, little is known concerning the horse's potential to develop tolerance or delayed hyperalgesia to opioid agonists, although their ability to induce ataxia and hyperexcitability has been known for decades. Opioids are believed to produce most, if not all of their clinically relevant analgesic effects by interacting with mu ($\mu$) and possibly kappa ($\kappa$) opioid receptors, although solid evidence for their analgesic efficacy in horses with clinical disease is sparce.[25] Opioid agonist-antagonists (butorphanol) and partial agonists (buprenorphine) produce morphinelike effects but are less potent than fentanyl, morphine, and methadone. Opioids are most effective when used as complementary or multimodal therapy in conjunction with other drugs including NSAIDs, alpha-2 agonists, and ketamine. Opioids require special licensing and record keeping; predispose to ileus, constipation, and colic; and can produce excitement (increased locomotor activity), agitation, disorientation, and ataxia in some horses. Large or repeated dosages of opioids may result in urine retention. Urine retention is an important postsurgical consideration in some horses. Fentanyl is a particularly potent, short-acting, $\mu$ opioid receptor agonist that can be administered by constant rate infusion. Alternatively, fentanyl transdermal patches are available but may need to be replaced every 24 to 36 hours in horses to maintain analgesia. Opioid antagonists (naloxone, nalmafene) are devoid of agonist activity and are used clinically to antagonize opioid effects.

## ALPHA-2 AGONISTS

Alpha-2 agonists (xylazine, detomidine, medetomidine, romifidine) produce stupor (sedation), ataxia, reluctance to move (muscle relaxation), and pain relief (analgesia) by differentially activating various alpha-2 receptors in the CNS and peripherally.[29] Individual drug effects vary dependent upon their alpha-2 versus alpha-1 selectivity; stimulation of CNS alpha-1 receptors causes arousal. Alpha-2 agonists are effective therapy for the acute treatment of superficial wounds, particularly those on the head and neck and mild to moderately severe visceral pain (colic). Sedation is attributed to activation of the CNS alpha-2A/D receptors in areas of the brain that are responsible for awareness, arousal, and vigilance. Clinically, the administration of alpha-2 agonists generally produces dose-dependent sedation, bradycardia, respiratory depression, and, rarely, violent behavior. Atropine or glycopyrrolate are effective therapy for brady-cardia and atrioventricular block. Respiratory stridor, snoring, irregular breathing patterns, and upper airway obstruction can occur in horses with upper airway diseases. Alpha-2 agonists promote sweating, urine production, and ileus, resulting in gas accumulation and the occasional development of colic. Their effects can be antagonized by the alpha-2 antagonists yohimbine, tolazoline, and atipamazole.

## NONTRADITIONAL, COMPLEMENTARY, AND ALTERNATIVE ANALGESIC THERAPIES

New drugs are continuously being developed for the treatment of acute and chronic pain. Gabapentin, an antiseizure drug that reduces calcium influx through N-type $Ca^{+2}$ channels thereby reducing cellular excitability, has been administered to horses to produce complementary analgesic effects, but its efficacy as analgesics is debat-able.[30,31] Tramadol, a mild mu opioid agonist, is purported to produce analgesia when administered IV or in the epidural space, but it is not effective after oral administration owing to poor bioavailability and relatively rapid elimination.[32] Ketamine is being promoted as pain therapy for the prevention of central sensitization and hyperalge-sia.[33] Capsaicin and similar analogs overstimulate C-fiber afferents resulting in acute

---

**Box 1**
**Alternative and complementary pain therapies**

Acupuncture

Biofeedback

Chiropractic

Herbalism

Homeopathy

Hydrotherapy

Kinesiology

Massage

Prolotherapy

Neural therapy

Reflexology

Static magnets

Herbal therapy

pain and hyperalgesia; however, repeated or prolonged treatment decreases chronic pain.[34,35] Sarapin, a drug with no known mechanism, has been advocated for nerve blocks in horses.[36] It is suggested that injection into the affected ligaments or tendons produces localized inflammation, triggering a "wound-healing" cascade, resulting in new collagen that shrinks as it matures. To date, no studies have confirmed these claims. Additionally, interventional techniques have been use to guide the administration of neurolytics (alcohol, phenol) for long-term pain relief in horses. Finally, alternative therapies, including but not limited to acupuncture, chiropractic, and neutraceuticals, are used for the treatment of pain in horses as adjuncts to more traditional regimens (**Box 1**).[24]

## SUMMARY

Pain is a multidimensional sensory phenomenon that has evolved as a protective method for maintaining homeostasis and facilitating tissue repair. Both excitatory and inhibitory physiologic and pathologic mechanisms are involved in its generation and maintenance. Untreated pain and nervous system changes (plasticity) that occur during chronic pain make pain much more difficult or impossible to effectively treat. Therapies directed toward the treatment of pain should be mechanism based and preventative whenever possible. Prospective, randomized clinical trials conducted in horses that suffer from naturally occurring pain will help to determine the current best approaches to effective pain therapy.[37]

## REFERENCES

1. Craig AD. Interoception: the sense of the physiological condition of the body. Curr Opin Neurobiol 2003;13:500–5.
2. Cox JJ, Reimann F, Nockolas AK, et al. An SCN9A channelopathy causes congenital inability to experience pain. Nature 2006;444:894–8.
3. Costigan M, Scholz J, Woolf CJ. Neuropathic pain: a maladaptive response of the nervous system to damage. Annu Rev Neurosci 2009;32:1–32.
4. Muir WW, Woolf CJ. Mechanisms of pain and their therapeutic implications. J Am Vet Med Assoc 2001;219:1346.
5. Craig AD. Why a soft touch can hurt. J Physiol 2010;588(Pt 1):13.
6. Latremoliere A, Woolf CJ. Central sensitization: a generator of pain hypersensitivity by central neural plasticity. J Pain 2009;10(9):895–926.
7. Costigan M, Woolf CJ. Pain: molecular mechanisms. J Pain 2000;1(Suppl 3):35–44.
8. Woolf CJ, Max MB. Mechanism-based pain diagnosis. Anesthesiology 2001;95:241.
9. Molony V, Kent JE. Assessment of acute pain in farm animals using behavioural and physiological measurements. J Anim Sci 1997;75:266–72.
10. Price J, Marques JM, Welsh EM, et al. Pilot epidemiological study of attitudes towards pain in horses. Vet Res 2002;151:570.
11. Elenkov IJ, Iezzoni DG, Daly A, et al. Cytokine dysregulation, inflammation and well-being. Neuroimmunomodulation 2005;12(5):255–69.
12. Loeser JD, Treede RD. The Kyoto protocol of IASP basic pain terminology. Pain 2008;137:473–7.
13. White JP, Cibelli M, Fidalgo AR, et al. Role of transient receptor potential and acid-sensing ion channels in peripheral inflammatory pain. Anesthesiology 2010;112:729–41.
14. da Cunha AF, Stokes AM, Chirgwin S, et al. Quantitative expression of the TRPV-1 gene in central and peripheral nervous tissue in horses. Int J Appl Res Vet Med 2008;6:15–9.

15. Sengupta JN. Visceral pain: the neurophysiological mechanism. Handb Exp Pharmacol 2009;194:31–74.
16. Woolf CJ. Pain: moving from symptom control toward mechanism-specific pharmacologic management. Ann Intern Med 2004;140:441–51.
17. Eide PK. Wind-up and the NMDA receptor complex from a clinical perspective. Eur J Pain 2000;4(1):5–15.
18. Heinricher MM, Tavares I, Leith JL, et al. Descending control of nociception: specificity, recruitment and plasticity. Brain Res Rev 2009;60(1):214–25.
19. Taylor PM. Equine stress response to anaesthesia. Br J Anaesth 1989;63:702–9.
20. Haussler KK, Hill AE, Frisbie DD, et al. Determination and use of mechanical nociceptive thresholds of the thoracic limb to assess pain associated with induced osteoarthritis of the middle carpal joint in horses. Am J Vet Res 2007;68(11):1167–76.
21. Jones E, Viñuela-Fernandez I, Eager RA, et al. Neuropathic changes in equine laminitis pain. Pain 2007;132(3):321–31.
22. Carstens E, Moberg GP. Recognizing pain and distress in laboratory animals. ILAR J 2000;41(2):62–71.
23. Flecknell P. Analgesia from a veterinary perspective. Br J Anaesth 2008;101(1): 121–4.
24. Fleming P. Nontraditional approaches to pain management. Vet Clin North Am Equine Pract 2002;18:83–106.
25. Kamerling SG. Narcotics and local anesthetics. Vet Clin North Am Equine Pract 1993;9(3):605–20.
26. Goodrich LR, Nixon AJ. Medical treatment of osteoarthritis in the horse—a review. Vet J 2006;171(1):51–69.
27. Bailey SR, Elliott J. The corticosteroid laminitis story: 2. Science of if, when and how. Equine Vet J 2007;39(1):7–11.
28. Bathe AP. The corticosteroid laminitis story: 3. The clinician's viewpoint. Equine Vet J 2007;39(1):12–3.
29. England GC, Clarke KW. Alpha 2 adrenoceptor agonists in the horse—a review. Br Vet J 1996;152(6):641–57.
30. Davis JL, Posner LP, Elce Y. Gabapentin for the treatment of neuropathic pain in a pregnant horse. J Am Vet Med Assoc 2007;231(5):755–8.
31. Terry RL, McDonnell M, Van Eps W, et al. Pharmacokinetic profile and behavioral effects of gabapentin in the horse. J Vet Pharmacol Therap 2010;33:485–94.
32. Dhanjal JK, Wilson DV, Robinson E, et al. Intravenous tramadol: effects, nociceptive properties, and pharmacokinetics in horses. Vet Anaesth Analg 2009;36(6): 581–90.
33. DeKock MF, Lavand'homme PM. The clinical role of NMDA receptor antagonists for the treatment of postoperative pain. Best Pract Res Clin Anaesthesiol 2007; 21(1):85–98.
34. White PF. Red-hot chili peppers: a spicy new approach to preventing postoperative pain. Anesth Analg 2008;107:6–8.
35. Seino KK, Foreman JH, Greene SA, et al. Effects of topical perineural capsaicin in a reversible model of equine foot lameness. J Vet Intern Med 2003;17(4):563–6.
36. Harkins JD, Mundy GD, Stanley SD, et al. Lack of local anaesthetic efficacy of Sarapin in the abaxial sesamoid block model. J Vet Pharmacol Ther 1997; 20(3):229–32.
37. White PF, Kehlet H. Improving postoperative pain management. Anesth 2010; 112:220–5.

# Effects of Stress on Pain in Horses and Incorporating Pain Scales for Equine Practice

Ann E. Wagner, DVM, MS

KEYWORDS

• Stress • Analgesia • Pain • Pain scale

## STRESS/HOMEOSTASIS

The stress response represents an animal's attempt to reestablish the body's homeostasis after injury, intense physical activity, or psychological strain. Two different neuroendocrine pathways may be activated in stressful situations: the hypothalamic-pituitary-adrenocortical axis, leading to increased cortisol levels, and the sympathoadrenomedullar system, leading to increased catecholamine levels (**Fig. 1**). The stress response may be evidenced physiologically by elevated heart and respiratory rates and by increased blood pressure and temperature, as well as by various behavioral changes.[1]

## STRESS-INDUCED ANALGESIA

The degree of pain perceived by an individual depends not only on the intensity of the nociceptive input but also on the psychological state of the individual at the time of that input.[2] Stress-induced analgesia (SIA) has been described by Butler and Finn[3] as "an in-built mammalian pain suppression response that occurs during or following exposure to a stressful or fearful stimulus." SIA has been described in soldiers suffering from battle wounds but experiencing little pain, even though similar injuries in an everyday, nonthreatening situation would be expected to cause extreme pain.[4] Perhaps a racehorse that suffers a serious leg injury during the excitement of a race, but keeps galloping despite its jockey's efforts to pull it up, is experiencing some degree of SIA.

Department of Clinical Sciences, College of Veterinary Medicine and Biomedical Sciences, Colorado State University, Fort Collins, CO 80523, USA
E-mail address: aewagner@colostate.edu

Vet Clin Equine 26 (2010) 481–492
doi:10.1016/j.cveq.2010.07.001
0749-0739/10/$ – see front matter © 2010 Elsevier Inc. All rights reserved.

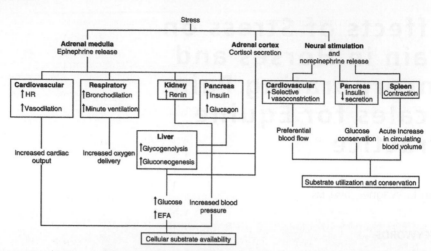

**Fig. 1.** The stress response. EFA, essential fatty acid; HR, heart rate. (*From* Muir WW, Hubbell JAE, editors. Equine anesthesia monitoring and emergency therapy. 2nd edition. St Louis (MO): Saunders Elsevier; 2009. p. 102; with permission.)

Experimental animal models demonstrating SIA typically involve exposure to a physical stressor, such as an inescapable electric foot shock or hot-plate stress, combined with a nociceptive test, such as the tail-flick test. Endogenous opioids are thought to mediate SIA through their effects on descending inhibitory pain pathways, including the amygdala, periaqueductal gray, and rostral ventromedial medulla. Work with transgenic mice has shown that genetic disruption of either β-endorphin or dynorphin, 2 endogenous opioids, abolishes the expression of SIA. Opioid antagonists such as naloxone and naltrexone have been shown to attenuate SIA in rodents.[4]

In addition to endogenous opioids, nonopioid mechanisms may also play a role in mediating SIA.[4] Neurotransmitters or neuropeptides that predominantly inhibit nociception include γ-aminobutyric acid (GABA), glycine, vasopressin, oxytocin, adenosine, and endocannabinoids, as well as endogenous opioids.[3] Benzodiazepine administration can attenuate SIA, probably through binding to GABA$_A$ receptors and promoting the inhibitory effects of GABA in the periaqueductal gray and amygdala. Recent evidence also suggests a role for another system, the endogenous cannabinoid system, in SIA; increased endocannabinoid levels in the amygdala occur in association with SIA in mice.[4] Results of various human studies have suggested that nonopioid-mediated SIA is associated with controllable stressors, such as an experimental phobic stressor, whereas opioid-mediated SIA results from uncontrollable stressors, such as a first-time parachute jump.[5–7]

## STRESS-INDUCED HYPERALGESIA

Although certain stressful stimuli can decrease pain perception, the converse may also occur. High levels of anxiety can actually enhance pain perception, leading to a separate phenomenon known as stress-induced hyperalgesia (SIH).[4] Apparently contradictory laboratory findings have been reported, with some experimental stressors producing decreased pain perception and others producing enhanced pain perception.[2] It is now becoming clear that fear and anxiety are different psychological states and have opposite effects on pain perception.[2,4] Fear is the immediate

with 0 representing no lameness and 5 indicating the worst lameness possible) and a verbal rating scale (VRS) described as follows[16]:

A = no lameness
B = difficult to observe; not consistently apparent regardless of circumstances
C = difficult to observe while walking or trotting in a straight line, consistently apparent under certain circumstances
D = consistently observable at a trot under all circumstances
E = obvious lameness with marked nodding, hitching, or shortened stride
F = minimal weight bearing in motion or at rest, inability to move.

However, interobserver agreement when using the NRS and VRS was only 56% and 60%, respectively, with some observers differing by up to 3 points on the 6-point scales. Even intraobserver agreement was only 58% and 60%, respectively, for the NRS and VRS. Therefore, the objectivity and reproducibility of the observational gait analysis may not be as reliable as most veterinarians think, especially if used as a measure of outcome.[16]

Other methods for assessment of lameness in horses include force plate gait analysis. Numerous studies reporting force plate analysis of horses under a variety of conditions have been published.[17–20] However, there are limitations even with this seemingly objective measurement technique, as different breeds of horses have different normal values for peak vertical force; for example, warmbloods load their front limbs with 118% of their body weight, whereas quarter horses load their front limbs with only 101%.[21] Therefore, breed differences must be taken into account when evaluating the results of force plate analysis. In addition, force plates are not available to most equine practitioners.

## LAMINITIS PAIN

Laminitis is thought to be one of the most excruciatingly painful conditions that can occur in horses. In 1948, the following system of rating degrees of lameness associated with laminitis was developed by Niles Obel.[22,23]

- Obel grade I: frequent shifting of weight between the feet, no discernible lameness at the walk, and bilateral lameness at the trot
- Obel grade II: no resistance to having a forelimb lifted, no reluctance to walk, but definite lameness at the walk
- Obel grade III: resistance to having a forelimb lifted and reluctance to walk
- Obel grade IV: horse walks only if forced.

A recent case report of a horse with laminitis used a modified composite pain score (MCPS) incorporating both the Obel Laminitis Pain Scale and a multifactorial descriptive numeric rating scale that quantitated observed behavioral and physiologic components. The numeric rating scale was as follows[22]:

1. No pain or distress; normal behavior
2. Mild pain; irritable, restless, decreased appetite
3. Mild pain; 2 plus resists handling
4. Mild to moderate pain; 3 plus standing in back of stall or with back to stall door
5. Moderate pain; 4 plus camped-out legs, increased digital pulses
6. Moderate to severe pain; 5 plus frequent recumbency, heart rate greater than 44 beats per minute, and/or respiratory rate greater than 24 breaths per minute
7. Moderate to severe pain; 6 plus sweating, muscle fasciculation, head tossing

8. Severe pain; 7 plus unwilling to move
9. Severe to extreme pain; 8 plus non–weight bearing when standing
10. Extreme pain; 9 or entirely recumbent, bordering on agony.

The investigators believe that the use of this MCPS facilitated the recognition of the horse's changing pain status and thus adjustments of therapy and found that multiple observers produced consistent, comparable scores that reflected changes in both the therapeutic interventions and the course of the disease.[22]

In another study of laminitis pain and its response to treatment, the association between heart rate, heart rate variability (HRV), endocrine levels, and behavioral pain measures was evaluated.[1] Cortisol and catecholamine levels were poorly associated with other pain indicators and did not change with treatment, but weight shifting and Obel grade decreased significantly with treatment. The low- and high-frequency components of HRV changed significantly with treatment, indicating a decrease in sympathetic influence and an increase in parasympathetic influence as pain subsided. The investigators concluded that determination of HRV may provide helpful complementary information for the assessment of pain but cautioned that it can be affected by other factors, such as movement, eating, and unfamiliar surroundings, and should not be relied on without appropriate control of such variables.[1]

## ORTHOPEDIC PAIN

A pain scale specific to orthopedic pain was developed and tested in an acute arthritis model using amphotericin B injection in the tarsocrural (hock) joint of horses.[14] This scale is a multifactorial NRS incorporating physiologic and behavioral data as well as response to treatment (**Table 1**). The physiologic parameters include heart rate, respiratory rate, bowel motility sounds, and rectal temperature; the behavioral parameters include appearance (reluctance to move, restlessness, agitation, anxiety), sweating, kicking at abdomen, pawing or pointing limbs, posture (weight distribution, comfort), head movement, and appetite; and the response-to-treatment parameters include interactive behavior and response to palpation of the painful area. Each parameter has a list of descriptors, which are used to assign a score from 0 to 3, with 0 being normal and 3 being farthest from normal; the maximum total possible score is 39.[14]

The investigators reported that high interobserver repeatability was obtained with this pain scale. Overall, the specificity and sensitivity of the composite pain scale were good. Regarding individual physiologic parameters, heart rate and respiratory rate were only moderately specific and moderately sensitive as indicators of orthopedic pain, bowel sounds had good-to-moderate specificity but weak sensitivity, and rectal temperature was neither specific nor sensitive. For individual behavioral parameters, appearance was not specific but was moderately sensitive, sweating had good specificity but was not sensitive, kicking at the abdomen was highly specific, pawing had good-to-moderate specificity and very good sensitivity, posture was specific and highly sensitive, head movement was not specific but was very sensitive, and appetite had good specificity but weak sensitivity. Interactive behavior was specific but not sensitive, and response to palpation was very specific and very sensitive.[14]

The investigators also looked at some additional physiologic criteria that were not included in the composite scale and found that noninvasive blood pressure (NIBP) measurement had a highly positive and significant association with the total composite pain score, such that for each increment of 1 unit in NIBP, the composite pain score increased by 0.18 units; mean NIBP was, therefore, a very specific and sensitive indicator of orthopedic pain. The level of blood cortisol was similarly positively associated with the composite pain score, such that for each increment of 1 unit in blood cortisol, the composite pain score increased by 0.095 units; cortisol was found to be a specific and moderately sensitive indicator of orthopedic pain. However, serum glucose value was neither a specific nor sensitive indicator of pain.[14]

To summarize, this study found that the most specific and sensitive behavioral indicators of orthopedic pain are response to palpation, posture, and (to a lesser extent) pawing. In addition, the only physiologic criterion that is beneficial in pain assessment is NIBP.[14]

A different group of investigators evaluated a behavior-based system for assessing postoperative pain in horses after arthroscopic surgery by comparing 12 horses that underwent arthroscopy with 6 pain-free control horses.[24] They used continuous videotaping, starting 24 hours before and continuing until 48 hours after surgery, noting certain behaviors and postures, and calculating activity time budgets for them. The pain-free horses spent more time eating, more time at the front of the stall, more time with the head above withers and ears forward, and less time exhibiting abnormal behaviors compared with the postarthroscopic horses. These investigators believe that activity budgets calculated from continuous videotaping may be a more sensitive way to identify pain-related behaviors compared with repeated, intermittent observations. They also pointed out that assessment of pain in postoperative horses must take into account the effects of anesthesia and fasting on behavior.[24]

## GASTROINTESTINAL/COLIC PAIN

A study was done to identify potential indicators of postoperative pain associated with abdominal exploratory surgery for colic.[25] Horses that had emergency surgery for acute colic were compared with horses that had anesthesia only for magnetic resonance imaging without surgery, as well as with horses that had no treatment at all. Physiologic data included heart rate, respiratory rate, and plasma cortisol level (**Fig. 2**). Behavior was assessed by 2 methods: the first was an NRS incorporating gross pain behaviors (pawing, sweating, looking at the flank, flehmen, and lying down/standing up repeatedly), head position, ear position, location in stall, spontaneous locomotion, response to open door, response to approach, lifting feet, and response to grain. The second method of behavioral evaluation involved calculating time budgets of behavior from video recordings of the horses. The behaviors that were recorded included activity (eg, eating, drinking, defecating, rolling, scratching, and pawing), locomotion, pain (flank gesture, Flehman, kick, stretch), and resting (stand or rest). The time budget was calculated by dividing the total duration of each behavior during a segment of video recording by the total time for that segment (**Table 2**).[25]

The investigators reported that horses that had undergone abdominal surgery spent significantly less time in locomotion than horses in the anesthesia-only or control group and that even though the surgery group spent significantly more time displaying painful behavior compared with the anesthesia-only or control group, it was a very small proportion of the total time evaluated. The NRS scores were also significantly higher in the surgery group. The investigators concluded that reduced locomotion, elevated plasma cortisol concentration, and elevated heart rate are potential indicators of postoperative pain in horses after abdominal surgery.[25]

**Table 1**
**Multifactorial numerical rating CPS**

| Physiologic Data | Criteria | Score/12 |
|---|---|---|
| Heart rate | Normal compared with initial value (increase <10%) | 0 |
| | 11%–30% increase | 1 |
| | 31%–50% increase | 2 |
| | >50% increase | 3 |
| Respiratory rate | Normal compared with initial value (increase <10%) | 0 |
| | 11%–30% increase | 1 |
| | 31%–50% increase | 2 |
| | >50% increase | 3 |
| Digestive sounds (bowel movements) | Normal motility | 0 |
| | Decreased motility | 1 |
| | No motility | 2 |
| | Hypermotility | 3 |
| Rectal temperature | Normal compared with initial value (variation <0.5°C) | 0 |
| | Variation <1°C | 1 |
| | Variation <1.5°C | 2 |
| | Variation <2°C | 3 |

| Response to treatment | Criteria | Score/06 |
|---|---|---|
| Interactive behavior | Pays attention to people | 0 |
| | Exaggerated response to auditory stimulus | 1 |
| | Excessive-to-aggressive response to auditory stimulus | 2 |
| | Stupor, prostration, no response to auditory stimulus | 3 |
| Response to palpation of the painful area | No reaction to palpation | 0 |
| | Mild reaction to palpation | 1 |
| | Resistance to palpation | 2 |
| | Violent reaction to palpation | 3 |

| Behavior | Criteria | Score/21 |
|---|---|---|
| Appearance (reluctance to move, restlessness, agitation, and anxiety) | Bright, lowered head and ears, no reluctance to move | 0 |
| | Bright and alert, occasional head movements, no reluctance to move | 1 |
| | Restlessness, pricked up ears, abnormal facial expressions, dilated pupils | 2 |
| | Excited, continuous body movements, abnormal facial expression | 3 |
| Sweating | No obvious signs of sweat | 0 |
| | Damp to the touch | 1 |
| | Wet to the touch, beads of sweat are apparent over the horse's body | 2 |
| | Excessive sweating, beads of water running off the animal | 3 |

*(continued on next page)*

| Table 1 (continued) | | |
| --- | --- | --- |
| **Physiologic Data** | **Criteria** | **Score/12** |
| Behavior | Criteria | Score |
| Kicking at abdomen | Quietly standing, no kicking | 0 |
| | Occasional kicking at abdomen (1–2 times/5 min) | 1 |
| | Frequent kicking at abdomen (3–4 times/5 min) | 2 |
| | Excessive kicking at abdomen (>5 times/5 min), intermittent attempts to lie down and roll | 3 |
| Pawing on the floor (pointing, hanging limbs) | Quietly standing, no pawing | 0 |
| | Occasional pawing (1–2 times/5 min) | 1 |
| | Frequent pawing (3–4 times/5 min) | 2 |
| | Excessive pawing (>5 times/5 min) | 3 |
| Posture (weight distribution, comfort) | Stands quietly, normal walk | 0 |
| | Occasional weight shift, slight muscle tremors | 1 |
| | Non–weight bearing, abnormal weight distribution | 2 |
| | Analgesic posture (attempts to urinate), prostration, muscle tremors | 3 |
| Head movement | No evidence of discomfort, head straight ahead for the most part | 0 |
| | Intermittent head movements laterally or vertically, occasional looking at flanks (1–2 times/5 min), lip curling (1–2 times/5 min) | 1 |
| | Intermittent and rapid head movements laterally or vertically, frequent looking at flank (3–4 times/5 min), lip curling (3–4 times/5 min) | 2 |
| | Continuous head movements, excessively looking at flank (>5 times/5 min), lip curling (>5 times/5 min) | 3 |
| Appetite | Eats hay readily | 0 |
| | Hesitates to eat hay | 1 |
| | Shows little interest in hay, eats very little, or takes hay in mouth but does not chew or swallow | 2 |
| | Neither shows interest in nor eats hay | 3 |
| | Total CPS | 39 |

*Abbreviation:* CPS, composite pain scale.

*From* Bussieres G, Jacques C, Lainay O, et al. Development of a composite orthopaedic pain scale in horses. Res Vet Sci 2008;85:296–7; with permission.

## WOUND SENSITIVITY

Cutaneous sensitivity is often evaluated by withdrawal response to a pinprick. However, repeated pinprick evaluations may result in tissue damage and worsen inflammation. Von Frey filaments, which are monofilaments of increasing diameter that apply gradually escalating force (varying from 0.004–447 g), were developed to provide a noninvasive, quantitative means of assessing the mechanical pain threshold

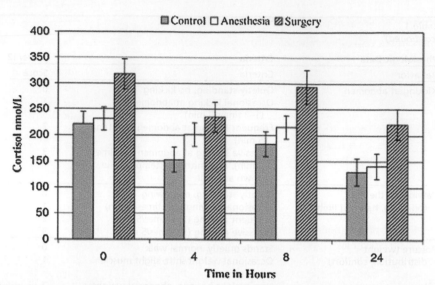

**Fig. 2.** Plasma cortisol concentration of stabled horses (comparison of control vs anesthesia only vs surgery). (*From* Pritchett LC, Ulibarri C, Oberst MC, et al. Identification of potential physiological and behavioral indicators of postoperative pain in horses after exploratory celiotomy for colic. Appl Anim Behav Sci 2003;80:38; with permission.)

of skin. The pain threshold is defined as the lowest force that produces discomfort or withdrawal. Von Frey filaments have been used in both experimental and clinical settings to assess wound sensitivity and detect hyperalgesia.[26,27]

To date, there has been only 1 study of horses that has made use of von Frey filaments.[28] To assess the potential preemptive effect of epidural ketamine on wound sensitivity in horses, a 10-cm skin incision was made on 1 lateral thigh and the sutured closed. The von Frey filaments were then applied at 1, 3, and 5 cm around the incision at predetermined time intervals to determine the nociceptive threshold. As would be expected, the nociceptive threshold was always lower on the incised thigh than on the contralateral, nonincised thigh. In addition, the untreated group had a significantly lower nociceptive threshold around the incision than did the epidural ketamine group, leading the investigators to conclude that the epidural ketamine produced a preemptive analgesic effect in this experimental model of wound hypersensitivity.[28]

Based on this limited information, von Frey filaments may prove to be useful in future studies of analgesic techniques for superficial or somatic pain, as well as in assessing clinical management of skin wounds or burns in horses.

**Table 2**
**Average time budgets of behavior of stabled horses measured by real-time video recording**

| Group | Active | Locomotion | Pain | Resting |
|---|---|---|---|---|
| Control | 22.6 ± 3.2a | 13.6 ± 2.1a | 0.0 ± 0.5a | 63.8 ± 3.1a |
| Anesthesia | 42.3 ± 3.3b | 14.0 ± 2.2a | 0.3 ± 0.05a | 43.3 ± 3.2b |
| Surgery | 11.1 ± 4.0c | 1.9 ± 2.6b | 3.9 ± 0.6b | 83.0 ± 3.8c |

a, b, c means with different letters within a column differ ($P<.05$) by the Bonferroni's t-test.
*Data From* Pritchett LC, Ulibarri C, Oberst MC, et al. Identification of potential physiological and behavioral indicators of postoperative pain in horses after exploratory celiotomy for colic. Appl Anim Behav Sci 2003;80:40.

## FACIAL EXPRESSION AS AN INDICATOR OF PAIN

Horse owners and others familiar with the equine species often believe that they can recognize certain facial expressions that seem to be associated with painful conditions. The eyes may be less focused, and the ears, down or back. Recently, the British Veterinary Association Animal Welfare Foundation funded a study to investigate how horses use facial expressions and how humans might learn to recognize equine facial expressions as a means to assess pain in horses. The study uses kinematic analysis of facial movements to develop a Horse Grimace Scale.[29] It is to be hoped that the results will become available within the next few years and will enhance caregivers' ability to recognize pain in their equine charges.

## SUMMARY

It is apparent that great effort is being made to improve recognition and quantitative evaluation of pain in horses. Management of stress and fear may have an important effect on an individual's perception of pain. Every insult and every situation is different, and as yet, there is no gold standard of equine pain measurement. As one investigator has stated, "Recognizing and classifying severity of pain always starts with observing the animal."[1] Even pain scoring systems that are intended to improve objectivity require excellent knowledge of equine behavior and physiology, as well as of individual temperament and surroundings. However, by applying some of the evaluation methods described in this article in the appropriate clinical situations, equine veterinarians can almost certainly improve their ability to recognize and manage pain in horses.

## REFERENCES

1. Riftmann TR, Stauffacher M, Bernasconi P, et al. The association between heart rate, heart rate variability, endocrine and behavioural pain measures in horses suffering from laminitis. J Vet Med 2004;51:218–25.
2. Rhudy JL, Meagher MW. Fear and anxiety: divergent effects on human pain thresholds. Pain 2000;84:65–75.
3. Butler RK, Finn DP. Stress-induced analgesia. Progress in Neurobiology 2009; 88(3):184–202.
4. Ford GK, Finn DP. Clinical correlates of stress-induced analgesia: evidence from pharmacological studies. Pain 2008;140:3–7.
5. Maier SF. Stressor controllability and stress-induced analgesia. Ann N Y Acad Sci 1986;467:55–72.
6. Janssen SA, Arntz A. No evidence for opioid-mediated analgesia induced by phobic fear. Behav Res Ther 1997;35:823–30.
7. Janssen SA, Arntz A. No interactive effects of naltrexone and benzodiazepines on pain during phobic fear. Behav Res Ther 1999;37:77–86.
8. Martenson ME, Cetas JS, Heinricher MM. A possible neural basis for stress-induced hyperalgesia. Pain 2009;142:236–44.
9. Marntell S, Nyman G, Funkquist P. Dissociative anaesthesia during field and hospital conditions for castration of colts. Acta Vet Scand 2006;47:1–11.
10. Bufalari A, Admi C, Angeli G, et al. Pain assessment in animals. Vet Res Commun 2007;31(Suppl 1):55–8.
11. Hansen B, Hardie E. Prescription and use of analgesics in dogs and cats in a veterinary teaching hospital: 258 cases (1983–1989). J Am Vet Med Assoc 1993;202:1485–94.

12. Dohoo SE, Dohoo IR. Postoperative use of analgesics in dogs and cats by Canadian veterinarians. Can Vet J 1996;37:546–51.

13. Price J, Marques JM, Welsh EM, et al. Pilot epidemiological study of attitudes towards pain in horses. Vet Rec 2002;151:570–5.

14. Bussieres G, Jacques C, Lainay O, et al. Development of a composite orthopaedic pain scale in horses. Res Vet Sci 2008;85:294–306.

15. Anonymous. Lameness exams; evaluating the lame horse. Available at: http://www.aaep.org/health_articles_view.php?id=280. Accessed February 15, 2010.

16. Hewetson M, Christley RM, Hunt ID, et al. Investigations of the reliability of observational gait analysis for the assessment of lameness in horses. Vet Rec 2006; 158:852–8.

17. Pratt GW Jr, O'Connor JT Jr. Force plate studies of equine biomechanics. Am J Vet Res 1976;37:1251–5.

18. Williams GE, Silverman BW, Wilson AM, et al. Disease-specific changes in equine ground reaction force data documented by use of principal component analysis. Am J Vet Res 1999;60:549–55.

19. Williams GE. Locomotor characteristics of horses with navicular disease. Am J Vet Res 2001;62:206–10.

20. McGuigan MP, Walsh TC, Pardoe CH, et al. Deep digital flexor tendon force and digital mechanics in normal ponies and ponies with rotation of the distal phalanx as a sequel to laminitis. Equine Vet J 2005;37:161–5.

21. Back W, MacAllister CG, van Heel MC, et al. Vertical frontlimb ground reaction forces of sound and lame warmbloods differ from those in quarter horses. J Eq Vet Sci 2007;27:123–9.

22. Dutton DW, Lashnits KJ, Wegner K. Managing severe hoof pain in a horse using multimodal analgesia and a modified composite pain scale. Eq Vet Educ 2009; 21:37–43.

23. Walsh DM, McGowan CM, McGowan T, et al. Correlation of plasma insulin concentration with laminitis score in a field study of equine Cushing's disease and equine metabolic syndrome. J Eq Vet Sci 2009;29:87–94.

24. Price J, Welsh EM, Waran NK. Preliminary evaluation of a behaviour-based system for assessment of post-operative pain in horses following arthroscopic surgery. Vet Anaesth Analg 2003;30:124–37.

25. Pritchett LC, Ulibarri C, Roberts MC, et al. Identification of potential physiological and behavioral indicators of postoperative pain in horses after exploratory celiotomy for colic. Appl Anim Behav Sci 2003;80:31–43.

26. Pedersen JL, Gall TS, Kehlet H. Peripheral analgesic effects of ketamine in acute inflammatory pain. Anesthesiology 1998;89:58–66.

27. Potgatzki EM, Gebhart GF, Brennan TJ. Characterization of Adelta- and C-fibers innervating the plantar rat hindpaw one day after an incision. J Neurophysiol 2002;10:721–31.

28. Redua MA, Valadao CA, Duque JC, et al. The pre-emptive effect of epidural ketamine on wound sensitivity in horses tested by using von Frey filaments. Vet Anaesth Analg 2002;29:200–6.

29. Anonymous. Facial expression of pain in horses. Available at: http://www.bva-awf.org.uk/headlines/facial_expression_of_pain_in_horses_2009-asp. Accessed March 6, 2010.

# Opioid Analgesia in Horses

R. Eddie Clutton, BVSc, MRCVS, DVA, MRCA

## KEYWORDS

• Opioid • Analgesic • Anesthesia • Horses

Opioid analgesics have been the foundation of human pain management for centuries, and their value in animals has increased since Yoxall[1] proposed that it was the veterinarian's duty to alleviate pain whenever it may occur. Compared with other domesticated species, the horse has benefitted less from the increased understanding of opioid pharmacology in animals. This situation has occurred because early literature was overlooked, whereas later work, which examined adverse side effects rather than analgesia, concluded that analgesic and excitatory doses were irreconcilably close. More recent studies have indicated a widening role for opioid analgesics in equine pain management, and radioligand studies have revealed a basis for the equine response pattern to opioid analgesics.[2]

## MORPHINE AND OPIOID ANALGESICS: EXCITATORY EFFECTS

The excitatory effects of morphine (fear of which is an important factor limiting the veterinary use of opioid drugs in horses[3]) were first described in 1899.[4] In 1917 Milks[5] reported that 2 to 5 grains of morphine provided "maximal analgesia with a minimum of excitement." Fröhner[6] reported that excitement combined with sensory and motor depression characterized all cases when morphine doses of 0.4, 0.75, 1.5, and 10 g were given to horses. These early reports omitted body mass data for the animals described, but an assumption that test animals weighed 600 kg indicates the doses studied were considerably greater than those used in contemporary practice. Amadon and Craigie[7] described minimal analgesic and excitant morphine doses of 0.2 and 0.5 mg/kg, respectively in pain-free horses, and ensured that veterinary scientists thereafter focused on the excitatory and locomotor side effects of the drug rather than its analgesic properties. To complicate matters, the term excitation when applied to opioid-induced side effects in horses was subsequently used indiscriminately. For example, in one study, excitation involved "continuous head nodding, digging, shifting of limbs, vocalizing, trotting and even galloping",[8] whereas in another the signs of excitement included muzzle tremors, muscle twitching, head jerks, head pressing, and a raised tail.[9]

Easter Bush Veterinary Centre, University of Edinburgh, Easter Bush, Roslin, Midlothian EH25 9RG, Scotland, UK
E-mail address: e.clutton@ed.ac.uk

Vet Clin Equine 26 (2010) 493–514
doi:10.1016/j.cveq.2010.07.002
0749-0739/10/$ – see front matter © 2010 Elsevier Inc. All rights reserved.

vetequine.theclinics.com

Morphine, meperidine, pentazocine, methadone, and hydromorphone were studied in varying numbers[1–9] of pain-free horses in what has probably become the most cited reference on opioid-induced locomotion in horses.[10] The study revealed 3 important points: (1) that opioids induce eating behavior at low doses and dose-dependent locomotor activity with incoordination at high doses; (2) that there is marked individual variation in responses; and (3) that the median effective value for morphine for increasing locomotion in pain-free animals is 0.91 mg/kg. This dose is considerably greater than the doses used to produce analgesia.

The opioid antagonist naloxone (15 μg/kg) entirely prevented locomotor responses to the μ-agonist fentanyl in pain-free horses, whereas a higher dose (20 μg/kg) reduced those of morphine by 75%.[11] This finding indicates that opioid-induced locomotion is mediated via opioid receptors. The propensity of an opioid analgesic to promote locomotion may be greater with μ- compared with κ-agonists.[12] although κ-agonism more commonly causes ataxia and staggering.[13,14] However, the evidence is confusing. The κ-agonist butorphanol (50 μg/kg intravenously [IV]) increased locomotion compared with fentanyl (5 μg/kg), although given later in the same animals, fentanyl antagonized the locomotor effect of butorphanol.[15] In contrast, another study showed that the κ-agonist U50,488H increased the intensity of fentanyl-induced locomotion.[16] Although the role of opioid receptor subtypes involved in drug-induced locomotion remains unclear, much evidence points to the role of dopamine because dopamine antagonists reduce the locomotor response in most species studied. Acepromazine has antidopaminergic effects and 0.16 mg/kg IV partly blocked the locomotor effects of fentanyl (20 μg/kg) and morphine (2.4 mg/kg) in horses.[11] In another study, acepromazine (0.1 mg/kg) injected IV before etorphine gave better relaxation than xylazine 3.0 mg/kg intramuscularly (IM).[17] However, the participation of dopamine is not straightforward: the dopamine antagonists NNC 01-0756 and eticlopride not only failed to inhibit alfentanil-induced locomotion after 20 μg/kg IV, but appeared to stimulate locomotion in their own right.[18]

Wide dose ranges tested in small study groups make it difficult to determine whether different receptors mediate different types of excitatory behaviors. However, κ-agonism might be associated with yawning, because this was seen with butorphanol (50 μg/kg IV)[15] and U50,488H (30, 60, and 120 μg/kg).[16] A sample of the range of side effects produced by high-dose opioid analgesics in pain-free horses is summarized in **Table 1**. This table illustrates a wide variation in response to fixed drug doses between studies, which in turn reflects the variation observed between horses within the same study.[10] Analysis of individual studies further reveals that a given animal frequently reacted differently in response to the same drug given under identical conditions. In one study of buprenorphine[26] 3 μg/kg caused signs of severe excitation, whereas doses of 5 and 10 μg/kg IV given later produced only hallucinations. Although this might reflect a true dose effect, it raises the question whether some horses and ponies used extensively in opioid research became opioid dependent and/or tolerant, despite reported washout periods between trials.

## DO OPIOID DRUGS PRODUCE ANALGESIA IN HORSES?

The use of opioid analgesics in horses can be justified when the benefits of their analgesic and sedative properties outweigh the disadvantages of potential side effects. However, demonstrating the analgesic properties of opioid analgesics is not straightforward (at least under experimental conditions) because of inconsistent results.[12] This finding may indicate biologic variability amongst the animals studied, inconsistent drug effects, or the use of flawed pain models.

*Opioid Analgesia: Experimental Studies*

Most experimental studies on the analgesic properties of opioid analgesics in horses have tested: (1) superficial analgesia by focusing a radiant light source onto the black painted skin overlying the distal limb or withers; the increasing time taken for the animal to respond by lifting the limb or twitching the skin in response to local heating (the withdrawal reflex latency) is taken to indicate an increasing level of analgesia; (2) visceral analgesia, using accelerometry to detect an animal's reaction to the increasing pressure in a rubber balloon implanted in the cecum; and (3) deep pain, by heating of an element implanted in the lateral surface of the humerus and recording the withdrawal reflex latency.[28] An alternative method (dental dolorimetry) involves recording the minimum electrical current applied to the canine tooth pulp nerve that elicits a head-lift or jaw-opening response.[29]

One or more of these techniques in combination have been used to show and/or compare the analgesic effects of the κ-agonist U50,488H,[30] fentanyl (0.22 mg/kg), meperidine (4.4 mg/kg), methadone (0.22 mg/kg), oxymorphone (0.033 mg/kg), pentazocine (2.2 mg/kg), xylazine (2.2 mg/kg),[28] butorphanol (0.22 mg/kg), flunixin (2.2 mg/kg), levorphanol (0.033 mg/kg), morphine (0.66 mg/kg), xylazine (2.2 mg/ kg),[21] butorphanol (0.05, 0.1, 0.2, and 0.4 mg/kg IV), and pentazocine (2.2 mg/kg IV)[31] in small (3–6) groups of horses or ponies. However, the assumption that increasing withdrawal reflex latencies indicate increasing degrees of analgesia alone is flawed. First, an animal's inclination to lift its feet is probably affected by drug-induced ataxia, if present. Alternatively, opioid-induced stepping behavior may complicate the interpretation of limb withdrawal.[31] Many analgesic studies have incorporated $\alpha_2$ agonist drugs (eg, xylazine[21,28] or detomidine[32,33]) and have concluded that opioid analgesics provide less analgesia than $\alpha_2$ agonists used alone, or contribute little analgesia to $\alpha_2$ agonist/opioid combinations. This finding is not surprising. All 3 tests for analgesia rely on motor responses as the experimental end point, which is likely to be delayed, if not by the sedative, then by the widely recognized muscle-relaxing properties of $\alpha_2$-agonist drugs. These and other factors may explain the wide variation in drug effects as well as discrepancies between the analgesic properties of opioids identified under experimental, compared with clinical, circumstances.[30] Furthermore, both heat and electrical current produce phasic pain of short duration that responds less to analgesics than tonic pain.[34] New techniques using electrophysiologic methods to investigate the pharmacologic modulation of nociception (eg, the nociceptive withdrawal reflex [NWR] and temporal summation) have been used in experimental equine pain research.[35] The NWR enables the examination of drug effects on evoked activity in A$\beta$ and A$\delta$ fibers, whereas temporal summation provides information on drug-related changes in the gain of the nociceptive system and modulation of central integration mechanisms. These methodologies may reveal the analgesic potential of opioid analgesics more accurately than previous methods.[36]

*Opioid Analgesia: Clinical Studies*

Discrepancies between experimental and clinical experiences may also be related to a belief that the risk of adverse opioid-mediated reactions is inversely proportional to the extent of the recipient's pain.[37] There is a paucity of literature supporting this subject. In one study, the responses of 66 horses with abdominal pain to butorphanol (0.1 mg/kg IV) were considered to be excellent (a pronounced analgesic effect was produced for a period adequate to permit specific therapy) or good (a noticeable analgesic effect with minor indications of pain).[38] In one case report[39] sublingual

**Table 1**
**Behavioral side effects associated with opioid analgesic use in pain-free Equidae**

| References | Dose | n | Effect |
|---|---|---|---|
| **Morphine** | | | |
| [19] | 70 µg/kg[a] | Unstated | Locomotor stimulation during recovery from general anesthesia (unsubstantiated) |
| [10] | 100 µg/kg | 5 ponies | Sham feeding, drinking and facial grimacing |
| [20] | 120 µg/kg | Unstated | Dysphoria, then euphoria |
| [10] | 0.3 mg/kg | 4 horses | 1 of 5 showed increased locomotor activity[b] |
| | 0.6 mg/kg | 4 horses | 4 of 5 showed increased locomotor activity; mean step rate = 30 steps per 2 minutes |
| [21] | 0.66 mg/kg | 8 ponies | 1 unaffected, 7 were restless |
| [10] | 1.2 mg/kg | 4 horses | Mean step rate = 50 steps per 2 minutes (mean) Marked propensity to eat from the hay rack; animals swiped at hay as they passed manger, but unable to chew or swallow prehended food |
| | 2.4 mg/kg | | Mean step rate =100 steps per 2 minutes (mean) Loss of coordination; walked as if oblivious to surroundings; played with, rather than drank, offered water; continued to eat large amounts of hay Incoordination and collapse |
| **Meperidine** | | | |
| [10] | 1.0 mg/kg | 1 horse | No effect |
| | 2.5 mg/kg | | Modest increase in locomotor activity |
| | 5.0 mg/kg | | Incoordination, shaking, immobility, then a good locomotor response |
| **Pentazocine** | | | |
| [10] | 0.25 mg/kg | 6 horses | Tendency to eat |
| | 0.5 mg/kg | 6 horses | Tendency to eat |
| | 1.0 mg/kg | 6 horses | Hay eating increased, incoordination |
| | 2.0 mg/kg | 10 horses | Severe incoordination, reluctance to walk |
| **Methadone** | | | |
| [10] | 0.1 mg/kg | 4 horses | Dose-dependent increase in stepping rate |
| | 0.5 mg/kg | | Poor coordination |
| | 1.0 mg/kg | | Tended to go down |
| **Fentanyl** | | | |
| [15] | 5 µg/kg | 4 ponies | Increased locomotion |
| [11] | 20 µg/kg | 3 horses | Increased locomotion |
| [16] | 20 µg/kg | 6 horses | Head bobbing, food snatching, cribbing |
| **Alfentanyl** | | | |
| [22] | 4 and 10 µg/kg | 6 horses | No effect |
| | 20 and 40 µg/kg | | Box walking, bizarre eating behaviors, head tossing, and shaking |
| **Butorphanol** | | | |
| [15] | 50 µg/kg | | Yawning |
| [23] | 0.1–0.13 mg/kg | | Staggering and ataxia |
| [24] | 0.1 mg/kg | | Box walking |
| [25] | 0.2 mg/kg | | Apprehension, increased locomotor activity, ataxia |
| [21] | 0.22 mg/kg | | Nodding, pacing, pawing, body swinging, head shaking, shivering |

(continued on next page)

| References | Dose | n | Effect |
|---|---|---|---|
| **Table 1**<br>*(continued)* | | | |
| Buprenorphine | | | |
| [26] | 3 µg/kg | 10 horses | Head nodding, pawing, chewing, facial rictus, a violent and potentially dangerous excitation crisis |
| | 5 and 10 µg/kg | | Marked ataxia, CN system excitation, or hallucinations in 3 animals |
| [8] | 5 and 10 µg/kg | 6 horses | Continuous head nodding, digging, shifting of limbs, vocalizing, trotting, galloping |
| [27] | 10 µg/kg | 6 horses | Continuous head nodding, head shaking, neighing, pawing, shifting of ground support, and restlessness |

[a] All doses intravenous unless otherwise stated.
[b] A statistically significant increase in the number of steps taken in a 2-minute sampling period.

buprenorphine (6 µg/kg) was given twice daily to a filly with traumatic head and neck injuries and in which signs of pain were unresponsive to phenylbutazone. After administration, "the filly became sedated and noticeably more comfortable. The neck muscles relaxed and the filly moved its head and neck more freely. Mild euphoria was displayed by the filly's tranquil and affectionate temperament. No signs of excitement of the central nervous system were seen." This report supports the view that opioids are beneficial when given to horses with real (ie, nonexperimental) pain.

## OPIOID ANALGESICS AND STANDING SURGICAL ANESTHESIA
### Do Opioids Enhance the Sedative Effects of $\alpha_2$ Agonists?

It seems so. Morphine (0.1 mg/kg), methadone (0.1 mg/kg), butorphanol (50 µg/kg), but not meperidine (1.0 mg/kg) improved the sedative effects of intravenous detomidine (10 µg/ kg) in 3 ponies and a thoroughbred and decreased responses to external stimuli.[9] In another study, the inclusion of butorphanol (50 µg/kg, IV) to one of 2 romifidine doses (40 and 80 µg/kg, IV) reduced responses in 4 pain-free ponies and one thoroughbred when the animals' coronets were touched, their ears tickled, a cloth was flapped in front, and hands were clapped behind them. However, the height of the muzzle from the ground was not lessened by the addition of butorphanol, which indicates that low-dose romifidine does not measurably relax the cervical muscles.[40] When the effects of intravenous detomidine (30 µg/kg), xylazine (1.1 mg/kg), and xylazine (1.1 mg/kg) with morphine (0.75 mg/kg up to 300 mg) were compared in 99 horses undergoing bronchoalveolar lavage, no significant differences between treatments were found. However, those assessing the level of sedation considered it to be unnecessarily deep. Opioids conferred no benefit because all animals were overdosed.[41]

### Do Opioid Analgesics Enhance the Experimentally Determined Analgesic Effects of $\alpha_2$ Agonists?

Three studies indicate an additive or synergistic effect, although one, using dental dolorimetry, concluded that xylazine (1.1 mg/kg IV) alone prevented motor responses to electrocution equal to that induced with xylazine/morphine (0.75 mg/kg IV), xylazine/butorphanol (0.04 mg/kg IV), or xylazine/nalbuphine (0.75 mg/kg IV) combinations.[29] In contrast, observers grading analgesia in the face of electrical and pressure stimuli applied to the body wall produced by xylazine (0.66 mg/kg IV) combined with one of 2 morphine doses (0.12 or 0.66 mg/kg IV) opined that analgesia was considerably improved when xylazine was combined with the higher morphine dose.[20] Detomidine (10 μg/kg IV) alone, or combined with butorphanol (25 μg/kg) or levomethadone (100 μg/kg),[33] caused a significant temporary increase in the nociceptive threshold (established electrically and pneumatically), although butorphanol and levomethadone both increased the threshold and prolonged antinociception compared with detomidine alone. The same results were found in a similar study examining the same drugs[32] but these investigators expressed concern that the stimulus applied (electrical or mechanical) might influence the interpretation of drug effects, because although both butorphanol and levomethadone increased the reaction threshold to a similar degree, the threshold increase was more apparent when the coronary band was heated.

### Do the Analgesic Properties of Opioids Compare with α₂ Agonists?

The contemporary popularity of multimodal pain therapy challenges the need to compare the analgesic effects of individual $\alpha_2$ agonist and opioid drugs, because most practitioners now recognize the benefits of using several analgesic drugs in combination. Nevertheless, one study comparing the effects of xylazine (2.2 mg/kg IM), pentazocine (1 mg/kg IM), and meperidine (2.2 mg/kg IM) injected 10 minutes after colic signs had been induced by cecal balloon inflation[42] concluded that xylazine was the only drug that provided consistent analgesia. A similar tendency to attribute the suppression of colic signs to a pure analgesic, rather than a sedative or muscle-relaxing effect, was apparent in a study comparing butorphanol (0.1 mg/kg) with detomidine (20 or 40 μg/kg), intravenous flunixin (1.0 mg/kg) and xylazine (0.5 mg/kg) in 152 horses presenting with colic.[43] Butorphanol was considered unsatisfactory as an analgesic 90% of the time, whereas detomidine was considered to be superior.

## OPIOID ANALGESICS AND TOTAL INTRAVENOUS ANESTHESIA

The evidence that the beneficial effects of opioids in standing surgical techniques may extend to those performed under total intravenous anesthesia (TIVA) is not compelling. Love and colleagues[44] studied the effects of preoperative butorphanol (0.1 mg/kg IV) on postcastration pain in 20 ponies and concluded that a single preoperative dose does not provide adequate postoperative analgesia for open castration in colts. In another study of colt castration (n = 36)[45] the analgesic effects of butorphanol alone (0.05 mg/kg IM before surgery, then every 4 hours for 24 hours), phenylbutazone alone (4.4 mg/kg IV, before surgery and then 2.2 mg/kg by mouth, every 12 hours for 3 days) or butorphanol and phenylbutazone at the aforementioned dosages were similar. However, every horse in the study received preoperative intratesticular lidocaine, which may have obscured differences between treatments. One study[46] compared the effects of butorphanol (50 μg/kg IV), morphine (0.1 mg/kg IV), or saline given with romifidine (100 μg/kg IV) in 54 ponies undergoing field castration and found sedation was significantly better in ponies receiving butorphanol compared with saline. Quality of anesthesia was better in the butorphanol group compared with the morphine and control groups. Quality of induction and recovery were not significantly different between groups, nor were recovery time and the number of repeated anesthetic doses required during surgery. This finding indicates that butorphanol at least improves the quality of some TIVA anesthetic techniques.

## OPIOID ANALGESICS AND INHALATIONAL ANESTHESIA
### The Effects of Opioid Analgesics on Minimum Alveolar Concentration

The sparing effects of morphine (and those of other opioids) on inhalational agents are less obvious in horses compared with other species.[12] The minimum alveolar concentration (MAC) (ie, the end-tidal concentration of inhaled anesthetic preventing purposeful responses to a specified noxious stimulus in 50% of a test population) is lowered by opioid drugs in most species studied. However, in horses most studies reveal opioid drugs exert either a negligible or a MAC-increasing effect and considerable individual variation. For example, in an investigation of the MAC of halothane in 7 ponies[47] acepromazine (0.05 mg/kg) reduced MAC by 36.9% (mean), whereas butorphanol (0.05 mg/kg) did not significantly change the mean group MAC value, although it increased it in 3 ponies, decreased it in 1, and was without effect in the remaining three. In another study[48] the MAC of isoflurane was unaffected by low-dose morphine (0.25 mg/kg) but was increased significantly by a higher dose (2.0 mg/kg). Again, the effects were highly variable; MAC was reduced by 19% in one horse, and increased by 56% in another. No significant changes in MAC of halothane were identified before and during the infusion of alfentanil (another opioid-3 agonist) given at 3 constant rate infusions[49] and the investigators concluded that plasma alfentanil concentrations known to be effective in human beings and dogs did not induce an appreciable change in halothane MAC in horses. In a fourth study[50] butorphanol (0.022 mg/kg and 0.044 mg/kg) decreased the MAC of halothane by 9% or 10%, depending on the dose; however, this was not a statistically significant effect, and in 2 ponies, MAC increased. These studies suggest that opioid drugs at certain doses stimulate rather than depress CN activity in horses anesthetized with experimental techniques and stimulated electrically.

### The Benefits of Opioid Analgesics During Inhalation Anesthesia

Opioids are used in other species during inhalational anesthesia to reduce the requirement for volatile anesthetic, and thus preserve cardiopulmonary function. This situation may not apply in horses given their variable effect on MAC. However, numerous studies show that intraoperative opioids given to horses undergoing surgical procedures have negligible cardiopulmonary effect and improve the quality of recovery (see later discussion), whereas at least 2 studies indicate an analgesic and anesthetic-sparing effect. In one study[51] involving 45 horses anesthetized for arthroscopy with halothane, 31 horses received preoperative butorphanol (50 μg/kg IV), whereas the remainder did not. The mean dose of vaporized halothane, the vaporizer dial setting, and the dose of dobutamine required to correct hypotension were significantly lower in butorphanol recipients, whereas mean arterial blood pressure was significantly higher. In a retrospective study of 82 surgical cases[52] butorphanol appeared to deepen isoflurane anesthesia without adversely affecting cardiovascular variables. Furthermore, it appeared to obtund sympathetic stimulation arising from surgery.

### Opioid Analgesics in Experimental versus Clinical Inhalation Anesthesia

Studies showing MAC increase by opioid analgesics do not confirm the absence of an analgesic effect[12] during inhalation anesthesia for several reasons. First, electrical stimulation is probably qualitatively different from surgical nocistimulation. Second, even under general anesthesia, opioid stimulation may obfuscate more subtle signs of antinociception. Extradural (rather than systemic) morphine (0.1 mg/kg) reduces the MAC of halothane by 14% during pelvic limb stimulation.[53] Third, MAC studies are performed on horses anesthetized with the drug being evaluated and no other, which contrasts with a typical general anesthetic for animals undergoing surgery. Fourth, the use of movement as an index of inadequate CN depression (ie, MAC) has been challenged.[54]

### Opioid Analgesics, Recovery from General Anesthesia, and Box-walking

Concerns have been raised[12] that opioid-induced locomotor activity may adversely affect recovery quality from anesthesia, whereas others have warned that opiates may prolong recovery when given before animals have recovered consciousness.[55] In support of these concerns, Steffey and colleagues[48] described poor recoveries in horses that had received 2.0 mg/kg morphine characterized by strong running or galloping movements made while horses were still in lateral recumbency; preoperative butorphanol (0.1 mg/kg IV) significantly prolonged recovery from a TIVA technique used for colt castration.[44]

However, several studies have indicated that morphine does not impair recovery quality after general anesthesia in clinical cases. One study, involving 25 horses undergoing minor orthopedic or soft-tissue surgery, found no differences in recovery quality between horses receiving saline, butorphanol (50 µg/kg), or morphine (0.02 or 0.05 mg/kg).[19] A retrospective study of 84 horses undergoing surgery found no significant differences in the incidence of postoperative box-walking between horses receiving (n = 51) and not receiving morphine.[56] Of the 2 horses that box-walked (one from each group) that which had received morphine (120 µg/kg IV) was identified as a habitual box-walker. In the United Kingdom, one study (n = 8427) revealed that 1.1% of racehorses box-walk spontaneously and without anesthetic and/or surgical provocation.[57] Furthermore, Mircica and colleagues[56] found recovery quality was better in horses receiving morphine. Box-walking was similarly absent in a prospective study of 22 horses undergoing elective surgical procedures in which 11 received preinduction morphine (0.15 mg/kg) followed by its infusion (0.1 mg/kg/h) during halothane anesthesia.[58] In this study, morphine recipients recovered better than those not receiving morphine, with quality differences increasing with the duration of anesthesia. In a fourth study involving 38 thoroughbred horses undergoing upper airway surgery[59] no box-walking was observed in any horse but recovery quality was significantly better in horses that received morphine (0.1 [n = 13] and 0.2 [n = 12] mg/kg). Meperidine (2 mg/kg IM) injected at the end of 3 different anesthetic techniques in 128 horses undergoing surgery and/or radiography did not affect recovery scores, nor the time to achieve sternal recumbency or standing.[60]

The use of intraoperative opioids also reduces the need for postoperative analgesics. In one study[61] analgesia was supplemented in 68 of 203 horses anesthetized with halothane using butorphanol (up to 0.1 mg/kg) treated postoperatively with phenylbutazone (4 mg/kg), flunixin (1 mg/kg), or carprofen (0.7 mg/kg). The need for additional postoperative analgesia was significantly reduced in horses receiving butorphanol.

### Reconciling Opioid-induced Locomotion Versus Improved Recovery Quality

One explanation for the absence of locomotor activity and improved recovery quality in surgical cases compared with experimental horses is that the former receive sedatives (eg, $\alpha_2$ agonists), which may obscure any stimulant effects that high-dose morphine or other opioids may exert, whereas drugs with antidopaminergic activity (eg, acepromazine) may depress the neural processes promoting adverse reactions.[62] Second, $\alpha_2$-agonist or phenothiazine drugs may potentiate the sedative and/or analgesic properties of opioid analgesics. Third, opioid doses used in clinical studies are substantially less than those used in deliberate attempts to experimentally produce side effects. Fourth, surgical pain may reveal the principal pharmacologic quality of morphine (ie, analgesia) more reliably than laboratory nocistimulation (ie, the drug performs better when real pain is present). These possibilities feature in one study[48] in which 6 pain-free horses anesthetized only with isoflurane had undesirable and dangerous recoveries after receiving high- (2.0 mg/kg) but not low- (0.25 mg/kg) dose morphine. Clinical anecdotes attributing postoperative box-walking to opioid analgesics may have described horses suffering from inadequate analgesia. Increased locomotor activity is a common sign of pain in horses, particularly those with gastrointestinal pain. Postoperative gastrointestinal pain is not uncommon in horses deprived of analgesia. In one study[63] horses not receiving phenylbutazone after arthroscopy were more likely to show signs of postoperative abdominal discomfort than those receiving the drug. Such signs could have been attributed to opioid analgesics, had they been given. In another study[59] 3 (of 12 horses) not receiving morphine showed signs of postoperative abdominal discomfort, whereas 25 (of 25) morphine recipients did not. In a study examining the postoperative effects of morphine[56] one horse ran obsessively around the recovery box after standing, and could be halted with difficulty only after 5 minutes. In this case, a misdiagnosis of opioid-induced locomotion could not be made because the horse had not received opioid analgesics. One multicenter study examining the role of opioids in controlling colic pain[43] graded abdominal discomfort using signs that included sweating, exaggerated body movement, heart and respiratory rates, continuous moving, stomping or pawing, weight-shifting, and exaggerated responses to noise. The same study simultaneously used sweating, excitation, cardiovascular or respiratory abnormalities, instability, and abnormal reactions to sight, sound, or touch as indicators of opioid-induced side effects. This study illustrates the potential to confuse signs of inadequate analgesia and the side effects of an opioid analgesic. The ability of veterinary surgeons to distinguish signs of pain from excitatory opioid effects in horses should not be assumed. The lack of consensus in the UK veterinary profession about whether a horse feels pain after castration suggests that equine pain behaviors are not well recognized or fully appreciated.[3]

## DOES MORPHINE CAUSE POSTOPERATIVE COLIC?

The gastrointestinal effects of morphine that are held to predispose to postanesthetic colic (PAC) have contributed to the unpopularity of opioid analgesics in horses.[3] Opioid-induced dysfunction in chronically instrumented bowel loops in small numbers of pain-free Equidae has been convincingly shown, although the clinical relevance of such studies at times seems obscure. For example, morphine (0.5 and 1.0 mg/kg) and fentanyl (10 or 50 μg, IV) initially stimulated, but then inhibited cecocolic electrical and mechanical activity for up to 3 hours in 3 pain-free ponies, whereas naloxone (0.5 mg/kg IV) elicited marked propulsive activity in the colonic segment.[64] Other opioid drugs behave similarly: meperidine (250 mg) and especially methadone (10 mg) decreased the total electrical activity of a chronically instrumented bowel loop in 3 ponies.[65] However, effects are often variable, and seem at odds with clinical observations. In one study[66] butorphanol (0.1 mg/kg) meperidine (1.0 mg/kg) and pentazocine (0.3 mg/kg) increased the duration of migrating myoelectric complexes (MMCs) in the jejunum of 4 pain-free ponies, but although metoclopramide (30 μg/kg) had no effect on MMCs it produced clinical signs of colic, whereas the opioid analgesics did not.

Morphine exerts a constipative effect in normal horses as in other species. In one study[67] morphine (0.5 mg/kg) given twice daily to 5 pain-free horses for 6 days decreased propulsive motility and moisture content in the gastrointestinal tract lumen. The investigators concluded that the effects observed may predispose treated horses to ileus and constipation although they did not reveal the medical indications for 6 days of morphine therapy in pain-free animals.

The volume of references to the adverse effects of μ-agonists on equine gastrointestinal function contrasts with that on μ-antagonist activity. Nevertheless, naloxone (0.75 mg/kg IV) produced rapid onset diarrhea, restlessness, abdominal checking, tachycardia, tachypnoea, and diaphoresis in 8 adult previously pain-free thoroughbreds, which the investigators concluded was an acute abdominal distress syndrome similar to spasmodic colic.[68] This finding confirms the complexity of equine gastrointestinal pharmacology and supports the possibility that inadequate analgesia may have been responsible for signs previously attributed to morphine.

### Nonopioid Causes of PAC in Horses

Other causes of gastrointestinal dysfunction may contribute to PAC in horses. Recent changes in management[69–72] such as exercise, diet, and transport may increase risk in hospitalized horses.[73] Prolonged starvation (18 hours) has also been implicated.[74] Sympathetic nervous stimulation as part of the stress response to anesthesia, surgery, and nocistimulation decreases gastrointestinal motility in human beings[75] and probably has similar effects in horses.[76] Many drugs used to ameliorate the stress response also depress gut motility, including $\alpha_2$-agonist drugs, which are almost universally used for preanesthetic medication[77,78] and nonsteroidal antiinflammatory drugs (NSAIDs),[79] which are commonly used for analgesic and antiendotoxic effects. The combination of xylazine and ketamine (arguably one of the most popular means of inducing anesthesia in horses) produced the longest period of hypomotility in one myoelectrical study of equine intestinal activity.[80] These findings challenge the justification for implicating opioid drugs as a principal cause of postoperative colic, which is unsupported by epidemiologic studies.

### Postoperative Colic: Epidemiologic Studies

One study[73] linked morphine with a 4-fold increase in risk of PAC after orthopedic surgery compared with the use of butorphanol, or abstinence from opioid analgesia. In this study, 14 horses develop colic after a total of 496 operations. However, despite a population dose range of 0.08 to 0.3 mg/kg, 13 of the 14 cases that subsequently developed colic received only 0.1 mg/kg. The study also failed to clarify the factors determining morphine dose. It is therefore possible that severe orthopedic pain contributed to postoperative gastrointestinal dysfunction in some of the horses that developed colic. Another link between morphine and an increased prevalence of PAC was identified in a different center,[81] but the association disappeared when analyses were stratified by procedure, indicating that the operation type was a greater risk factor than the opioid analgesic. This study, which examined the anesthetic records of 553 horses (342 undergoing magnetic resonance imaging [MRI]; 211 having nonabdominal [predominantly orthopedic] surgery), found 20 cases developed PAC,[81] representing 7.1% of surgical and 1.5% of MRI cases. Increased risk was associated with isoflurane, and the use of benzyl penicillin and/or ceftiofur for antibiosis. Factors reducing risk were romifidine for preanesthetic medication, prolonged anesthesia, and sedation within 2 days of general anesthesia. Perianesthetic morphine administration was not associated with increased risk. A multicenter case-control study[82] looking at the prevalence of and risk factors associated with PAC in 861 horses undergoing nonabdominal surgery found that the center involved and the operation type increased risk, nonseptic orthopedic cases being at greatest risk. Preoperative food deprivation (horses that were not starved were more likely to develop colic) and opioid drugs were confounding factors. In this study, 45 horses developed colic. Although the use of opioid analgesics increased risk when compared with surgeries in which none were used, there were no significant differences between butorphanol or morphine use. The prevalence of PAC in those centers using butorphanol exclusively was the same as those using only morphine. In one study[60,61] of 38 thoroughbreds undergoing upper airway surgery, the prevalence of decreased appetite for up to 4 postoperative days in horses not receiving morphine (8 of 12) was similar with those receiving morphine at 0.1 mg/kg (7 of 13) or 0.2 mg/kg (7 of 12). However, 3 (of 12) horses not receiving morphine showed signs of postoperative discomfort consistent with colic. No horses receiving morphine developed PAC. Butorphanol also seems to confer benefit. Doses up to 100 µg/kg were used in a proportion of 203 horses under-going surgery and randomly allocated to receive flunixin, carprofen, or phenylbuta-zone. Signs of mild colic were observed in 18 horses but were unassociated with use of butorphanol. Butophanol ensured a reduced requirement for postoperative NSAID therapy.[59] In another study[56] there were no significant differences in the inci-dence of postoperative gastrointestinal complications between horses receiving (n = 51) and not receiving (n = 33) morphine at 100 to 170 µg/kg.

The literature indicates a multifactorial cause for PAC and an equivocal contribution by morphine and other opioid analgesics. However, even unequivocal evidence for an opioid-associated risk would have to be weighed against the better recoveries that opioid analgesics promote. In 5 studies[56,59,73,81,82] investigating opioid-induced morbidities in a total of 2240 horses, PAC occurred in 100. None of these died directly from postoperative colic and only 2 required surgical treatment. In contrast, fractures in recovery, some of which are related to poor-quality recoveries, are the second greatest cause of postoperative equine mortality.[83]

### Opioid Analgesics in the Control of Gastrointestinal Pain

Some authorities, although acknowledging the efficacy of opioids as analgesics, have condemned their use in equine colic because they cause excitation.[21] Others have suggested the ability of opioids to stimulate forceful contractions in an already dis-tended bowel supports a relative contraindication for their use in colicky horses with that condition.[12] In 1946 Milks wrote, "Small doses [of morphine] are usually sedative to the horse so that the drug is especially indicated in strong persistent pain such as enteritis. It may often be extremely useful in spasmodic colic and produces its action here by arresting the irregular and violent peristalsis which is the cause of the pain."[84] Later support for the role of morphine in colic pain emerged in a study that recorded gastrointestinal electrical potentials from 2 ponies that devel-oped colic naturally.[85] The investigators recommended the use of morphine because "it provided concomitant antispasmodic action on the small bowels while stimulating colonic activity." This recommendation contrasts with the conclusion of a study[78] examining the effects of xylazine (0.5 mg/kg) detomidine (12.5 µg/kg) and a xylazine (0.5 mg/kg)-butorphanol (0.05 mg/kg) combination on equine duodenal motility that concluded that "the profound suppressive effect of a routine dose of detomidine or xylazine - butorphanol combination on equine duodenal motility must be considered when using these agents for management of colic, especially when encouragement of intestinal motility is desirable."

In the clinical situation, the effective management of pain overrides theoretic concerns with the effects of opioid analgesics on gastrointestinal function for at least 2 reasons: (1) it allows the safer diagnosis of surgical versus medical colic; and (2) it is humane.

## CARDIOVASCULAR EFFECTS OF OPIOID DRUGS IN HORSES

The cardiovascular effects of opioid analgesics in horses seem to depend on the drug, dose, administration route, and coadministered drugs, although the recipient's level of consciousness is important because cardiovascular hyperdynamism is often linked with central nervous (CN) stimulation. Morphine can cause hypotension in human beings by initiating histamine release with peripheral vasodilatation and tachycardia. The likelihood of this is said to be greatest when high doses are given rapidly IV. Morphine has caused urticarial lesions in horses, which may be linked to this finding, although associated cardiovascular effects are unreported. This is not the case with meperidine, which has caused severe reactions when given IV (1 mg/kg) in both conscious and unconscious horses.[86] In general, opioid drugs seem not to depress cardiovascular variables in anesthetized horses to the same (modest) extent that they do in other species,[20] although all studies conducted in this area have involved small numbers of pain-free horses or ponies.

### Cardiovascular Effects of Opioid Analgesics in Conscious Horses

Intravenous morphine (0.12 mg/kg), meperidine (1.1 mg/kg), oxymorphone (0.03 mg/kg), methadone (0.12 mg/kg), and pentazocine (0.9 mg/kg) caused similar levels of cardiovascular stimulation[87] linked with dysphoria and euphoria. Heart rate (HR) increased after injection but returned to baseline within 30 minutes. Systolic (SAP), mean (MAP), and diastolic (DAP) arterial pressures increased significantly although transiently. In another study[21] morphine (0.66 mg/kg IM) caused excitation and increased all cardiovascular variables for at least 4 hours. Buprenorphine (10 µg/kg IV) also stimulated 6 pain-free horses, causing a sustained (120- minute) increase in HR, SAP, MAP, and DAP and cardiac index.[27] However, in another buprenorphine study several effects did not coincide with CN system activity: 3 µg/kg IV caused a marked and lasting hypertension without a corresponding HR increase. In one horse that became sedated DAP, but not SAP, increased without a concomitant increase in HR.[26]

Cardiovascular and CN stimulation are variably linked in horses receiving butorphanol. Intravenous doses of 0.1, 0.2, and 0.4 mg/kg caused predominantly excitatory signs yet did not significantly affect HR, MAP, or DAP.[88] In another study[23] IV butorphanol (0.1–0.13 mg/kg) caused gross behavioral disturbances although the HR was unaltered in 4 of 7 animals. Although these studies suggest that the depressant effect of butorphanol on HR overcomes the chronotropy of CN stimulation, another study[21] found 0.22 mg/kg increased HR. Furthermore, neither HR nor MAP changed from pre-injection values when butorphanol (0.05 mg/kg) was injected IV in horses anesthetized with halothane undergoing minor orthopedic or soft-tissue surgery.[19]

### Cardiovascular Effects of Opioid Analgesics with $\alpha_2$ Agonists

The cardiovascular effects of opioid/$\alpha_2$ agonist combinations are unpredictable because the latter have complex time- and dose-dependent effects, whereas their sedative properties ameliorate any opioid-induced CN stimulation in nonpainful horses. Most studies indicate the hemodynamic effects of $\alpha_2$ agonists prevail over those of opioid analgesics. For example, in one study, butorphanol (50 µg/kg, IV) added to one of 2 romifidine doses (40 and 80 µg/kg, IV) had no effect on HR and MAP compared with those of romifidine alone.[40] In another study,[20] 2 doses of morphine (0.12 and 0.66 mg/kg) given to horses presedated with xylazine (0.66 mg/kg) caused similar significant decreases in cardiac output (Qt) and increases in central venous pressure, SAP, MAP, DAP, and pulmonary arterial pressure.

Detomidine (10 µg/kg) seems to ameliorate opioid-induced cardiovascular effects less than xylazine and romifidine.[9] When morphine (0.1 mg/kg), methadone (0.1 mg/kg), meperidine (1.0 mg/kg), or butorphanol (50 µg/kg) were administered IV to pain-free ponies and a thoroughbred sedated 6 minutes earlier with detomidine (10 µg/kg), marked tachycardia and hypertension followed morphine and meperidine injection, although cardiovascular changes were minimal within 5 minutes. This finding was not associated with excitation except in one pony whose HR rose to 70 beats per minute and MAP to 200 mm Hg. Despite preexisting sedation, meperidine caused marked excitation in one pony and increased HR to 100 beats per minute and MAP to 215 mm Hg.

### Cardiovascular Effects of Opioid Analgesics with Inhalant Anesthetics

Opioids seem to have little, if any, cardiovascular effects in anesthetized horses undergoing surgery. Neither HR nor MAP changed when intravenous morphine (20 and 50 µg/kg) or butorphanol (0.05 mg/kg) were given to horses anesthetized with halothane undergoing minor orthopedic or soft-tissue surgery.[19] The incidence of bradycardia, tachycardia, hypertension, and hypotension was similar in 84 horses anesthetized with halothane irrespective of whether morphine (100–170 µg/kg) was given or not (n = 33).[56] In another study[89] 19 of 38 horses anesthetized with halothane received preoperative morphine (0.15 mg/kg IV) followed by infusion (0.1 mg/kg/h). There were no significant differences in the MAP or HR of these animals compared with those receiving the same anesthetic without morphine. Butorphanol also exerted little measurable effect in horses anesthetized with isoflurane.[52] A retrospective evaluation of anesthetic records from 76 horses anesthetized for various operations revealed that butorphanol did not affect SAP, MAP, DAP, or HR, causing the investigators to conclude that butorphanol can be administered to horses during isoflurane anesthesia without adverse cardiovascular effects.

Pharmacologic relationships do not seem to allow the prediction of the effect of a drug. In one study of horses anesthetized with halothane not undergoing surgery[50] infused alfentanil caused dose-dependent increases in blood pressure, although HR did not change. In contrast, the related phenylpiperidine derivative sufentanil (1 and 2 µg/kg IV) transiently reduced MAP and HR in 6 different animals similarly anesthetized.[90]

It is possible that surgical nocistimulation during inhalation anesthesia offsets any opioid-induced cardiovascular depression, whereas general anesthesia obtunds sympathoadrenal responses arising from opioid-induced CN stimulation.

## RESPIRATORY EFFECTS OF OPIOID DRUGS IN HORSES

The respiratory effects of morphine and other opioid drugs in horses also seem to depend on whether recipients are conscious and excitable, or unconscious,[87] although this is not always predictable.

### Respiratory Effects of Opioid Analgesics in Conscious Horses

In one study, butorphanol (0.1, 0.2, and 0.4 mg/kg IV) caused excitatory signs but did not significantly affect respiratory rate (fr), arterial blood gas values, or arterial pH (pHa).[23] In contrast, buprenorphine (10 µg/kg IV) caused CN stimulation and increased fr although the arterial partial pressure of oxygen ($Pao_2$) and carbon dioxide ($Paco_2$) and hemoglobin saturation (as determined by pulse oximetry [$Spo_2$]) were unchanged.[27] Changes are usually minor and drug dependent. In a comparison of morphine (0.12 mg/kg IV), meperidine (1.1 mg/kg IV), oxymorphone (0.03 mg/kg IV), methadone (0.12 mg/kg IV), and pentazocine (0.9 mg/kg IV)[87] fr was unchanged or initially increased and then decreased minimally. Although $Paco_2$ decreased slightly, arterial and venous $O_2$ tensions and pH were unchanged. The fr was changed least by morphine, meperidine, and oxymorphone and most by methadone. In general, changes were linked with dysphoria and euphoria. In another study[21] comparing butorphanol (0.22 mg/kg), flunixin (2.2 mg/kg), levorphanol (0.033 mg/kg), and morphine (0.66 mg/kg), butorphanol, flunixin, and levorphanol produced no effect on fr or blood-gas values, whereas morphine increased fr for 4 hours without affecting blood gas values. One study[26] concluded that the modest respiratory effects (increased fr and minute expiratory ventilation with reduced tidal volume) of buprenorphine (3, 5, and 10 µg/kg IV) were not dose related, nor linked with CN excitation.

### Respiratory Effects of Opioid Analgesics with α2 Agonists

$α_2$ agonists seem to modestly potentiate the respiratory depressant effects of some, but not all, opioid drugs. Detomidine (10 µg/kg) given alone or followed with morphine (0.1 mg/kg), methadone (0.1 mg/kg), meperidine (1.0 mg/kg), or butorphanol (50 µg/kg) was studied in 3 ponies and a thoroughbred. Morphine caused modest falls in $Pao_2$ and rises in $Paco_2$, whereas meperidine increased only $Paco_2$.[9] The effect may depend on the $α_2$ agonist involved: butorphanol (50 µg/kg IV) had no effect on $Pao_2$ and pHa, but significantly increased $Paco_2$ for 20 minutes when added to romifidine (40 and 80 µg/kg, IV).[40]

The dose of opioid involved seems to be unimportant. Two doses of morphine (0.12 and 0.66 mg/kg) given to 9 horses sedated with xylazine (0.66 mg/kg) caused similar and significant decreases in fr whereas $Paco_2$, $Pao_2$, and pHa remained unchanged.[20]

### Respiratory Effects of Opioid Analgesics with Inhalant Anesthetics

Neither low morphine doses (20 and 50 µg/kg) nor butorphanol (0.05 mg/kg) caused significant changes from preinjection values for fr, $Paco_2$, $Pao_2$ and airway occlusion pressure in horses anesthetized with halothane.[19] In another study of horses anesthetized with halothane undergoing elective surgery, the preoperative injection of morphine (0.15 mg/kg IV) followed by infusion (0.1 mg/kg/h) did not cause significant differences in $Pao_2$ or $Paco_2$ when compared with horses from which morphine was withheld.[89]

These data do not support the widely held view[9,24] that high doses of intraoperative opioids depress ventilation in unconscious horses, a view to which this author subscribes.

## MORPHINE AND PULMONARY EDEMA

Despite its mild cardiopulmonary effects, morphine has been implicated in 2 cases of postoperative pulmonary edema.[91] Although the investigators identified numerous risk factors[92] in both cases, they concluded that fluid overload was worsened by a "morphine-induced reduction in urine production," and by "potential morphine-induced changes in pulmonary permeability." This reveals the most useful role of morphine in equine anesthesia: to assume responsibility for any untoward perioperative event.

## OPIOID ANALGESICS IN HORSES: RECOMMENDATIONS

Recommended doses of opioid analgesics in horses vary widely (**Table 2**) because the effective dose depends on numerous factors. Dosing should follow 4 general rules: (1) the more severe the pain (or the greater the surgical insult), the greater the dose of

**Table 2**
**Recommended doses of opioid analgesics in horses**

|  | Analgesia | Preoperative | Intraoperative | Postoperative |
|---|---|---|---|---|
| Morphine | 0.05–0.1 mg/kg IV or IM[a 24,93] 0.1–0.3 mg/kg IV[b] | 0.15 mg/kg[58,59] | 0.1 mg/kg/h[58,59] | 0.1–0.2 mg/kg[b] |
| Meperidine | 0.3–0.6 mg/kg IV[93] 1–2 mg/kg IM only[24] |  |  | 2 mg/kg IM[62,63] |
| Methadone | 0.05–0.1 mg/kg[93] 0.1 mg/kg IV or IM[24] |  |  |  |
| Butorphanol | 0.01–0.02 mg/kg[93] 0.05–0.1 mg/kg[24] |  |  | 13 μg/kg/h[94,b] |
| Buprenorphine | 10–20 μg/kg IV[93] 60 μg/kg IV or IM[24] |  |  |  |

[a] All doses intravenous unless stated otherwise.
[b] Author's preference.

opioid analgesic required, and the lower the risk of excitatory side effects; (2) in pain-free horses, giving appropriate doses of $\alpha_2$ agonists matched for duration of action eliminates the risk of excitation; acepromazine reduces, but does not eliminate, risk; (3) although opioid analgesics are described in terms of duration of action, they should be given to effect (ie, when the desired level of analgesia has waned below acceptable levels), and not by the clock; and (4) clinical signs of underdose (ie, pain) may mimic signs of overdosage.

## NEW TECHNIQUES FOR PERIOPERATIVE OPIOID ANALGESIA
### Extradural Opioid Analgesia

Extradural morphine injection consistently suppresses responses to experimental and clinical nocistimulation in horses without causing sensory, sympathetic nervous, or motor blockade. This subject is discussed elsewhere.

### Opioid Analgesics and Intraarticular Analgesia

Opioid receptors have been identified on peripheral terminals of sensory nerves, whereas opioid peptide ligands (principally β-endorphin and met-encephalin) have been discovered in immune cells from inflamed synovial tissue of human patients undergoing arthroscopic knee surgery.[95] The identification of opioid receptors in the equine synovia[96] has stimulated interest in producing intraarticular (IA) opioid analgesia in horses.

Initial studies showed an absence of tissue irritancy or systemic effects after IA morphine. No evidence of adverse local reactions or systemic effects were seen after IA morphine sulfate (1 mg) or buprenorphine hydrochloride (300 μg) injection into the middle carpal joints of 5 ponies. However, the vehicles of each drug were not detailed.[97] The disposition and local effects (15 mg in 5 mL saline) of morphine were also studied after injection into the tarsocrural joint of normal ponies.[98] Morphine remained detectable in synovial fluid 24 hours after injection, although systemic levels were unmeasureable after 6 hours. No adverse systemic effects were seen. The injection contained 0.1% w/v sodium metabisulfite but morphine did not irritate the joint any more than saline.

A later study[99] compared the analgesic efficacy of IA and intravenous morphine (0.05/mg both routes) in horses with experimentally induced radiocarpal synovitis. As might be expected from the predictable differences in effector site drug concentration, IA morphine resulted in significantly less lameness than intravenous morphine, although overall pain scores did not differ between treatments. The results indicate the potential usefulness of IA morphine after arthroscopic surgery, although further studies in clinical cases are needed. The analgesic effects of IA morphine (40 mg) were compared with the local anesthetic ropivacaine (40 mg) and a ropivacaine (20 mg)-morphine (200 mg) mixture injected intraarticularly in 12 horses with experimentally induced radiocarpal synovitis.[100] Ropivacaine produced approximately 3 hours of analgesia after a rapid onset, whereas morphine had a slower onset but a greater analgesic effect of longer duration (>24 hours). The combination combined the advantages of both drugs.

## Transdermal Fentanyl Analgesia

The fentanyl transdermal therapeutic system or patches has become popular in small animals and has recently been studied in horses. Plasma fentanyl concentration during transdermal administration depends on the properties of the skin and so may vary with the application site of the patches. An in vitro[101] study of equine skin from thoracic, inguinal, and dorsal metacarpal areas revealed similar values for fentanyl flux (over 48 hours) for thoracic and inguinal skin, which were greater than those from the dorsal metacarpus. Fentanyl penetration through inguinal skin was significantly slower compared with the other 2 sites. Two 100-μg/h fentanyl patches applied to the lateral necks of 3 horses weighing 352 to 459 kg[102] resulted in rapid absorption, with plasma fentanyl levels exceeding 2 ng/mL after 4 hours. Peak plasma concentrations (3.85 ng/mL) occurred at 6.7 hours, after which levels declined over 48 hours but remained greater than 1 ng/mL (which is held to represent an analgesic concentration in other species) for 54 hours. Plasma drug levels decreased rapidly after patch removal and no adverse behavioral responses were reported. In another study[103] 3 10-mg patches (equivalent to 60–67 μg/kg) were applied to the middorsal thorax and resulted, after a 2-hour lag period, in a rapid increase in plasma fentanyl concentration, which was a maximum at 12 hours and declined thereafter in a near-linear fashion. However, there was much individual variation. In 2 horses, plasma concentrations failed to reach 1 ng/mL. In the remaining four it was greater than 1 ng/mL for at least 40 hours and longer than 72 hours in two of these. No adverse effects attributable to fentanyl were observed, indicating that the dose tested was safe in healthy adult horses. However, it failed to achieve plasma fentanyl concentrations generally considered to be analgesic in about one-third of horses. The clinical efficacy of transdermal fentanyl was investigated in 9 horses whose pain was unresponsive to phenylbutazone (n = 3) or flunixin (n = 6) and which subsequently received between 39 and 110 μg/kg of transdermal fentanyl.[104] One 10-mg patch was applied per 150 kg of body mass to the lateral cervical and/or lateral or medial proximal antebrachial area. After administration, mean time to serum fentanyl concentrations greater than 1 ng/mL was 14 hours. Serum fentanyl concentrations 1 ng/mL or greater were maintained in all but one horse for at least 18 hours. No adverse effects were observed. Pain scores were significantly decreased after fentanyl and NSAID administration but improvement was minimal in horses with orthopedic disease, and lameness scores did not change in the 3 horses with septic physitis or osteomyelitis. That transdermal fentanyl is less effective at relieving orthopedic pain compared with soft-tissue pain has been observed elsewhere.[105]

## SUMMARY

A questionnaire-based study of UK equine veterinarians' attitudes to analgesics (which confused the terms potency with efficacy) revealed the most important determinant of choice was the perceived potency of a drug.[3] Fears of adverse gastrointestinal and locomotor effects were also important. These fears have been generated by studies that lack external validity, having been conducted on small numbers of pain-free horses or ponies, exposed to artificial, rather than surgical or traumatic, nocistimulation and not receiving the range of drugs that would be the case in the perioperative or trauma setting. Similarities between equine pain behaviors and opioid side effects make it possible that some adverse reactions attributed to drugs were signs of inadequate analgesia. Despite increasing evidence of their clinical usefulness, unenlightened assertions concerning opioid analgesics continue to be made. The statement "Opioids are not widely used in horses because they can cause CN system excitation, sympathetic stimulation, and can stimulate locomotion" was recently used to justify an experimental study of the analgesic activity of tramadol in pain-free horses.[106] To show that the margin between the analgesic and stimulant effects of opioid analgesics in horses is probably much broader than hitherto proposed requires (1) an improved ability to recognize equine pain; (2) a precise and valid equine pain scoring system; (3) the use of effective, not excessive, opioid doses; (4) a large number of animals with actual, rather than experimentally induced, pain.

## REFERENCES

1. Yoxall AT. Pain in small animals–its recognition and control. J Small Anim Pract 1978;19:423–38.
2. Hellyer PW, Bai L, Supon J, et al. Comparison of opioid and alpha-2 adrenergic receptor binding in horse and dog brain using radioligand autoradiography. Vet Anaesth Analg 2003;30:172–82.
3. Price J, Marques M, Welsh EM, et al. Pilot epidemiological study of attitudes towards pain in horses. Vet Rec 2002;151:570–5.
4. Guinard L. Encyclopedie cadeac veterinaire, "effets apparents du morphinisme chez les solipèdes" therapeutique et pharmacodynamie, Tome 1. 401, Paris, 1899.
5. Milks HJ. Opium-morphine. In: Practical veterinary pharmacology and therapeutics. New York: The Macmillan Company; 1917. p. 139–46.
6. Frohner E. Morphinum hydrochloricum. Salzsaures morphium. In: Lehrbuch der arzneiverordnungslehre fur tierarzte. Stuttgart (Germany): Verlag von Ferdin & Enke; 1921. p. 62–70.
7. Amadon RS, Craigie AH. The actions of morphine on the horse. Preliminary studies: diacetylmorphine (heroin), dihydrodesoxymorphine-D (desomorphine) and dihydroheterocodeine. J Am Vet Med Assoc 1937;91:674–8.
8. Carregaro AB, Luna SP, Mataqueiro MI, et al. Effects of buprenorphine on nociception and spontaneous locomotor activity in horses. Am J Vet Res 2007;68: 246–50.
9. Clarke KW, Paton BS. Combined use of detomidine with opiates in the horse. Equine Vet J 1988;20:331–4.
10. Combie J, Dougherty J, Nugent E, et al. The pharmacology of narcotic analgesics in the horse. IV. Dose and time response relationships for behavioral responses to morphine. meperidine, pentazocine, anileridine, methadone, and hydromorphone. J Equine Med Surg 1979;3:377–85.

11. Combie J, Shultz T, Nugent EC, et al. Pharmacology of narcotic analgesics in the horse: selective blockade of narcotic-induced locomotor activity. Am J Vet Res 1981;42:716–21.
12. Bennet RC, Steffey EP. Use of opioids for pain and anesthetic management in horses. Vet Clin North Am Equine Pract 2002;18(1):47–60.
13. Tobin T, Combie J, Miller JR, et al. The pharmacology of narcotic analgesics in the horse. II. Studies on the detection, pharmacokinetics, urinary clearance times and behavioral effects of pentozocine and fentanyl in the horse. Ir Vet J 1979;33:169–76.
14. Kamerling SG, DeQuick DJ, Weckman TJ, et al. Dose-related effects of ethylketazocine on nociception, behaviour and autonomic responses in the horse. J Pharm Pharmacol 1985;38:40–5.
15. Nolan AM, Besley W, Reid J, et al. The effects of butorphanol on locomotor activity in ponies: a preliminary study. J Vet Pharmacol Ther 1994;17:323–6.
16. Mama KR, Pascoe PJ, Steffey EP. Evaluation of the interaction of mu and kappa opioid agonists on locomotor behavior in the horse. Can J Vet Res 1992;57:106–9.
17. Bogan JA, Mackenzie G, Snow DH. An evaluation of tranquilizers for use with etorphine as neuroleptanalgesic agents in the horse. Vet Rec 1978;103:471–2.
18. Pascoe PJ, Taylor PM. Effects of dopamine antagonists on alfentanil-induced locomotor activity in horses. Vet Anaesth Analg 2003;30:165–71.
19. Nolan AM, Chambers JP, Hale GJ. The cardiorespiratory effects of morphine and butorphanol in horses anaesthetized under clinical conditions. J Vet Anaesth 1991;18:19–24.
20. Muir WW, Skarda RT, Sheehan WC. Hemodynamic and respiratory effects of xylazine-morphine sulfate in horses. Am J Vet Res 1979;40:1417–20.
21. Kalpravidh M, Lumb WV, Wright M, et al. Effects of butorphanol, flunixin, levorphanol, morphine, and xylazine in ponies. Am J Vet Res 1984;45:217–23.
22. Pascoe PJ, Black WD, Claxton JM, et al. The pharmacokinetics and locomotor activity of alfentanil in the horse. J Vet Pharmacol Ther 1991;14:317–25.
23. Sellon DC, Monroe VL, Roberts MC, et al. Pharmacokinetics and adverse effects of butorphanol administered by single intravenous injection or continuous intravenous infusion in horses. Am J Vet Res 2001;62:183–9.
24. Hall LW, Clarke KW. Trim CM veterinary anaesthesia. 10th edition. London: WB Saunders; 2001. p. 255.
25. Kohn CW, Muir WW. Selected aspects of the clinical pharmacology of visceral analgesics and gut motility modifying drugs in the horse. J Vet Intern Med 1988;2:85–91.
26. Szoke MO, Blais D, Cuvelliez SG, et al. Effects of buprenorphine on cardiovascular and pulmonary function in clinically normal horses and horses with chronic obstructive pulmonary disease. Am J Vet Res 1998;59:1287–91.
27. Carregaro AB, Neto FJ, Beier SL, et al. Cardiopulmonary effects of buprenorphine in horses. Am J Vet Res 2006;67:1675–80.
28. Pippi NL, Lumb WV. Objective tests of analgesic drugs in ponies. Am J Vet Res 1979;40:1082–6.
29. Brunson DB, Majors LJ. Comparative analgesia of xylazine, xylazine/morphine, xylazine/butorphanol, and xylazine/nalbuphine in the horse, using dental dolorimetry. Am J Vet Res 1987;48:1087–92.
30. Kamerling S, Weckman T, Donahoe J, et al. Dose related effects of the kappa agonist U-50,488H on behaviour, nociception and autonomic response in the horse. Equine Vet J 1988;20:114–8.

31. Kalpravidh M, Lumb WV, Wright M, et al. Analgesic effects of butorphanol in horses: dose-response studies. Am J Vet Res 1984;45:211–7.
32. Stucki F, Armbuster S, Moens Y, et al. Comparative studies on analgesia provoked by butorphanol or L-polamidone in detomidine sedated horses. Proceedings of the Association of Veterinary Anaesthesia & European Society of Laboratory Animal Veterinarians, Newcastle (UK), 1999.
33. Schatzman U, Armbruster S, Stucki F, et al. Analgesic effect of butorphanol and levomethadone in detomidine sedated horses. J Vet Med A Physiol Pathol Clin Med 2001;48:337–42.
34. Le Bars D, Gozariu M, Cadden SW. Animal models of nociception. Pharmacol Rev 2001;53:597–652.
35. Spadavecchia C, Spadavecchia L, Andersen OK, et al. Quantitative assessment of nociception in horses by use of the nociceptive withdrawal reflex evoked by transcutaneous electrical stimulation. Am J Vet Res 2002;63:1551–6.
36. Spadavecchia C, Arendt-Nielsen L, Andersen OK, et al. Comparison of nociceptive withdrawal reflexes and recruitment curves between the forelimbs and hind limbs in conscious horses. Am J Vet Res 2003;64:700–7.
37. Muir WW. Drugs used to produce standing chemical restraint in horses. Vet Clin North Am Large Anim Pract 1981;3(1):17–44.
38. Stout RC, Priest GT. Clinical experience using butorphanol tartrate for relief of abdominal pain in the horse. In: Moore JN, White NA, Becht JL, editors, Equine colic research. Proceedings of the second symposium at the University of Georgia, vol. 2. Lawrenceville (NJ): Veterinary Learning Systems; 1986. p. 68–70.
39. Walker AF. Sublingual administration of buprenorphine for long-term analgesia in the horse. Vet Rec 2007;160:808–9.
40. Clarke KW, England GC, Goossens L. Sedative and cardiovascular effects of romifidine alone and in combination with butorphanol in the horse. J Vet Anaesth 1991;18:25–9.
41. Dyson DH, Pascoe PJ, Viel L, et al. Comparison of detomidine hydrochloride, xylazine, and xylazine plus morphine in horses: a double blind study. J Equine Vet Sci 1987;7:211–6.
42. Lowe JE. Xylazine, pentazocine, meperidine and dipyrone for relief of balloon induced equine colic: a double blind comparative evaluation. J Equine Med Surg 1978;2:286–91.
43. Jochle W, Moore JN, Brown J, et al. Comparison of detomidine, butorphanol, flunixin meglumine and xylazine in clinical cases of equine colic. Equine Vet J Suppl 1989;7:111–6.
44. Love EJ, Taylor PM, Clark C, et al. Analgesic effect of butorphanol in ponies following castration. Equine Vet J 2009;41:552–6.
45. Sanz MG, Sellon DC, Cary JA, et al. Analgesic effects of butorphanol tartrate and phenylbutazone administered alone and in combination in young horses undergoing routine castration. J Am Vet Med Assoc 2009;235:1194–203.
46. Corletto F, Raisis AA, Brearley JC. Comparison of morphine and butorphanol as pre-anaesthetic agents in combination with romifidine for field castration in ponies. Vet Anaesth Analg 2005;32:16–22.
47. Doherty TJ, Geiser DR, Rohrbach BW. Effect of acepromazine and butorphanol on halothane minimum alveolar concentration in ponies. Equine Vet J 1997;29:374–6.
48. Steffey EP, Eisele JH, Baggot JD. Interactions of morphine and isoflurane in horses. Am J Vet Res 2003;64:166–75.

49. Pascoe PJ, Steffey EP, Black WD, et al. Evaluation of the effect of alfentanil on the minimum alveolar concentration on halothane in horses. Am J Vet Res 1993;54:1327–32.
50. Matthews NS, Lindsay SL. Effect of low dose butorphanol on halothane minimum alveolar concentration in ponies. Equine Vet J 1990;22:325–7.
51. Caure S, Cousty M, Tricaud C. Effects of adding butorphanol to a balanced anaesthesia protocol during arthroscopic surgery in horses. Vet Rec 2010;166:324–8.
52. Hofmeister EH, Mackey EB, Trim CM. Effect of butorphanol administration on cardiovascular parameters in isoflurane-anesthetized horses – a retrospective clinical evaluation. Vet Anaesth Analg 2008;35:38–44.
53. Doherty TJ, Goiser DR, Rohrbach BW. Effects of high-volume epidural morphine, butorphanol and ketamine on halothane MAC in the horse. J Vet Anaesth 1995;22:37.
54. Rampil IJ, Laster MJ. No correlation between quantitative electroencephalographic measurements and movement response to noxious stimuli during isoflurane anesthesia in rats. Anesthesiology 1992;77:920–5.
55. Hall LW, Clarke KW. Veterinary anaesthesia. 8th edition. London: Bailliere Tindall; 1983. p. 242.
56. Mircica C, Clutton RE, Blissitt KJ. Problems associated with perioperative morphine in horses: a retrospective case analysis. Vet Anaesth Analg 2003; 30:147–55.
57. McBride SD, Long L. Management of horses showing stereotypic behaviour, owner perception and the implications for welfare. Vet Rec 2001;148:799–802.
58. Clark L, Clutton RE, Blissitt KJ, et al. Effects of peri-operative morphine administration on recovery from halothane anaesthesia in horses. Vet Anaesth Analg 2008;35:22–9.
59. Love EJ, Lane JG, Murison PJ. Morphine administration in horses anaesthetized for upper respiratory tract surgery. Vet Anaesth Analg 2006;33:179–88.
60. Taylor PM. Effect of postoperative pethidine on the anaesthetic recovery period in the horse. Equine Vet J 1986;18:70–2.
61. Johnson CB, Taylor PM, Young SS, et al. Postoperative analgesia using phenylbutazone, flunixin or carprofen in horses. Vet Rec 1993;133:336–8.
62. Lal H. Narcotic dependence, narcotic action and dopamine receptors. Life Sci 1978;17:483–96.
63. Raekallio M, Taylor PM, Bennett RC. Post operative analgesia after arthroscopy in horses abstract. Proceedings, 5th International Congress of Veterinary Anesthesia. Guelph (Canada); 1994. p. 145.
64. Roger T, Bardon T, Ruckebusch Y. Colonic motor responses in the pony: relevance of colonic stimulation by opiate antagonists. Am J Vet Res 1985;46:31–6.
65. Davies JV, Getting EL. Effect of spasmolytic analgesic drugs on the motility patterns of the equine small intestine. Res Vet Sci 1983;34:334–9.
66. Sojka JE, Adams SB, Lamar CH, et al. Effect of butorphanol, pentazocine, meperidine, or metoclopramide on intestinal motility in female ponies. Am J Vet Res 1988;49:527–9.
67. Boscan P, Van Hoogmoed LM, Farver TB, et al. Evaluation of the effects of the opioid agonist morphine on gastrointestinal tract function in horses. Am J Vet Res 2006;67:992–7.
68. Kamerling SG, Hamra JG, Bagwell CA. Naloxone-induced abdominal distress in the horse. Equine Vet J 1990;22:241–3.
69. Tinkler MK, White NA, Lessard P, et al. Prospective study of equine colic incidence and mortality. Equine Vet J 1997;29:448–53.

70. Tinkler MK, White NA, Lessard P, et al. Prospective study of equine colic risk factors. Equine Vet J 1997;29:454–8.
71. Cohen ND, Gibbs PG, Woods AM. Dietary and other management factors associated with colic in horses. J Am Vet Med Assoc 1999;215:53–60.
72. Hillyer MH, Taylor FG, Proudman CJ, et al. A case control study of simple colonic obstruction and distension colic in the horse. Equine Vet J 2002;34:455–63.
73. Senior JM, Pinchbeck GL, Dugdale AH, et al. Retrospective study of the risk factors and prevalence of colic in horses after orthopaedic surgery. Vet Rec 2004;155:321–5.
74. Jones RS, Edwards GB, Brearley JC. Commentary on prolonged starvation as a factor associated with post operative colic. Equine Vet Educ 1991;3:16–8.
75. Steinbrook RA. Epidural anesthesia and gastrointestinal motility. Anesth Analg 1998;86:837–44.
76. Little D, Redding WR, Blikslager AT. Risk factors for reduced fecal output in horses: 37 cases (1997–1998). J Am Vet Med Assoc 2001;218:414–20.
77. Roger T, Ruckebusch Y. Colonic $\alpha_2$-adrenoreceptor-mediated responses in the pony. J Vet Pharmacol Ther 1987;10:310–8.
78. Merritt AM, Burrow JA, Harless CS. Effect of xylazine, detomidine, and a combination of xylazine and butorphanol on equine duodenal motility. Am J Vet Res 1998;59:619–23.
79. Van Hoogmoed L, Rakestraw PC, Snyder JR, et al. In vitro effects of nonsteroidal anti-inflammatory agents and prostaglandins I2, E2, and F2-alpha on contractility of taenia of the large colon of horses. Am J Vet Res 1999;60:1004–9.
80. Lester GD, Bolton JR, Cullen LK, et al. Effects of general anesthesia on myoelectric activity of the intestine in horses. Am J Vet Res 1992;53:1553–7.
81. Andersen MS, Clark L, Dyson SJ, et al. Risk factors for colic in horses after general anaesthesia for MRI or nonabdominal surgery: absence of evidence of effect from perianaesthetic morphine. Equine Vet J 2006;38:368–74.
82. Senior JM, Pinchbeck GL, Allister R, et al. Reported morbidities following 861 anaesthetics given at four equine hospitals. Vet Rec 2007;160:407–8.
83. Johnston GM, Taylor PM, Holmes MA, et al. Confidential enquiry of perioperative equine fatalities (CEPEF-1): preliminary results. Equine Vet J 1995;27:193–200.
84. Milks HJ. Practical veterinary pharmacology, materia medica and therapeutics. 5th edition. Chicago: Eger Inc; 1946. p. 158–84.
85. Phaneuf LP, Grivel ML, Ruckebusch Y. Electromyoenterography during normal gastro-intestinal activity, painful or non-painful colic and morphine analgesia, in the horse. Can J Comp Med 1972;36:138–44.
86. Clutton RE. Unexpected responses following intravenous pethidine injection in two horses. Equine Vet J 1987;19:72–3.
87. Muir WW, Skarda RT, Sheehan WC. Cardiopulmonary effects of narcotic agonists and a partial agonist in horses. Am J Vet Res 1978;29:1632–5.
88. Robertson JT, Muir WW, Sams R. Cardiopulmonary effects of butorphanol tartrate in horses. Am J Vet Res 1981;42:41–4.
89. Clark L, Clutton RE, Blissitt KJ, et al. Effects of peri-operative morphine administration during halothane anaesthesia in horses. Vet Anaesth Analg 2005;32:10–5.
90. Van Dijk P, Nyks SK. Changes in heart rate, mean arterial pressure, blood biochemistry, plasma glucose, plasma lactate and some plasma enzymes during sufentanil halothane anaesthesia in horses. J Vet Anaesth 1998;25:13–8.
91. Kaartinen MJ, Pang DS, Cuvelliez SG. Post-anesthetic pulmonary edema in two horses. Vet Anaesth Analg 2010;37:136–43.

92. Senior M. Post-anaesthetic pulmonary oedema in horses: a review. Vet Anaesth Analg 2005;32:193–200.
93. Muir WW. Standing chemical restraint in horses. In: Muir WW, Hubbell JA, editors. Equine anesthesia. Monitoring and emergency therapy. St Louis (MO): Mosby-Year Book; 1991. p. 247–80.
94. Sellon DC, Roberts MC, Blikslager AT, et al. Effects of continuous rate intravenous infusion of butorphanol on physiologic and outcome variables in horses after celiotomy. J Vet Intern Med 2004;18:555–63.
95. Stein C. The control of pain in peripheral tissue by opioids. N Engl J Med 1995; 332:1685–90.
96. Sheehy JG, Hellyer PW, Sammonds GE, et al. Evaluation of opioid receptors in synovial membranes of horses. Am J Vet Res 2001;62:1408–12.
97. Manning M, Wilson D, Hendrickson D et al. The effects of intrarticular administration of morphine and buprenorphine on the middle carpal joints of ponies abstract. Proceedings, 5th International Congress of Veterinary Anesthesia. Guelph (Canada); 1994. p. 155.
98. Raekallio M, Taylor PM, Johnson CB, et al. The disposition and local effects of intra-articular morphine in normal ponies. J Vet Anaesth 1996;23:23–6.
99. Lindegaard C, Thomsen MH, Larsen S, et al. Analgesic efficacy of intra-articular morphine in experimentally induced radiocarpal synovitis in horses. Vet Anaesth Analg 2010;37:171–85.
100. Santos LC, de Moraes AN, Saito ME. Effects of intraarticular ropivacaine and morphine on lipopolysaccharide-induced synovitis in horses. Vet Anaesth Analg 2009;36:280–6.
101. Mills PC, Cross SE. Regional differences in transdermal penetration of fentanyl through equine skin. Res Vet Sci 2007;82:252–6.
102. Matthews NS, Peck KE, Mealey KL. Transdermal fentanyl: absorption and plasma levels in horses abstract. Proceedings, 6th International Congress of Veterinary Anaesthesiology. Thessaloniki (Greece); 1997. p. 116.
103. Orsini JA, Moate PJ, Kuersten K, et al. Pharmacokinetics of fentanyl delivered transdermally in healthy adult horses – variability among horses and its clinical implications. J Vet Pharmacol Ther 2006;29:539–46.
104. Thomasy SM, Slovis N, Maxwell LK, et al. Transdermal fentanyl combined with nonsteroidal anti-inflammatory drugs for analgesia in horses. J Vet Intern Med 2008;18:550–4.
105. Wegner K, Franklin RP, Long MT, et al. How to use fentanyl transdermal patches for analgesia in horses. Proceedings of the American Association of Equine Practitioner 2002;48:291–4.
106. Dhanjal JK, Wilson DV, Robinson E, et al. Intravenous tramadol: effects, nociceptive properties and pharmacokinetics in horses. Vet Anaesth Analg 2009; 36:581–90.

# Alpha-2 Agonists as Pain Therapy in Horses

Alexander Valverde, DVM, DVSc

**KEYWORDS**

- Epidural • Constant rate infusion • Xylazine • Romifidine
- Detomidine • Medetomidine • Dexmedetomidine • Clonidine

Alpha-2 agonists, such as xylazine, clonidine, romifidine, detomidine, medetomidine, and dexmedetomidine, are potent analgesic drugs that also induce physiologic and behavioral changes, such as hypertension, bradycardia, atrioventricular block, excessive sedation and ataxia, all of which can potentially limit their systemic use as analgesics in some clinical cases. Therefore it is of utmost importance to know the individual properties of each of the alpha-2 agonists to select the ideal drug for each clinical condition, based on the duration of action of analgesia and behavioral changes.

Since the last review on this subject from this Journal,[1] the use of medetomidine and dexmetomidine has been introduced for equine anesthesia/analgesia, and although not approved in this species, their increased specificity for alpha-2 receptors may offer some potential advantages over the traditional alpha-2 agonists. Similarly, other routes of administration and benefits of alpha-2 agonists are recognized in the human and laboratory animal literature, which may prove useful in the equine patient if validated in the near future. This review presents this relevant information.

## PHARMACOLOGY OF ADRENERGIC RECEPTORS

Adrenergic receptors are subdivided into alpha and beta. Both alpha and beta are further classified into alpha-1, alpha-2, beta-1, and beta-2. Alpha receptors are located postsynaptically (alpha-1 and alpha-2) and presynaptically (alpha-2) at sympathetic neuroeffector junctions of many organs (**Fig. 1**). Beta receptors are located postsynaptically and in general mediate decreased activity of the effector cells (beta-2: vasodilation, bronchodilation, uterine relaxation) or increased activity (beta-1: heart automaticity and contractility). Postsynaptic activation of alpha receptors mediate increased activity of the effector cells.

Department of Clinical Studies, Ontario Veterinary College, University of Guelph, Guelph, 50 Stone Road, ON, Canada N1G 2W1
E-mail address: valverde@uoguelph.ca

Vet Clin Equine 26 (2010) 515–532
doi:10.1016/j.cveq.2010.07.003
0749-0739/10/$ – see front matter © 2010 Elsevier Inc. All rights reserved.

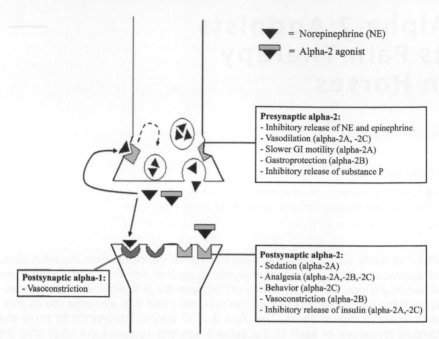

▼ = Norepinephrine (NE)

▼ = Alpha-2 agonist

**Presynaptic alpha-2:**
- Inhibitory release of NE and epinephrine
- Vasodilation (alpha-2A, -2C)
- Slower GI motility (alpha-2A)
- Gastroprotection (alpha-2B)
- Inhibitory release of substance P

**Postsynaptic alpha-1:**
- Vasoconstriction

**Postsynaptic alpha-2:**
- Sedation (alpha-2A)
- Analgesia (alpha-2A,-2B,-2C)
- Behavior (alpha-2C)
- Vasoconstriction (alpha-2B)
- Inhibitory release of insulin (alpha-2A,-2C)

**Fig. 1.** Adrenergic receptors are subdivided into alpha and beta. Both alpha and beta are further classified into alpha-1, alpha-2, beta-1, and beta-2. Alpha receptors are located post-synaptically (alpha-1 and alpha-2) and presynaptically (alpha-2) at sympathetic neuroeffector junctions of many organs.

Activation of the presynaptic alpha-2 receptor inhibits the release of norepinephrine (NE) into the synaptic cleft and autoregulates its actions on the effector cells. The net effect of activation of alpha-2 adrenergic receptors is modulation of sympathetic nervous system activity by inhibition of NE. Manifestations of this response include decreased cardiac output due to decreased inotropy and decreased heart rate, as well as a reduction in systemic vascular resistance. Conversely, the activation of post-synaptic alpha receptors mediates an increase in systemic vascular resistance. Actions at centrally located alpha-2 adrenergic receptors mediate sedation, anxiolysis, analgesia, and hypnosis. It has also been shown that the alpha-1 agonistic activity can reduce the alpha-2 mediated analgesia, and it has been suggested that coadministration of an alpha-1 antagonist (prazosin) with the alpha-2 agonist may enhance analgesic potency.[2] The alpha-2/alpha-1 selectivity for alpha-2 agonists is 160 for xylazine, 220 for clonidine, 260 for detomidine, and 1620 for medetomidine or dexmedetomidine,[3] and is unknown for romifidine but higher than for xylazine. As selectivity for alpha-2 receptors increases, the greater specificity results in higher potency, especially at central alpha-2 adrenoceptors. Medetomidine is considered 10 times, 7 times, and 6 times more potent than xylazine, clonidine, and detomidine, respectively.[4] However, other nonadrenergic mechanisms are probably implicated in analgesic actions of alpha-2 agonists because the rank potency order of spinal depressant actions on in vitro preparations is the same as their rank analgesic potencies in vivo: dexmedetomidine (medetomidine) > clonidine > detomidine > xylazine,[5–7] which does not coincide precisely with alpha-2 agonists of intermediate specificity. It has also been suggested that differences between the actions of these ligands are attributable to an action at alpha-1 receptors.[5]

Alpha-2 agonists activate 3 distinct subtypes of alpha-2 adrenergic receptors: alpha-2A, alpha-2B, and alpha-2C. Despite the higher affinity of detomidine and medetomidine for the alpha-2 receptors compared with xylazine, the former drugs cannot discriminate between the different receptor subtypes.[8] The alpha-2A adrenergic receptor is the primary mediator involved in alpha-adrenergic spinal analgesia for endogenous NE as well as exogenous adrenergic agonists.[9] These receptors are G-protein–coupled receptors that decrease neuronal excitation by several mechanisms, including opening of rectifying potassium channels, decrease of presynaptic calcium influx, and inhibition of adenylyl cyclase.[9] The activation of alpha-2 receptors by an agonist induces the receptor to interact with a $G_i$ type of G protein and inhibits the actions of adenylyl cyclase, decreasing the synthesis of cyclic adenosine monophosphate from adenosine triphosphate. Besides analgesia, the alpha-2A receptor promotes hypnosis, sedation, inhibition of insulin secretion, neuroprotection, and sympatholysis.[10–12] Alpha-2B receptors are involved in spinal analgesia and vasoconstriction of peripheral arteries.[12,13] Alpha-2C receptors are involved in pain modulation, mood- and stimulant-induced locomotor activity, regulation of epinephrine outflow from the adrenal medulla, and modulation of cognition.[2,12–14]

## PHARMACOKINETICS OF ALPHA-2 AGONISTS

Alpha-2 agonists administered intravenously (IV) in clinical doses have elimination half-lives of less than 1.5 hours and relatively small volumes of distribution of 0.5 to 1.6 L/kg. Elimination half-lives are slightly longer when administered intramuscularly (IM).[15–19]

Based on similar sedative effects, equipotent IV doses of these drugs are: 5 to 10 µg/kg of medetomidine, 3.5 µg/kg of dexmedetomidine, 20 to 40 µg/kg of detomidine, 80 to 120 µg/kg of romifidine, 1 mg/kg of xylazine, and 25 µg/kg of clonidine.[20–24]

## ANALGESIC ACTIONS AND ROUTE OF ADMINISTRATION

The analgesic effects of alpha-2 agonists result from spinal and supraspinal actions (**Table 1**). Alpha-2 receptors are found on primary afferent terminals in peripheral and spinal nerve endings, at the level of the superficial laminae of the dorsal horn of the spinal cord, and centrally in the brainstem. Therefore, administration of alpha-2 agonists in any of these locations offers the possibility of analgesic actions, which may also be synergistic with other groups of analgesic drugs. There is good evidence for primary analgesic actions as well as opioid-sparing effects; for example, epidural coadministration of alpha-2 agonists in combination with opioids contribute to the potency and efficacy of opioids and allow for administration of lower doses to achieve analgesia.[9,14,25]

In the horse, systemic and epidural administration are currently the most common routes for alpha-2 agonists (**Table 2**), but in humans the intra-articular, intercostal infiltration, and intravenous regional routes have also been used.[26–30]

### Systemic Administration

The most commonly recognized cardiovascular effects of alpha-2 agonists are a decrease in heart rate, an initial increase in systemic vascular resistance and blood pressure followed by a decrease, an initial decrease in cardiac output and respiratory rate followed by recovery to baseline, and transient decreases in $PaO_2$.[21,23,31,32] The biphasic effects on blood pressure are caused by initial increases in vascular resistance from postsynaptic alpha-2B receptor stimulation that induces hypertension, followed by decreased sympathetic discharge from presynaptic alpha-2A receptor

**Table 1**
**Analgesic effects from agonistic actions on alpha-2 receptors**

| | Site of Action | Mechanism |
|---|---|---|
| Spinal | Superficial laminae of dorsal horn | Receptors 2A, 2B, 2C<br>Presynaptic: inhibits release of substance P from C fibers and to less extent A-delta fibers<br>Postsynaptic: inhibit dorsal horn wide dynamic-range neurons<br>Increases concentrations of acetylcholine in cerebrospinal fluid |
| Supraspinal | Brainstem | Receptors 2A, 2B, 2C<br>Sedation and behavioral effects that may contribute to analgesia are related to 2A and 2C receptors, respectively |
| Intra-articular | Joint capsule | Receptors 2A |
| Local anesthetic effect | Spinal cord, local infiltration | Blockade of C and A-delta fibers (more specific for xylazine) |

stimulation that decreases NE release and presynaptic alpha-2C receptor stimulation that decreases epinephrine release from the adrenal glands, resulting in a decrease in vascular resistance and blood pressure.[33] The use of higher doses of alpha-2 agonists results in a more prolonged increase in vascular resistance and as a result cardiac output can be more adversely affected, resulting in hypotension despite the increased vascular resistance.

Reported sedative effects of alpha-2 agonists in horses include decreased awareness, ptosis of the head, lower lip, and eyelids, ataxia, and a wide stance,[17,24,31,32,34,35] and are mediated through alpha-2A receptors.[33]

Both sedative and physiologic effects of alpha-2 agonists have been correlated with plasma concentrations, and have been shown to be of greater magnitude and observed earlier after IV than after IM administration, although the duration of these changes may be shorter after IV administration.[16] It is not clear, however, whether the analgesic effects endure and correlate with the duration of the sedative and physiologic changes. Horses administered clonidine (25 μg/kg, IV) showed peak sedative and analgesic effects at 20 minutes and 30 minutes, respectively. Analgesia was assessed using a heat source to elicit hoof withdrawal reflexes and, despite lowering of the head associated with the sedation for up to 2.5 to 3 hours, significant analgesia was present for a shorter period (45 minutes) and was only considered submaximal at peak effect.[20] In another study using a model of nociceptive withdrawal reflex (NWR) that limits the influence of the animal's behavior over analgesia, administration of equipotent IV doses of xylazine (1 mg/kg), detomidine (20 μg/kg), or romifidine (80 μg/kg) resulted in similar increases in thresholds to elicit the NWR in hind- and forelimbs and therefore equipotent analgesic effects.[34] Analgesia peaked at 10 to 40 minutes after injection (first for xylazine and last for romifidine) and lasted 60 minutes for xylazine and 90 minutes for detomidine, and was still present at 120 minutes for romifidine.[34] Of note, sedation was significant and present for the duration of action of analgesia for xylazine and detomidine, but shorter (90 minutes) for romifidine.[34] It seems from these studies that sedation and analgesia do not correlate, because one study reports shorter duration of analgesia than sedation[20] and another study reports similar or more prolonged analgesia than sedation.[34] Differences could be due to the properties of the individual alpha-2 agonist, the pain model used and site of nociceptive stimulation,

**Table 2**
Doses of alpha-2 agonists used in horses for standing sedation and analgesia

| | Sedative/Analgesic Full Dose (IV) (mg/kg) | Sedative/Analgesic Dose for Intraoperative Use (IV) (mg/kg) | CRI for Intraoperative Use (mg/kg/h) | Epidural Dose (mg/kg) |
|---|---|---|---|---|
| Xylazine | 1[24] | Usually lower than the full dose | 2.4–3.9[a] 2.1–4.2[115] | 0.17–0.25[72–75] |
| Clonidine | 0.025[20] | | NA | 0.005[83] |
| Romifidine | 0.08–0.12[22,24] | | 0.018[100] | |
| Detomidine | 0.02–0.04[22–24] | | 0.007–0.022[a] 0.0085–0.011[93,102] | 0.01–0.06[76–78] |
| Medetomidine | 0.005–0.01[21,23] | | 0.004–0.006[a] 0.0035–0.005[17,31,58,105] | NA |
| Dexmedetomidine | 0.0035[21] | | NA | NA |
| Detomidine/butorphanol | | 0.01/0.02[91] 0.02/0.02[92,94] 0.01/0.05[98] 0.015/0.03[93] | Followed by 0.036 of detomidine alone[91] Followed by 0.0085 of detomidine alone[92] | NA |
| Detomidine/buprenorphine | | 0.01/0.006[95] | Followed by 0.006–0.0096 of detomidine alone[95] | NA |
| Detomidine/morphine | | 0.01/0.1[98] | 0.012/0.07[97] | 0.03/0.2[77,78] 0.01/0.1 |
| Detomidine/methadone | | 0.01/0.1[98] | | NA |
| Medetomidine/morphine | | 0.005/0.05[31] | Followed by 0.005/0.03[31] | NA |
| Xylazine/morphine | | 0.66/0.12[99] 0.66/0.66[99] | 0.58/0.07[97] | NA |

[a] Dose calculated from available pharmacokinetic data (CRI = Therapeutic dose × Clearance) assuming therapeutic plasma concentrations of 2150–3440 ng/mL for xylazine, 10–30 ng/mL for detomidine, 1.0–1.5 ng/mL for medetomidine; and clearances of 18.9 mL/kg/min for xylazine, 12.4 mL/kg/min for detomidine, and 66.7 mL/kg/min for medetomidine.[15–19]

and the end points used to assess sedation and analgesia. For example, with use of electrical stimulation (coronary band, withers or perineal region, digital nerves) or pin pressure of the cannon bone, contradictory results have been reported for all alpha-2 agonists; romifidine resulted in less degree of analgesia than detomidine or was as potent as detomidine; xylazine was less potent than detomidine or similar to detomidine and romifidine; detomidine was longer acting than xylazine and romifidine; and romifidine was longer acting than xylazine and detomidine.[34,36–38]

The analgesic effects of alpha-2 agonists have also been demonstrated in visceral pain models, including colorectal, cecal, and duodenal distension.[39–44] The analgesic effects are related to the spinal and supraspinal effects of alpha-2s, including central sedative effects that decrease awareness of the horse but also peripheral relaxation of the intestine by inhibition of phasic and tonic motor activity.[41] In a model of cecal distension, xylazine was more effective than opioids (morphine, butorphanol, pentazocine, meperidine) and nonsteroidal anti-inflammatories (NSAIDs) (dipyrone, flunixin).[40,42] Similar results were also demonstrated in clinical cases of colic where xylazine or detomidine were more effective than butorphanol and flunixin in decreasing signs of pain, such as sweating, kicking, pawing, lip curling, attitude, head and body movement, and increased autonomic responses (pulse rate and respiratory rate).[45] Due to the effectiveness of alpha-2 agonists in pain therapy for visceral conditions, it is important to properly assess the health status of the patient to avoid underestimating the severity of the condition when analgesia is present that could mask clinical signs and the integrity of viscera, especially if longer-acting alpha-2 agonists are used.

Alpha-2 agonists can decrease intestinal motility, which may predispose to ileus. Studies in rats using clonidine have implicated activation of presynaptic alpha-2A subtype receptors as responsible for the slower motility.[46–48] In horses, xylazine-induced vasoconstriction of the cecal vasculature decreased arterial blood flow to the lateral cecal artery to a greater extent than systemic reductions in cardiac output, decreasing local normal motility for up to 120 minutes with a full sedative dose (1.1 mg/kg, IV) and for 30 minutes with a low dose (0.275 mg/kg).[49,50]

The following effects on gastrointestinal motility have been reported in the horse: detomidine (10–30 μg/kg, IV) and to a lesser extent xylazine (0.5–1.0 mg/kg, IV), decreased gastric emptying[51]; detomidine (12.5 μg/kg, IV) and to a lesser extent xylazine (0.5 mg/kg, IV), decreased duodenum motility[52]; xylazine (1.1 mg/kg), decreased motility of jejunum and pelvic flexure[53]; and romifidine (80–120 μg/kg, IV), decreased motility of the small intestine, cecum, and left ventral colon.[54] Unfortunately, the effects of the different alpha-2 agonists on gastrointestinal motility and on different segments of the gastrointestinal tract have not been compared in one single study in horses so as to better assess which alpha-2 agonists are less detrimental. In dogs, medetomidine inhibited the motility of the gastric antrum and small intestine to a greater degree and for a longer period than xylazine.[55] In the latter study, medetomidine also affected the motility of the stomach and duodenum to greater extent than for the jejunum and ileum, due to its higher alpha-2 specificity.[55] Also in dogs, medetomidine and clonidine affected the motility of the colon and, as happened for cranial segments of the gastrointestinal tract, the effects were more prolonged with the more selective alpha-2 agonist, medetomidine.[56] It is important that future studies in horses determine whether different segments of the gastrointestinal tract are affected to the same extent, and which alpha-2 agonists result in a higher risk of decreased motility in both the presence and absence of pain.

Despite the adverse effects on gastrointestinal motility, administration of alpha-2 agonists results in a beneficial effect to the stomach. In rats, stimulation of presynaptic alpha-2B receptors induces a gastroprotective effect by regulating gastric acid secretion and by inhibiting chemically (including NSAIDs) and physically (stress) induced gastric mucosal lesions.[46,48,57] These benefits have not been evaluated in horses, and may prove useful in the colic horse that requires analgesia and has the predisposition for ulceration during hospitalization.

Other considerations in horses administered alpha-2 agonists include the effects of these drugs on urine output. Alpha-2 agonists administered for sedation or during anesthesia increase urine production, due to hyperglycemia from hypoinsulinemia[17,58–61] mediated through alpha-2A and -2C receptors,[62] and due to a reduced secretion rate of arginine vasopressin.[63] Patients should be monitored for urine output, hydration status, and comfort to avoid excessive bladder distension.

Equipotent sedative doses of xylazine, romifidine, and detomidine increase intrauterine pressure for up to 30 minutes, as a result of increased uterine contractions.[64] Electrical activity of the myometrium in the last trimester was observed to increase shortly (3–5 minutes) after IM injection of 20 or 40 µg/kg of detomidine, but with no effect after 60 µg/kg, and lasted for 50 to 70 minutes without any adverse effects, and is therefore considered safe.[65] In a study in which 8 mares during 10 pregnancies were administered detomidine (20 µg/kg, IV) once a week from days 14 to 60 of pregnancy and thereafter once a month until parturition, no side effects could be associated with administration, although 1 case of abortion was reported at 167 days.[66] In a similar study, detomidine (15 µg/kg) administered to pregnant mares at 3-week intervals during the last trimester of pregnancy to assess maternal and fetal electrocardiographs showed reductions in heart rate in both, but alterations in conduction were detected only in mares, and there were no adverse outcomes of pregnancy.[67] Another study has also demonstrated that despite systemic cardiovascular effects associated with alpha-2 agonists, it appears that based on color Doppler ultrasonographic examinations local uterine and ovarian perfusion is not affected by detomidine or xylazine.[68] In view of these findings, alpha-2 agonists are safe in pregnant animals, but close monitoring is advised.

## Epidural

The epidural analgesic effects of alpha-2 agonists involve a spinal cholinergic mechanism of action in which acetylcholine concentrations increase in cerebrospinal fluid (CSF) because of release from the dorsal horn.[69] Spinal presynaptic alpha 2-receptor binding blocks the release of substance P from C fibers, whereas postsynaptic actions inhibit dorsal horn wide dynamic-range neurons, similar to effects elicited by opioids but not antagonized by opioid antagonists.[70,71] The degree of analgesia induced by epidural xylazine of the perineal and caudal region compares to the actions of epidural local anesthetics. Alpha-2 agonists preferentially block conduction of C fibers; however, A-delta fibers are also affected, and it appears that xylazine has a greater effect than other alpha-2 agonists. Doses of 0.17 to 0.25 mg/kg of xylazine provide surgical analgesia/anesthesia of the perineal region within 15 to 30 minutes and for up to 3.5 hours.[72–75] The epidural dose of xylazine is lower than recommended systemic doses and, despite systemic absorption from the epidural space, results in less behavioral (sedation, ataxia) and cardiovascular changes but provides prolonged analgesia. Epidural detomidine requires doses similar to systemic ones, which results in significant ataxia and sedation from systemic absorption from the epidural space, and is shorter acting than epidural xylazine.[73,76] Epidural doses of 30 to 60 µg/kg of detomidine have been reported to produce analgesia within 10 to 25 minutes for approximately 2.5 hours,[76] and both degree and duration of analgesia (6–12 hours) are enhanced when combined with morphine.[77,78] In the author's experience, lower doses of detomidine (10–20 µg/kg) are routinely used epidurally in combination with morphine (0.1 mg/kg) to provide analgesia of pelvic limbs/perineal area, and appear to be as effective as the reported higher doses but provide less systemic absorption and, therefore, sedation. For repetitive administration an epidural catheter can be placed to facilitate injections and long-term management.[79]

Administration of alpha-2 agonists in combination with local anesthetics by the epidural route enhances sensory and motor blockade induced by the latter.[80–82] The effects of epidural xylazine on motor function are well established in horses and laboratory animals, and can be readily recognized as tail relaxation, anal sphincter relaxation, and hindlimb weakness.[7,75,83] Therefore, epidural combinations of alpha-2 agonists with local anesthetics in horses should consider a reduction in the dose of local anesthetic to avoid excessive ataxia from motor blockade, particularly for xylazine.

Other factors that enhance ataxia from epidural injections include systemic absorption when epidural doses are similar to systemic doses (detomidine) and rostral epidural spread is facilitated by dilution of the alpha-2 agonist with diluents (saline or local anesthetic), or epidural catheters that are placed too rostral. For example, clonidine induced recumbency from excessive ataxia in horses after epidural injection into sacral segments through an epidural catheter,[83] although it has not been reported to cause motor blockade, even at high doses, in humans.[84]

In halothane-anesthetized ponies, epidural xylazine reduces inhalant requirements (minimum alveolar concentration [MAC]) in a segmental manner, the reduction being greater near the site of administration: 43% MAC reduction for the pelvic limb and 34% for the thoracic limb.[85] This latter study demonstrates that xylazine has the potential for providing analgesia in more rostral areas than the perineal and caudal area associated with the sacrococcygeal or first intercoccygeal space epidural injection. As happens with epidural opioids, it is likely that the low lipophilicity of xylazine (octanol/buffer coefficient of 0.15)[86] and the low molecular weight (220) facilitates greater bioavailability in CSF than in the epidural space, which promotes rostral spread with the CSF along the spinal cord.[87] In contrast, medetomidine and detomidine have low molecular weights (236 and 222, respectively) but high octanol/buffer coefficients (2.8 and 2.5, respectively)[86] that limit rostral spread and analgesic actions beyond the perineal and caudal area.

## Intra-Articular

Intra-articular administration of alpha-2 agonists mediate analgesia through several proposed mechanisms, including activation of peripheral alpha-2A receptors that inhibit the release of NE at peripheral afferent nociceptors, a local anesthetic effect that inhibits the conduction of nerve signal through C and A-delta fibers, stimulation of the release of enkephalin-like substances at peripheral sites, and modulation of the opioid-analgesic pathway.[5,26,88] There is no reported intra-articular use of alpha-2 agonists in horses, but the potential for this route is encouraging and studies are warranted.

## Intercostal and Intravenous Regional

Intercostal or local blocks and intravenous regional (Bier block) have not been documented in the horse; however, local anesthetic effects are well recognized for xylazine in horses after epidural administration. This local anesthetic effect probably involves blockade of mostly A-delta and to a less extent C fibers because nonselective alpha agonists, such as NE, have been shown to inhibit A-delta fiber transmission more effectively than C-fiber transmission.[89]

*Intraoperative Use*

Use of alpha-2 agonists for sedation or during anesthesia to provide analgesia are widely described in horses. For standing sedation, it is common to combine them with other drugs, mainly opioids, to induce neuroleptanalgesic effects that result in a better degree of sedation/analgesia, more prolonged effects, and ideally less adverse effects as a result of lower individual doses. Additive or synergistic effects are expected in neuroleptanalgesic combinations; however, these may be observed for the degree of sedation but not necessarily analgesia. In a dental dolorimetry model, full doses of xylazine (1.1 mg/kg, IV) alone or administered 5 minutes before an opioid (morphine [0.75 mg/kg, IV], nalbuphine [0.75 mg/kg, IV], butorphanol [0.04 mg/kg, IV]) did not result in additive analgesic effects, and the degree of analgesia was similar for all treatments.[90] However, in contrast to the latter study that used full doses in the combinations, using lower doses of each drug in clinical situations seems to provide the same or better degree of analgesia than each drug alone at a full dose, while sedation is still satisfactory.

During standing surgery, the most common combinations of alpha-2 agonists with opioids have typically included detomidine with butorphanol or buprenorphine or morphine or methadone, medetomidine/morphine, and xylazine with morphine or butorphanol, which have been used for minor surgical procedures and more invasive procedures such as laparoscopic surgery, paranasal sinus surgery, and condylar fracture repair.[31,91–99]

Sedative/analgesic effects of these drugs have been obtained by administering a single bolus with subsequent doses as needed during the procedure, and as a single bolus followed by a constant rate infusion (CRI). A CRI is more likely to provide a steady-state plasma concentration that prevents fluctuations in the degree of sedation and analgesia, and most important, profound transient effects on cardiorespiratory function and degree of ataxia. With the current available information on pharmacokinetics of alpha-2 agonists, it is possible to estimate ideal CRI of these drugs; data for detomidine,[15] medetomidine,[17] dexmedetomidine,[21] and xylazine[19] are available, whereas no information is published for romifidine although a CRI has been described.[100]

Detomidine and medetomidine alone or combined with an opioid have been used in this fashion to provide an ideal degree of analgesia in horses for standing surgery. In one study, an overall visual analog score (VAS) of 8.3/10 for sedation, analgesia, and behavior was achieved throughout the surgical procedure, and was considered satisfactory by surgeons and anesthetists.[31] The administration of these combinations by CRI has also been associated with acceptable cardiorespiratory function.[31,93,95]

In horses under inhalant anesthesia, the use of a CRI of alpha-2 agonists has also been studied and has focused on the inhalant sparing effect and cardiovascular interactions (**Table 3**). Xylazine (0.5–1 mg/kg, IV) decreased the MAC of halothane or isoflurane by approximately 20% to 35% in a dose- and time-dependent fashion.[60,101] Detomidine administered as an average CRI dose of 10.8 μg/kg/h to horses undergoing neurectomy under halothane anesthesia reduced MAC by 33%,[102] whereas a medetomidine CRI of 3.5 μg/kg/h reduced isoflurane end-tidal concentrations by 20% when compared with horses not receiving it during surgery[103] and by 28% in research ponies under desflurane anesthesia.[104] This sparing effect allows for an easier maintenance of an adequate anesthetic plane even at lower anesthetic concentrations than with other drugs that offer a similar degree of MAC reduction, such as lidocaine given by CRI.[105,106]

Due to the profound effects of alpha-2 agonists on cardiovascular function, several studies have assessed the safety of these drugs in combination with inhalant

**Table 3**
Doses of alpha-2 agonists used in horses for total (TIVA) or partial (PIVA) intravenous general anesthesia and analgesia

| | Sedative Dose (IV) (mg/kg) | Induction IV Anesthetic Drug (mg/kg) | Bolus for Intraoperative Use (IV) (mg/kg) | CRI for Intraoperative Use (mg/kg/h) |
|---|---|---|---|---|
| **TIVA (procedures of ≤60 minutes duration)** | | | | |
| Xylazine (X) | 1.1[116] | Ketamine (K) 2.2 | X 0.25 + K 0.25 To effect | NA |
| Xylazine | 0.75[115] | Guaifenesin (G) 75 Ketamine 2 | NA | X 2.1 + K 5.4 X 2.1 + K 7.2 X 2.1 + K 9 X 4.2 + K 5.4 |
| Xylazine | 1.1[116] | Tiletamine/zolazepam (TZ) 0.67 Ketamine 0.53 Detomidine (D) 0.013 (all mixed in the same syringe) | TZ 0.19 + K 0.15 + D 0.004 To effect | NA |
| Xylazine | 1.1[116] | Xylazine 0.5 mg/mL/guaifenesin 50 mg/mL/ketamine 1 mg/mL (Triple drip to effect) | NA | X 0.75 + G 75 + K 1.5 |
| **PIVA** | | | | |
| Medetomidine (M) | 0.005[107] | Diazepam 0.04 Ketamine 2.5 | NA | M 0.00125 + G 25 + K 1 + sevoflurane 1.5% |
| Xylazine | 1[58] | Diazepam 0.02 Ketamine 2 | Lidocaine (L) 2 | M 0.005 + L 0.05 + isoflurane 1.1% |
| Acepromazine | 0.03[102] | Guaifenesin 87 Thiamylal 4.9 | NA | D 0.011 + halothane 1.05% |
| Acepromazine Medetomidine | 0.03[105] 0.007 | Diazepam 0.02 Ketamine 2.2 | NA | M 0.0035 + isoflurane 1.1% |

anesthesia. Cardiac output and heart rate at 1.1% end-tidal isoflurane anesthesia in a group of horses undergoing arthroscopy with a CRI of medetomidine (5 µg/kg/h) and lidocaine (50 µg/kg/min) was similar to those in a group of horses with a CRI of lidocaine alone (50 µg/kg/min), but blood pressure was higher in the group that included medetomidine.[58] Another study in 2 groups of horses undergoing surgery and maintained at 1.1% end-tidal isoflurane demonstrated lower cardiac output and heart rate in horses that received a CRI of medetomidine at 3.5 µg/kg/h intraoperatively after sedation with 7 µg/kg IV than in horses that received a bolus and CRI of 2 mg/kg and 50 µg/kg/min, respectively of lidocaine intraoperatively after a sedative dose of 1 mg/kg of xylazine IV; however, horses in the lidocaine group also required rescue analgesia with ketamine and thiopental, and isoflurane concentrations had to be increased toward the end of the procedure to achieve the same degree of anesthetic depth and analgesia as the medetomidine group.[105] In another study, horses receiving romifidine at a CRI of 18 µg/kg/h required less isoflurane and had higher blood pressures during elective surgeries than horses without the CRI.[100] Horses undergoing neurectomy under halothane anesthesia (1.1%) and administered detomidine to maintain a steady plasma concentration of 25 ng/mL (average CRI of 11 µg/kg/h) had slower heart rates than horses under halothane alone (1.5%), whereas blood pressures and cardiac output were similar.[102] It is interesting that all of these studies were done in horses undergoing surgery; therefore the effects of surgical stimulation on autonomic responses have a significant impact on the cardiovascular variables measured. Based on these studies, the anesthetist should expect higher blood pressures and occasional lower heart rates; both parameters can be affected by the concurrent degree of surgical stimulation. The determined effects on cardiac output indicate that this variable may be reduced with alpha-2 agonist CRIs; however the measurements in any of the aforementioned studies should be considered within acceptable levels. Cardiac indices of 55 mL/kg/min for medetomidine under isoflurane anesthesia[58,105] and 31 mL/kg/min for detomidine under halothane anesthesia[102] were reported at 60 to 90 minutes of infusion in those studies. The more cardiovascular depressive effects of halothane in combination with alpha-2 agonists are probably best avoided, but inhalant anesthetics that better preserve cardiovascular function, such as sevoflurane and isoflurane, result in stable combinations.

Cardiac indices obtained from combinations of alpha-2 agonists with isoflurane are not different from values of 48 to 65 mL/kg/min reported in awake horses sedated with a bolus of medetomidine (5 µg/kg) and a CRI of medetomidine-morphine (5 µg/kg/h-30 µg/kg/h) for laparoscopic surgery.[31] Similarly, cardiac indices of 46 to 62 mL/kg/min or 49 to 53 mL/kg/min have been reported in horses anesthetized with sevoflurane alone (2.8%–3.1% end-tidal) and supported with dobutamine or with sevoflurane and a CRI of guaifenesin-ketamine-medetomidine (1.4%–1.6% end-tidal), respectively.[107] Therefore, inclusion of alpha-2 agonists does not exacerbate cardiovascular depression from inhalant anesthesia, because of the sparing effect on end-tidal concentrations that counteracts the depressive effects of each individual drug.

The impact of alpha-2 in the intraoperative period should also be considered for the recovery period, and even though they result in more prolonged recoveries, the quality is generally better.[58,59,105]

## ANTAGONISTS

Antagonism of alpha-2 agonists is mostly used to counteract overdosing. Yohimbine, tolazoline, idazoxan, and atipamezole are all recognized antagonists, and their use has been reported in horses except for idazoxan. Atipamezole has an alpha-2/alpha-1 selectivity of 8526, whereas idazoxan and yohimbine have ratios of 27 and 40, respectively. The affinity of atipamezole for alpha-2 receptors is 100 times higher than that of other antagonists.[108] In an experimental trial, detomidine's (10–20 μg/kg, IV) sedative and bradycardic effects were antagonized 15 minutes after administration with doses of 100 to 160 μg/kg of atipamezole IV within 2 minutes; however, recovery was never complete to baseline observations even at 20 minutes after reversal.[109] Higher doses of atipamezole of 160 to 200 μg/kg induced hyperexcitability in all horses for 6 to 10 minutes after injection.[109]

Ponies administered detomidine, 40 μg/kg IV and antagonized 20 minutes later with tolazoline (4 mg/kg, IV) had less sedation and analgesia within 15 to 60 minutes after administration than controls; however, sweating and salivation, and increased levels of cortisol, glucose, and free fatty acids were noted, indicating a stress response associated with tolazoline.[110]

Yohimbine is a less specific antagonist, and has been used in doses of 0.1 mg/kg IV to reverse xylazine and shorten time to recovery from injectable combinations used for general anesthesia, such as xylazine-ketamine, xylazine-thiopental, and xylazine-pentobarbital.[111–113] Doses of 0.075 to 0.15 mg/kg IV had a mean residence time of 106 to 119 minutes and a harmonic mean effective half-life of 53 to 76 minutes, which prevents relapse of sedation in horses.[114]

## SUMMARY AND CLINICAL RELEVANCE

Understanding the pharmacology of alpha-2 agonists is important for equine practitioners to better use the different available options. Old drugs like xylazine offer reliable effects, and its individual properties make this drug different from the other alpha-2 agonists, for example by the epidural route. Similarly, the newer alpha-2 agonists medetomidine and dexmedetomidine offer pharmacologic properties that make them ideal for CRI.

Ideal pain management with sole administration of alpha-2 agonists is not possible or desirable, as is the case for most drugs with analgesic actions; however, this group of drugs offer important analgesic properties despite their profound cardiovascular effects. Judicious use of these drugs should provide the equine practitioner and anesthetist with valuable means of treating pain in healthy and critical patients. Nontraditional applications of alpha-2 agonists such as intra-articular administration, intravenous regional administration, and validation of their usefulness as gastroprotective drugs merit investigation.

## REFERENCES

1. Daunt DA, Steffey EP. Alpha-2 adrenergic agonists as analgesic in horses. Vet Clin North Am Equine Pract 2002;18(1):39–46.
2. Gil DW, Cheevers CV, Kedzie KM, et al. α-1 adrenergic receptor agonist activity of clinical α-adrenergic receptor agonists interferes with α-2 mediated analgesia. Anesthesiology 2009;110(2):401–7.
3. Virtanen R, Savola JM, Saano V, et al. Characterization of the selectivity, specificity and potency of medetomidine as an $\alpha_2$-adrenoceptor agonist. Eur J Pharmacol 1988;150(1–2):9–14.
4. Virtanen R, MacDonald E. Comparison of the effects of detomidine and xylazine on some alpha 2-adrenoceptor-mediated responses in the central and peripheral nervous systems. Eur J Pharmacol 1985;115(2–3):277–84.

5. Faber ESL, Chambers JP, Evans RH. Depression of NMDA receptor-mediated synaptic transmission by four $\alpha_2$ adrenoceptor agonists on the in vitro rat spinal cord preparation. Br J Pharmacol 1998;124(3):507–12.

6. Virtanen R. Antinociceptive activity and mechanism of action of detomidine. J Vet Pharmacol Ther 1986;9(3):286–92.

7. Ossipov MH, Suarez LJ, Spaulding TC. A comparison of the antinociceptive and behavioural effects of intrathecally administered opiates, alpha-2-adrenergic agonists, and local anaesthetics in mice and rats. Anaesth Analg 1988;677(7): 616–24.

8. Schwartz DD, Clark TP. Affinity of detomidine, medetomidine and xylazine for alpha-2 adrenergic receptor subtypes. J Vet Pharmacol Ther 1998;21(2): 107–11.

9. Stone LS, MacMillan LB, Kitto KF, et al. The $\alpha_{2a}$ adrenergic receptor subtype mediates spinal analgesia evoked by $\alpha_2$ agonists and is necessary for spinal adrenergic-opioid synergy. J Neurosci 1997;17(18):7157–65.

10. Fagerholm V, Scheinin M, Haaparanta M. Alpha2A-adrenoceptor antagonism increases insulin secretion and synergistically augments the insulinotropic effect of glibenclamide in mice. Br J Pharmacol 2008;154(6):1287–96.

11. Ma D, Hossain M, Rajakumaraswamy N, et al. Dexmedetomidine produces it neuroprotective effect via the alpha 2A-adrenoceptor subtype. Eur J Pharmacol 2004;502(1–2):87–97.

12. Philipp M, Brede M, Hein L. Physiological significance of $\alpha_2$-adrenergic receptor subtype diversity: one receptor is not enough. Am J Physiol Regul Integr Comp Physiol 2002;283(2):R287–95.

13. Panzer O, Moitra V, Sladen RN. Pharmacology of sedative-analgesic agents: dexmedetomidine, remifentanil, ketamine, volatile anesthetics, and the role of peripheral mu antagonists. Crit Care Clin 2009;25(3):451–69.

14. Fairbanks CA, Stone LS, Kitto KF, et al. $\alpha_{2c}$-adrenergic receptors mediate spinal analgesia and adrenergic-opioid synergy. J Pharmacol Exp Ther 2002;300(1):282–90.

15. Grimsrud KN, Mama KR, Thomas SM, et al. Pharmacokinetics of detomidine and its metabolites following intravenous and intramuscular administration in horses. Equine Vet J 2009;41(4):361–5.

16. Mama KR, Grimsrud K, Snell T, et al. Plasma concentrations, behavioural and physiological effects following intravenous and intramuscular detomidine in horses. Equine Vet J 2009;41(8):772–7.

17. Bettschart-Wolfensberger R, Clarke KW, Vainio O, et al. Pharmacokinetics of medetomidine in ponies and elaboration of a medetomidine infusion regime which provides a constant level of sedation. Res Vet Sci 1999;67(1):41–6.

18. Salonen JS, Vaha-Vahe T, Vanio O, et al. Single-dose pharmacokinetics of detomidine in the horse and cow. J Vet Pharmacol Ther 1989;12(1):65–72.

19. Dyer DC, Hsu WH, Lloyd WE. Pharmacokinetics of xylazine in ponies: influence of yohimbine. Arch Int Pharmacodyn Ther 1987;289(1):5–10.

20. Dirikolu L, McFadden ET, Ely KJ, et al. Clonidine in horses: identification, detection, and clinical pharmacology. Vet Ther 2006;7(2):141–55.

21. Bettschart-Wolfensberger R, Freeman SL, Bowen IM, et al. Cardiopulmonary effects and pharmacokinetics of i.v. dexmedetomidine in ponies. Equine Vet J 2005;37(1):60–4.

22. Freeman SL, England GC. Investigation of romifidine and detomidine for the clinical sedation of horses. Vet Rec 2000;147(18):507–11.

23. Yamashita K, Tsubakishita S, Futaoka S, et al. Cardiovascular effects of medetomidine, detomidine and xylazine in horses. J Vet Med Sci 2000;62(10):1025–32.

24. England GC, Clarke KW, Goossens L. A comparison of the sedative effects of three alpha 2-adrenoceptor agonists (romifidine, detomidine and xylazine) in the horse. J Vet Pharmacol Ther 1992;15(2):194–201.

25. Monasky MS, Zinsmeister AR, Stevens CW, et al. Interaction of intrathecal morphine and ST-91 on antinociception in the rat: dose-response analysis, antagonism and clearance. J Pharmacol Exp Ther 1990;254(2):383–92.

26. Al-Metwalli RR, Mowafi HA, Ismail SA, et al. Effect of intra-articular dexmedetomidine on postoperative analgesia after arthroscopic knee surgery. Br J Anaesth 2008;101(3):395–9.

27. Tan PH, Buerkle H, Cheng JT, et al. Double-blind parallel comparison of multiple doses of apraclonidine, clonidine, and placebo administered intra-articularly to patients undergoing arthroscopic knee surgery. Clin J Pain 2004;20(4):256–60.

28. Tschernko EM, Klepetko H, Gruber E, et al. Clonidine added to the anesthetic solution enhances analgesia and improves oxygenation after intercostal nerve block for thoracotomy. Anesth Analg 1998;87(1):107–11.

29. Reuben SS, Steinberg RB, Madabhushi I, et al. Intravenous regional clonidine in the management of sympathetically maintained pain. Anesthesiology 1998; 89(2):527–30.

30. Gentili M, Houssel P, Osman M, et al. Intra-articular morphine and clonidine produce comparable analgesia but the combination is not more effective. Br J Anaesth 1997;79(5):660–1.

31. Solano AM, Valverde A, Desrochers, et al. Behavioural and cardiorespiratory effects of a constant rate infusion of medetomidine and morphine for sedation during standing laparoscopy in horses. Equine Vet J 2009;41(2):153–9.

32. Freeman SL, Bowen IM, Bettschart-Wolfensberger R, et al. Cardiovascular effects of romifidine in the standing horse. Res Vet Sci 2002;72(2):123–9.

33. Knaus AE, Muthig V, Schickinger S, et al. $\alpha_2$-adrenoceptor subtypes—unexpected functions for receptors and ligands derived from gene-targeted mouse models. Neurochem Int 2007;51(5):277–81.

34. Rohrbach H, Korpivaara T, Schatzmann U, et al. Comparison of the effects of the alpha-2 agonists detomidine, romifidine and xylazine on nociceptive withdrawal reflex and temporal summation in horses. Vet Anaesth Analg 2009; 36(4):394–5.

35. Figueiredo JP, Muir WW, Smith J, et al. Sedative and analgesic effects of romifidine in horses. Intern J Appl Res Vet Med 2005;3(3):249–58.

36. Moens Y, Lanz F, Doherr MG, et al. A comparison of the antinociceptive effects of xylazine, detomidine and romifidine on experimental pain in horses. Vet Anaesth Analg 2003;30(3):183–90.

37. Hamm D, Turchi P, Jöchle W. Sedative and analgesic effects of detomidine and romifidine in horses. Vet Rec 1995;136(13):324–7.

38. Jöchle W, Hamm D. Sedation and analgesia with Domosedan (detomidine hydrochloride) in horses: dose response studies on efficacy and its duration. Acta Vet Scand 1986;82(Suppl):69–84.

39. Elfenbein JR, Sanchez LC, Robertson SA, et al. Effect of detomidine on visceral and somatic nociception and duodenal motility in conscious adult horses. Vet Anaesth Analg 2009;36(2):162–72.

40. Kohn CW, Muir WW 3rd. Selected aspects of the clinical pharmacology of visceral analgesics and gut motility modifying drugs in the horse. J Vet Intern Med 1988;2(2):85–91.

41. Roger T, Ruckebusch Y. Colonic alpha 2-adrenoceptor-mediated responses in the pony. J Vet Pharmacol Ther 1987;10(4):310–8.

42. Muir WW, Robertson JT. Visceral analgesia: effects of xylazine, butorphanol, meperidine, and pentazocine in horses. Am J Vet Res 1985;46(10):2081–4.
43. Kalpravidh M, Lumb WV, Wright M, et al. Effects of butorphanol, flunixin, levorphanol, morphine, and xylazine in ponies. Am J Vet Res 1984;45(2):217–23.
44. Pippi NL, Lumb WV. Objective tests of analgesic drugs in ponies. Am J Vet Res 1979;40(8):1082–6.
45. Jöchle W, Moore JN, Brown J, et al. Comparison of detomidine, butorphanol, flunixin meglumine and xylazine in clinical cases of equine colic. Equine Vet J Suppl 1989;7:111–6.
46. Gyires K, Zádori ZS, Shujaa N, et al. Pharmacological analysis of alpha(2)-adrenoceptor subtypes mediating analgesic, anti-inflammatory and gastroprotective actions. Inflammopharmacology 2009;17(3):171–9.
47. Zádori ZS, Shujaa N, Fülöp K, et al. Pre- and postsynaptic mechanisms in the clonidine- and oxymetazoline-induced inhibition of gastric motility in the rat. Neurochem Int 2007;51(5):297–305.
48. Fülöp K, Zádori Z, Rónai AZ, et al. Characterisation of alpha2-adrenoceptor subtypes involved in gastric emptying, gastric motility and gastric mucosal defence. Eur J Pharmacol 2005;528(1–3):150–7.
49. Rutkowski JA, Eades SC, Moore JN. Effects of xylazine butorphanol on cecal arterial blood flow, cecal mechanical activity, and systemic hemodynamics in horses. Am J Vet Res 1991;52(7):1153–8.
50. Clark ES, Thompson SA, Becht JL, et al. Effects of xylazine on cecal mechanical activity and cecal blood flow in healthy horses. Am J Vet Res 1988;49(5):720–3.
51. Sutton DG, Preston T, Christley RM, et al. The effects of xylazine, detomidine, acepromazine and butorphanol on equine solid phase gastric emptying rate. Equine Vet J 2002;34(5):486–92.
52. Merritt AM, Burrow JA, Hartless CS. Effect of xylazine, detomidine, and a combination of xylazine and butorphanol on equine duodenal motility. Am J Vet Res 1998;59(5):619–23.
53. Adams SB, Lamar CH, Masty J. Motility of the distal portion of the jejunum and pelvic flexure in ponies: effects of six drugs. Am J Vet Res 1984;45(4):795–9.
54. Freeman SL, England GC. Effect of romifidine on gastrointestinal motility, assessed by transrectal ultrasonography. Equine Vet J 2001;33(6):570–6.
55. Nakamura K, Hara S, Tomizawa N. The effects of medetomidine and xylazine on gastrointestinal motility and gastrin release in the dog. J Vet Pharmacol Ther 1997;20(4):290–5.
56. Maugeri S, Ferrè JP, Intorre L, et al. Effects of medetomidine on intestinal and colonic motility in the dog. J Vet Pharmacol Ther 1994;17(2):148–54.
57. Gyires K, Müllner K, Fürst S, et al. Alpha-2 adrenergic and opioid receptor-mediated gastroprotection. J Physiol 2000;94(2):117–21.
58. Valverde A, Rickey E, Sinclair M, et al. Comparison of cardiovascular function and quality of recovery in isoflurane-anaesthetised horses administered a constant rate infusion of lidocaine or lidocaine and medetomidine during elective surgery. Equine Vet J 2010;42(3):192–9.
59. Bettschart-Wolfensberger R, Larenza MP. Balanced anesthesia in the equine. Clin Tech Equine Pract 2007;6(2):104–10.
60. Stoffoy EP, Pascoe PJ, Woliner MJ, et al. Effects of xylazine hydrochloride during isoflurane-induced anesthesia in horses. Am J Vet Res 2000;61(10):1225–31.
61. Tranquilli WJ, Thurmon JC, Neff-Davis CA, et al. Hyperglycemia and hypoinsulinemia during xylazine-ketamine anesthesia in thoroughbred horses. Am J Vet Res 1984;45(1):11–4.

62. Peterhoff M, Sieg A, Brede M, et al. Inhibition of insulin secretion via distinct signalling pathways in α2-adrenoceptor knockout mice. Eur J Endocrinol 2003; 149(4):343–50.

63. Alexander SL, Irvine CH. The effect of the alpha-2-adrenergic agonist, clonidine, on secretion patterns and rates of adrenocorticotropic hormone and its secretagogues in the horse. J Neuroendocrinol 2000;12(9):874–80.

64. Schatzmann U, Jozzfck H, Stauffer JL, et al. Effects of alpha 2-agonists on intrauterine pressure and sedation in horses: comparison between detomidine, romifidine and xylazine. Zentralbl Veterinarmed A 1994;41(7):523–9.

65. Jedruch J, Gajewski Z, Kuussaari J. The effect of detomidine hydrochloride on the electrical activity of uterus in pregnant mares. Acta Vet Scand 1989;30(3): 307–11.

66. Katila T, Oijala M. The effect of detomidine (Domosedan) on the maintenance of equine pregnancy and foetal development: ten cases. Equine Vet J 1988;20(5): 323–6.

67. Luukkanen L, Katila T, Koskinen E. Some effects of multiple administration of detomidine during the last trimester of equine pregnancy. Equine Vet J 1997;29(5): 400–2.

68. Araujo RR, Ginther OJ. Vascular perfusion of reproductive organs in pony mares and heifers during sedation with detomidine or xylazine. Am J Vet Res 2009; 70(1):141–8.

69. Klimscha W, Tong C, Eisenach JC. Intrathecal alpha 2-adrenergic agonists stimulate acetylcholine and norepinephrine release from the spinal cord dorsal horn in sheep. An in vivo microdialysis study. Anesthesiology 1997;87(1):110–6.

70. Sabbe MB, Grafe MR, Mjanger E, et al. Spinal delivery of sufentanil, alfentanil and morphine in dogs: physiologic and toxicologic investigations. Anesthesiology 1994;81(4):899–920.

71. Sabbe MB, Penning JP, Ozaki GT, et al. Spinal and systemic action of the alpha 2 receptor agonist dexmedetomidine in dogs. Antinociception and carbon dioxide response. Anesthesiology 1994;80(5):1057–72.

72. Skarda RT, Muir WW 3rd. Analgesic, hemodynamic, and respiratory effects of caudal epidurally administered xylazine hydrochloride solution in mares. Am J Vet Res 1996;57(2):193–200.

73. Skarda RT, Muir WW 3rd. Comparison of antinociceptive, cardiovascular, and respiratory effects, head ptosis, and position of pelvic limbs in mares after caudal epidural administration of xylazine and detomidine hydrochloride solution. Am J Vet Res 1996;57(9):1338–45.

74. Grubb TL, Riebold TW, Huber MJ. Comparison of lidocaine, xylazine, and xylazine/lidocaine for caudal epidural analgesia in horses. J Am Vet Med Assoc 1992;201(8):1187–90.

75. LeBlanc PH, Caron JP. Clinical use of epidural xylazine in the horse. Equine Vet J 1990;22(3):180–1.

76. Skarda RT, Muir WW 3rd. Caudal analgesia induced by epidural or subarachnoid administration of detomidine hydrochloride solution in mares. Am J Vet Res 1994;55(5):670–80.

77. Goodrich LR, Nixon AJ, Fubini SL, et al. Epidural morphine and detomidine decreases postoperative hindlimb lameness in horses after bilateral stifle arthroscopy. Vet Surg 2002;31(3):232–9.

78. Sysel AM, Pleasant SR, Jacobson JD. Efficacy of an epidural combination of morphine and detomidine in alleviating experimentally induced hindlimb lameness in horses. Vet Surg 1996;25(6):511–8.

79. Valverde A, Gunkel CI. Pain management in horses and farm animals. J Vet Emerg Crit Care 2005;15(4):295–307.

80. Hutschala D, Mascher H, Schmetterer L, et al. Clonidine added to bupivacaine enhances and prolongs analgesia after brachial plexus block via a local mechanism in healthy volunteers. Eur J Anaesthesiol 2004;21(3):198–204.

81. Eisenach JC, De Kock R, Klimscha W. Alpha2-adrenergic agonists for regional anesthesia: a clinical review of clonidine (1984–1995). Anesthesiology 1996; 85(3):655–74.

82. Butterworth JF, Strichartz GR. The alpha sub 2-adrenergic agonists clonidine and guanfacine produce tonic and phasic block of conduction in rat sciatic nerve fibers. Anesth Analg 1993;76(2):295–301.

83. Dória RG, Valadão CA, Duque JC, et al. Comparative study of epidural xylazine or clonidine in horses. Vet Anaesth Analg 2008;35(2):166–72.

84. Eisenach J, Lysak SZ, Viscorni CM. Epidural clonidine analgesia following surgery: phase 1. Anesthesiology 1989;71(5):640–6.

85. Doherty TJ, Geiser DR, Rohrbach BW. The effect of epidural xylazine on halothane minimum alveolar concentration in ponies. J Vet Pharmacol Ther 1997; 20(3):246–8.

86. Timmermans PB, Brands A, Van Zwieten PA. Lipophilicity and brain disposition of clonidine and structurally related imidazolines. Naunyn Schmiedebergs Arch Pharmacol 1977;300(3):217–26.

87. Valverde A. Epidural analgesia and anesthesia in dogs and cats. Vet Clin North Am Small Anim 2008;38(6):1205–30.

88. Yoshitomi T, Kohjitani A, Maeda S, et al. Dexmedetomidine enhances the local anesthetic action of lidocaine via an alpha-2A adrenoceptor. Anesth Analg 2008;107(1):96–101.

89. Kawasaki Y, Kumamoto E, Furue H, et al. Alpha 2 adrenoceptor-mediated presynaptic inhibition of primary afferent glutamatergic transmission in rat substantia gelatinosa neurons. Anesthesiology 2003;98(3):682–9.

90. Brunson DB, Majors LJ. Comparative analgesia of xylazine, xylazine/morphine, xylazine/butorphanol, and xylazine/nalbuphine in the horse, using dental dolorimetry. Am J Vet Res 1987;48(7):1087–91.

91. Russell TM, MacLean AA. Standing surgical repair of propagating metacarpal and metatarsal condylar fractures in racehorses. Equine Vet J 2006;38(5):423–7.

92. van Hoogmoed LM, Galuppo LD. Laparoscopic ovariectomy using the Endo-GIA stapling device and Endo-catch pouches and evaluation of analgesic efficacy of epidural morphine sulfate in 10 mares. Vet Surg 2005;34(6): 646–50.

93. Cruz AM, Kerr CL, Bouré LP, et al. Cardiovascular effects of insufflation of the abdomen with carbon dioxide in standing horses sedated with detomidine. Am J Vet Res 2004;65(3):357–62.

94. Latimer FG, Eades SC, Pettifer G, et al. Cardiopulmonary, blood and peritoneal fluid alterations associated with abdominal insufflation of carbon dioxide in standing horses. Equine Vet J 2003;35(3):283–90.

95. van Dijk P, Lakveld DP, Rijkenhuizen AB, et al. Hormonal, metabolic and physiological effects of laparoscopic surgery using a detomidine-buprenorphine combination in standing horses. Vet Anaesth Analg 2003;30(2):71–9.

96. Schumacher J, Dutton DM, Murphy DJ, et al. Paranasal sinus surgery through a frontonasal flap in sedated, standing horses. Vet Surg 2000;29(2):173–7.

97. Moon PF, Suter CM. Paravertebral thoracolumbar anaesthesia in 10 horses. Equine Vet J 1993;25(4):304–8.

98. Clarke KW, Paton BS. Combined use of detomidine with opiates in the horse. Equine Vet J 1988;20(5):331–4.

99. Muir WW, Skarda RT, Sheehan WC. Hemodynamic and respiratory effects of xylazine-morphine sulfate in horses. Am J Vet Res 1979;40(10):1417–20.

100. Kuhn M, Köhler L, Fenner A, et al. Isofluran-Reduktion und Beeinflussung kardiovaskulärer und pulmonaler Parameter durch kontinuierliche Romifidin-Infusion während der Narkose bei Pferden—Eine klinische Studie. Pferdeheilkunde 2004;20(6):511–6 [in German].

101. Bennett RC, Kollias-Baker C, Steffey EP, et al. The influence of morphine on the halothane sparing effect of xylazine: II, xylazine and morphine concentrations. Vet Anaesth Analg 2000;27(1):56.

102. Wagner AE, Dunlop CI, Heath RB, et al. Hemodynamic function during neurectomy in halothane anesthetized horses with or without constant dose detomidine infusion. Vet Surg 1992;21(3):248–55.

103. Neges K, Bettschart-Wolfensberger R, Müller J, et al. The isoflurane sparing effect of a medetomidine constant rate infusion in horses. Vet Anaesth Analg 2003;30(2):93–4.

104. Bettschart-Wolfensberger R, Jäggin-Schmucker N, Lendl C, et al. Minimal alveolar concentration of desflurane in combination with an infusion of medetomidine for the anaesthesia of ponies. Vet Rec 2001;148(9):264–7.

105. Ringer SK, Kalchofner K, Boller J, et al. A clinical comparison of two anaesthetic protocols using lidocaine or medetomidine in horses. Vet Anaesth Analg 2007;34(4):257–68.

106. Doherty TJ, Frazier DL. Effect of intravenous lidocaine on halothane minimum alveolar concentration in ponies. Equine Vet J 1998;30(4):300–3.

107. Yamashita K, Satoh M, Umikawa A, et al. Combination of continuous intravenous infusion using a mixture of guaifenesin-ketamine-medetomidine and sevoflurane anesthesia in horses. J Vet Med Sci 2000;62(3):229–335.

108. Virtanen R, Savola JM, Saano V. Highly selective and specific antagonism of central and peripherals alpha 2-adrenoceptors by atipamezole. Arch Int Pharmacodyn Ther 1989;297:190–204.

109. Ramseyer B, Schmucker N, Schatzmann U, et al. Antagonism of detomidine sedation with atipamezole in horses. J Vet Anaesth 1998;25(1):47–51.

110. Carroll GL, Matthews NS, Hartsfield SM, et al. The effect of detomidine and its antagonism with tolazoline on stress-related hormones, metabolites, physiologic responses and behavior in awake ponies. Vet Surg 1997;26(1):69–77.

111. Kitzman JV, Wilson RC, Hatch RC, et al. Antagonism of xylazine and ketamine anesthesia by 4-aminopyridine and yohimbine in geldings. Am J Vet Res 1984;45(5):875–9.

112. Hsu WH, Mcgruder JP, Lu ZX. The effect of yohimbine on xylazine/thiopental anesthesia in ponies. Vet Med 1985;80:69–72.

113. McGruder JP, Hsu WH. Antagonism of xylazine-pentobarbital anesthesia by yohimbine in ponies. Am J Vet Res 1985;46(6):1276–81.

114. Jernigan AD, Wilson RC, Booth NH, et al. Comparative pharmacokinetics of yohimbine in steers, horses and dogs. Can J Vet Res 1988;52(2):172–6.

115. Mama KR, Wagner AE, Steffey EP, et al. Evaluation of xylazine and ketamine for total intravenous anesthesia in horses. Am J Vet Res 2005;66(6):1002–7.

116. Muir WW, Lerche P, Robertson JT, et al. Comparison of four drug combinations for total intravenous anesthesia of horses undergoing surgical removal of an abdominal testis. J Am Vet Med Assoc 2000;217(6):869–73.

# Local Anesthetics as Pain Therapy in Horses

Thomas J. Doherty, MVB, MSc*, M. Reza Seddighi, DVM, PhD

**KEYWORDS**

• Lidocaine • Anesthesia • Antinociception • Horse

Despite the introduction of new drugs and techniques, it is recognized that many human patients experience moderate to severe pain postoperatively. In addition, it is now understood that postoperative pain can result in undesirable sequelae, such as chronic pain.[1] Although anthropomorphizing can lead to erroneous conclusions, it appears reasonable to assume that horses may also develop chronic pain after an episode of acute postoperative pain, and a recent study indicates that acute laminitis may lead to neuropathic pain.[2] Presently, the arsenal of analgesic drugs for use in the equine patient is limited. Systemic use of opioids is restricted because of adverse effects such as behavioral changes[3] and ileus.[4] The epidural administration of local anesthetics is mainly limited to pain relief of the perineum because of the need to maintain motor function, although morphine can be administered by this route without causing motor block. However, many clinicians see epidural drug administration as invasive and carrying the risk of infection. Consequently, equine practitioners continue to rely heavily on less efficacious drugs, primarily nonsteroidal anti-inflammatory drugs, for pain control. Thus, there is a need for safe and inexpensive alternative pain therapies for horses.

Studies in human patients and laboratory animals have demonstrated that systemically administered local anesthetics, such as lidocaine and its congener mexiletine, can reduce the intensity of postoperative and neuropathic pain, although the mechanisms of lidocaine's actions are uncertain. Mexiletine is rarely used clinically, primarily because it has significant side effects. Recent studies indicate that systemic lidocaine may have potential as an analgesic and as a supplement to general anesthesia in horses.

## HISTORICAL PERSPECTIVE ON THE SYSTEMIC USE OF LOCAL ANESTHETICS

The intravenous (IV) administration of the local anesthetic procaine, for analgesic purposes, was initially described by Gordon in 1943,[5] and further reports on its use

The authors have nothing to disclose.
Department of Large Animal Clinical Sciences, College of Veterinary Medicine, The University of Tennessee, 2407 River Drive, Knoxville, TN 37996, USA
* Corresponding author.
E-mail address: tdoherty@utk.edu

in human patients followed.[6,7] Lidocaine (lignocaine) is an amide local anesthetic that is primarily used systemically as an antiarrhythmic drug; however, the use of IV lidocaine for anesthetic and analgesic purposes was first reported over 50 years ago.[8,9] In 1954, De Clive-Lowe and colleagues[10] described their experiences with the administration of lidocaine in association with succinylcholine for general anesthesia in 1,000 human patients. It was later reported that the incidence of postoperative pain was significantly less in patients that were administered lidocaine perioperatively and, surprisingly, the analgesic effects were still evident on the third postoperative day.[11] In spite of those early clinical studies demonstrating the anesthetic and analgesics effects of IV lidocaine, there was no further interest in the topic for over 30 years, presumably due to concerns of toxicity.

## REDISCOVERY OF LIDOCAINE'S ANTINOCICEPTIVE EFFECTS

Renewed interest in the systemic administration of local anesthetics began in 1986, when it was demonstrated that intra-abdominal instillation of bupivacaine decreased the duration of postoperative colonic ileus in human patients.[12] This research was soon followed by a study that demonstrated the efficacy of IV lidocaine in decreasing the duration of colonic stasis.[13] Importantly, these studies showed that local anesthetics were efficacious at blood concentrations less than those considered to be toxic; however, it is important to note that bupivacaine is not administered intravenously because of its narrow therapeutic index.

The systemic administration of lidocaine for neuropathic pain has been the focus of numerous studies,[14,15] but the efficacy of lidocaine for the treatment of acute postoperative pain has gained attention of late. The analgesic effects of sodium ($Na^+$) channel blockers, such as lidocaine and mexiletine, have been demonstrated in studies in rats[16,17] and human volunteers.[18,19] In human patients, IV lidocaine decreases postoperative pain,[18,20] is antihyperalgesic[21] and anti-inflammatory,[22] improves bowel function postoperatively,[23] and facilitates rehabilitation.[24]

Although it was initially established that IV lidocaine has analgesic effects in patients with chronic neuropathic pain[14,15] and is efficacious for the treatment of visceral pain,[25] the results of its efficacy in postoperative pain were conflicting. It is now understood that differences in study findings are related to the timing of the lidocaine administration, and perhaps the dose of lidocaine administered and the type of noxious stimulus. The intraoperative administration of large doses of lidocaine resulted in analgesia and morphine-sparing effects.[10,11] Intraoperative administration of lidocaine, followed by a constant infusion for 24 hours postoperatively, resulted in significant analgesia on the first and second postoperative day.[26] In contrast to the aforementioned findings, administering a small dose of lidocaine, by infusion, in the postoperative period did not produce analgesic effects.[27,28]

## ORIGINS OF POSTOPERATIVE PAIN

Current understanding of pain mechanisms has progressed from the Cartesian concept that pain resulted from the direct transmission from peripheral receptors and fibers, via the spinal cord, to a pain center in the brain. It is now understood that nociceptive input is transmitted to the spinal cord, or specific cranial nerves, by myelinated A$\delta$ and unmyelinated C-fibers. The signal crosses the synaptic junction in the dorsal horn of the spinal cord via a series of chemical interactions before being transmitted by nociceptive-specific or nonspecific wide dynamic range (WDR) neurons.

It is recognized that tissue injury may induce changes in the responsiveness of the nociceptive system by causing peripheral and central sensitization.[29] Generally, postoperative pain is believed to result from the interaction of three sources: (1) trauma at the surgical site, which generates impulses in peripheral neurons; (2) peripheral sensitization of nerve fibers at the surgical site due to the effects of inflammatory mediators; and (3) central sensitization of the spinal cord subsequent to prolonged barrage from nociceptive inputs. Although the trauma of incision and tissue manipulation activates central pathways implicated in sensitization, its influence may be restricted to the intraoperative period.[30] It is currently understood that local anesthetics can be used perioperatively to affect all three aforementioned sources of postoperative pain.

Peripheral sensitization involves (1) lowering of the response threshold in primary afferent fibers, (2) an increase in response magnitude to suprathreshold stimuli, (3) an increase in spontaneous activity, and (4) an increase in receptive field size.[29] Decrease in tissue pH after surgical incision may also contribute to postoperative pain and hyperalgesia.[31] In addition, inflammatory mediators and the increased temperature at the surgical site increase the activity of the transient receptor potential vanilloid type 1 (TRPV1) receptor, resulting in the generation of action potentials that may be perceived as pain.[32] Neuronal excitability is amplified by chemokines and cytokines, such as tumor necrosis factor $\alpha$ (TNF-$\alpha$), interleukin (IL)-6, and prostaglandin $E_2$ (PGE$_2$), which, together with nerve growth factor, increases the expression or activity of voltage-gated Na$^+$ channels (VGSCs).[33]

In central sensitization there is a decrease in the pain threshold as a result of exposure to excessive and prolonged nociceptive input altering the responsiveness of the central nervous system (CNS).[34] Thus, after development of central sensitization, an innocuous stimulus is perceived as noxious.[35] Secondary hyperalgesia, another consequence of central sensitization, is an exaggerated response to stimuli applied to undamaged tissue surrounding the site of injury.[36] The process of central sensitization involves a number of neurotransmitters and receptors including the N-methyl-D-aspartate (NMDA) receptor.

The idea that inhalational anesthesia does not protect against central sensitization was proposed by Crile[37] in 1913. He claimed that patients who had regional anesthesia of the surgical site, in addition to inhalational anesthesia, experienced a reduction in postoperative pain. This concept of preemptive analgesia was reintroduced in 1983 by Woolf,[38] who provided evidence, based on animal studies, to support Crile's observations.

## MECHANISMS OF LIDOCAINE-INDUCED ANTINOCICEPTION

The mechanisms by which systemic lidocaine suppresses postoperative pain are uncertain; however, a number of mechanisms have been proposed for its antinociceptive effect (**Box 1**). Local anesthetics were initially considered to block only Na$^+$ channels; however, there is an increasing body of evidence that these drugs also modulate a wide range of ion channels, receptors, and nociceptive pathways in the CNS. Interestingly, some of these effects occur at concentrations of local anesthetic much less than those required for Na$^+$ channel blockade.[22] At clinically relevant blood concentrations of lidocaine, there is little or no effect on impulse conduction in uninjured peripheral nerves. The plasma concentration (2-5μg/mL) of lidocaine that is efficacious in alleviating pain is profoundly less than what is required to block electrically evoked peripheral nerve conduction in nociceptive C and Aδ fibers, as this would require plasma concentrations of approximately 250μg/mL.[39]

### Action at Sodium Channels

VGSCs transmit electrical signals along sensory neurons to the CNS by generation of rapid action potentials. VGSCs are transmembrane proteins with gated pores. Opening

---

**Box 1**
**Reported effects of systemic lidocaine**

Antinociceptive and minimum alveolar concentration-sparing mechanisms

   Blockade of sodium channels

   Blockade of calcium channels

   Blockade of potassium channels

   Blockade of presynaptic muscarinic receptors

   Blockade or activation of transient receptor potential vanilloid type 1 receptors

   Blockade of N-methyl-D-aspartate receptors

   Activation of γ-aminobutyric acid receptors

   Activation of glycine receptors

Anti-inflammatory mechanisms

   Inhibition of sequestration, migration, and activation of polymorphonuclear cells (PMNs).

   Inhibition of PMN adherence to endothelial cells

   Inhibition of $Na^+- H^+$ exchanger in PMNs

   Suppression of histamine release from mast cells

   Inhibition of nuclear factor κB

   Decrease in chemotactic factors and cytokines

   Decrease in albumin extravasation and microvascular permeability

   Inhibition of sensory neurons with resultant decreases in release of substance P

   Decrease in release of proinflammatory lipoxygenase products

   Inhibition of the release of toxic oxygen metabolites

   Decreased expression of inducible nitric oxide synthase

---

and closing of these pores is controlled by changes in transmembrane voltage gradients.[40] Lidocaine binds to a receptor site within the α-subunit of the channel, thereby blocking $Na^+$ conduction and preventing the generation of an action potential.[41]

### Interaction of lidocaine with sodium channels

Lidocaine is a weak base and is available commercially as a salt. The salt form dissolves in an aqueous solution into the nonionized (lipid soluble) and ionized (hydrophilic) forms. The nonionized form of lidocaine crosses the axonal membrane more readily, becomes protonated (**Fig. 1**), and then attaches to the binding site for local anesthetics, located on the inside of the sodium channel,[42,43] resulting in blockade of sodium transfer across the channel. The ionization constant (pKa) of lidocaine is 7.9 and, at physiologic pH (7.4), 79% of lidocaine exists in the ionized form.[44] Thus, if the pH of the solution was closer to the pKa, more of the nonionized form would be present, and the onset of nerve block would be more rapid. Sodium bicarbonate is sometimes added to the lidocaine solution to increase pH and, thereby, decrease the onset time and increase the duration of the nerve block,[45] in addition to decreasing pain on injection.[46] However, there is no evidence that the efficacy of systemically administered lidocaine is decreased by the magnitude of pH change that might occur clinically; therefore, concurrent administration of sodium bicarbonate to acidotic animals cannot be recommended for the purpose of increasing the efficacy of lidocaine.

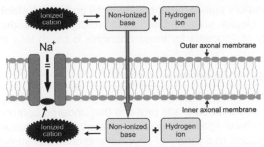

**Fig. 1.** Mechanism of action of lidocaine for $Na^+$ channel blockade. The nonionized form of lidocaine crosses the axonal membrane and becomes ionized (protonated). The ionized form binds to the cytoplasmic side of the $Na^+$ channel, thereby blocking $Na^+$ transfer across the membrane.

## Sodium channel subtypes

There are at least nine different VGSC subtypes in the nervous system and numerous sensory neuronal channels have been implicated in pain mechanisms. The various $Na^+$ channel subtypes are encoded by different genes and changes in gene expression, resulting in upregulation of channels, may occur following tissue injury.[47] VGSCs subtypes $Na_v1.8$ and $Na_v1.9$ have been identified in nociceptive dorsal root ganglion (DRG) neurons.[48] The subtype $Na_v1.7$ is considered to play a crucial role in nociception because humans lacking functional $Na_v1.7$ channels are insensitive to noxious stimuli[49] and a $Na_v1.7$ knockout mouse model has deficits in response to inflammatory stimuli.[50] Although $Na_v1.3$ is not normally expressed in adult sensory neurons, its expression is upregulated as a consequence of chronic inflammation or nerve injury.[51]

## Blockade of ectopic discharges

Under physiologic conditions, primary afferent neuronal inputs, which encode nociceptive information from the periphery to the spinal cord, are generated only after stimulation of peripheral receptors by chemical, heat, mechanical stimuli, or a combination thereof. However, injury to a peripheral nerve can cause a primary afferent input to be generated spontaneously without activation of peripheral receptors. These spontaneous discharges are often referred to as ectopic discharges. Ectopic discharges in injured nerves result primarily from the activation of $Na^+$ channels,[52] and studies in numerous animal preparations indicate that the systemic administration of lidocaine, at clinically relevant concentrations, can silence ectopic discharges in injured nerves.[16,53]

## Action at Calcium Channels

Synaptic transmission in the dorsal horn is triggered by calcium ($Ca^{++}$) channel opening, and $Ca^{++}$ channels can propagate action potentials, as has been demonstrated in heat nociceptive neurons in mammalian skin.[54] Voltage-gated $Ca^{++}$ channels closely resemble $Na^+$ channels in structure and, not surprisingly, are blocked by local anesthetics; although a greater concentration of local anesthetic is necessary when compared with that needed for $Na^+$ channel blockade.[55]

## Action at Potassium Channels

Potassium ($K^+$) channels are expressed in many areas of the nervous system and have a role in neuronal plasticity. In peripheral neurons, $K^+$ channels contribute to the decay phase of the action potential and have a role in maintaining the resting membrane potential. A specific $K^+$ channel, $K_v4.2$, is thought to play a significant role in transmitting inflammatory pain in peripheral neurons and is important in neuronal plasticity.[56] Lidocaine blocks voltage-gated and voltage-independent $K^+$ channels, although the affinity of lidocaine for these channels is much less than its affinity for $Na^+$ channels.[57]

### Inhibition of G Protein-Coupled Receptors

Lidocaine is known to inhibit G protein-coupled receptors (GPCRs), which make up a large superfamily of transmembrane proteins that undergo conformational changes after binding extracellular ligands, resulting in regulation of intracellular enzymes.[58] These receptors respond to a variety of physical and chemical stimuli, neurotransmitters, neuropeptides, hormones, and glycoproteins. Sensory neuron-specific GPCRs are expressed exclusively on nociceptive neurons and are implicated in the modulation of nociception.[59] Lidocaine interacts with the signaling of GPCRs to modulate $K^+$ and $Ca^{++}$ channel function.[60]

### Activation of TRPV1 Receptors

The TRPV1 receptor is a nonselective cation channel that is expressed by sensory neurons and in small-diameter DRG neurons, and was initially identified as the receptor for capsaicin.[61,62] It is now believed that these channels are sensory transducers that participate in the generation and modulation of nociception evoked by chemical, thermal, and mechanical stimuli.

Lidocaine may activate and sensitize TRPV1, and this activation can contribute to the release of neurotransmitters resulting in nociceptive modulation.[63] There is also evidence that TRPV1 and transient receptor potential ankyrin-1 receptors are coexpressed in small-diameter noxious sensory neurons (Aδ and C-fibers),[64] and their activation by systemic lidocaine modulates nociception.

### Inhibition of NMDA Receptors

Hypersensitivity in either inflammatory or neuropathic pain is predominantly mediated by N-methyl-D-aspartate (NMDA) receptors.[65,66] At the spinal cord, lidocaine reduces the postsynaptic depolarization mediated by NMDA receptors.[67,68] Lidocaine's inhibition of activated NMDA receptors in vitro is thought to be due to inhibition of protein kinase C (PKC).[69] In rats, small concentrations of lidocaine inhibited the depolarizations detected in spinal root recordings resulting from the direct chemical activation of NMDA receptors.[68,70] The wind-up phenomenon that contributes to central sensitization after repeated or intense noxious stimulation is suppressed by lidocaine applied directly to the spinal cord.[71] Systemic administration of lidocaine suppressed neuronal activity, including C-afferent fiber-evoked activity, in rat spinal cord.[72]

### Anti-Inflammatory Effects

The anti-inflammatory effects of local anesthetics are another important mechanism for their antinociceptive actions (see Box. 1). Inflammatory products, such as $PGE_2$, 5-hydroxytryptamine, and adenosine, augment the excitability of neurons by enhancing inward currents on $Na^+$ channels expressed on primary afferent neurons.[73] These changes result in peripheral and central sensitization. Interestingly, the effects of lidocaine on inflammatory cells such as polymorphonuclear granulocytes (PMNs) are not caused by $Na^+$ channel blockade because $Na^+$ channels are not expressed on PMNs.[74]

Although there is ample evidence, from in vitro and in vivo studies, for the anti-inflammatory properties of lidocaine, the molecular mechanism underlying these anti-inflammatory effects are not well described. Proposed mechanisms include effects on cyclic adenosine monophosphate, GPCRs, nicotinamide adenine dinucleotide, $Na^+- H^+$ exchanger, and PKC.[22] In lipopolysaccharide-stimulated macrophages, lidocaine significantly decreased inducible nitric oxide synthase expression by suppression of nuclear factor κB activation.[75] In human surgical patients, perioperative lidocaine administration significantly decreased the ex vivo production of IL-1ra and IL-6.[76]

### Miscellaneous Effects of Lidocaine

Gamma-aminobutyric acid (GABA) and glycine are the main inhibitory neurotransmitters in the CNS.[77] There is ample evidence for the modulating effect of lidocaine on glycine signaling. Indeed, it is suggested that lidocaine may exert some of its antinociceptive activity through glycinergic pathways.[63,78] Intravenous lidocaine activates the strychnine-sensitive glycine receptors in WDR neurons in rats, resulting in inhibition of transmission of noxious and nonnoxious information.[63] Excitation of GABAergic/glycinergic inhibitory interneurons, via TRPV1 receptors, after IV administration of lidocaine, may also have a role in suppression of WDR neuronal activities.[63]

Lidocaine can inhibit substance P binding to neural cells,[79] neurokinin receptor-mediated postsynaptic depolarizations,[68] and glutamate-evoked activity in spinal dorsal horn neurons.[80]

## ANESTHETIC AND ANTINOCICEPTIVE EFFECTS OF LIDOCAINE IN THE HORSE

Systemically administered lidocaine has recently gained popularity in equine practice for its volatile anesthetic sparing effects, its presumed antinociceptive actions, and for treatment of ileus. However, to date, there are only a few studies of the effects of intravenously administered lidocaine in either anesthetized or conscious horses.

### Anesthetic-Sparing Effects of Lidocaine

In an experimental setting, lidocaine decreased the minimum alveolar concentration (MAC) of halothane in ponies.[81] In clinical studies of horses undergoing surgery, lidocaine alone[82–84] and in combination with ketamine[85] decreased the required end-tidal concentration of isoflurane. Lidocaine combined with ketamine and morphine decreased the end-tidal concentration of sevoflurane required to maintain a surgical plane of anesthesia in horses.[86] These findings are consistent with those of a study in which lidocaine caused a dose-dependent decrease in the bispectral index in anesthetized horses.[87]

The mechanism by which lidocaine decreases the volatile anesthetic MAC is uncertain, but is probably not simply due to its antinociceptive properties, and may involve multiple receptor types (see **Box 1**) such as NMDA, $GABA_A$, acetylcholine, and glycine.[88] The magnitude of MAC reduction with lidocaine in ponies is dose-dependent.[81] Small doses of lidocaine (eg, 0.05 mg/kg/min) reduce the MAC by about 20%,[81] and this is consistent with findings in clinical studies that used lidocaine at doses no greater than 0.05 mg/kg/min.[82,83] A greater dose of lidocaine (eg, 0.1 mg/kg/min) reduces the MAC of a volatile anesthetic by at least 35%.[81]

In a surgical model, lidocaine (3.0 mg/kg) was administered IV to horses anesthetized with xylazine and ketamine.[89] In that study, there was no difference between the lidocaine and saline treatments in regards to the number of supplementary injections of xylazine and ketamine needed to maintain a surgical plane of anesthesia. However, the study could not be tightly controlled because the horses were not weighed before anesthesia, thus drug doses had to be estimated. The study did not evaluate the analgesic effect of lidocaine in the postoperative period.

Adverse effects of lidocaine administration were not reported in any of the afore-mentioned studies; nevertheless, there is evidence that the intraoperative administration of lidocaine may decrease the quality of recovery.[90] However, in the authors' experience, this effect can be readily overcome by decreasing the plasma concentration of lidocaine at the time of awakening by (1) stopping the infusion before the end of surgery or (2) decreasing the infusion rate over time or (3) delaying the horse's first attempt to stand by inducing sedation.

### Antinociceptive Effects of Lidocaine

The effects of intravenously administered lidocaine on electroencephalography (EEG) parameters were investigated in anesthetized ponies.[91] Under halothane anesthesia, ponies were given a loading dose of lidocaine (5.0 mg/kg, [IV]) over 15 minutes and an infusion of 0.1 mg/kg/min. Lidocaine administration abolished measured EEG changes which are indicative of noxious stimulation during castration; based on these findings, the authors concluded that lidocaine is antinociceptive.

In 2005, Robertson and colleagues[92] investigated the antinociceptive effects of systemically administered lidocaine in response to visceral and somatic stimuli in conscious horses. Somatic antinociception was assessed using a thermal stimulus, by applying a heat source over the withers. Visceral antinociception was evaluated by the response to colorectal and duodenal distension. Lidocaine was administered as a loading dose of 2.0 mg/kg over 20 minutes and a constant rate infusion (CRI) of 0.05 mg/kg/min. The resulting plasma concentrations of lidocaine during delivery of the noxious stimuli ranged from 0.7 to 1.2 μg/mL. Lidocaine treatment did not have a significant effect on the response to colorectal or duodenal distension in the horses of that study, which was surprising, given that lidocaine dose-dependently inhibited cardiovascular responses to colorectal distension in rats.[25] Lidocaine treatment significantly increased the thermal threshold, and this was contrary to the findings in studies using human volunteers, where systemic lidocaine has no effect on thermal thresholds.[93]

### Potential Role in Treating Laminitis-Induced Pain

There is a clinical report that intravenously administered lidocaine provided analgesia in horses suffering from chronic laminitis.[94] A recent study has demonstrated that the histopathological changes in the sensory nerves innervating the forelimb of horses suffering from chronic laminitis were consistent with those reported in previously characterized neuropathic pain states.[2] Thus, it seems plausible that systemic lidocaine, which has been shown to be effective for the treatment of neuropathic pain,[14,15] would be beneficial in the treatment of laminitis.

## OTHER POTENTIAL BENEFITS OF SYSTEMIC LIDOCAINE

Besides its anesthetic and antinociceptive effects, lidocaine has properties that make its use desirable in the surgical patient, particularly in the horse undergoing abdominal surgery.

### Effect on the Incidence of Post-Operative Ileus

A number of studies with human patients have established that the perioperative use of lidocaine reduces the duration of postoperative ileus (POI).[13,23,95] The effect of intraoperative administration of lidocaine on the incidence and severity of POI has not been investigated widely in horses; however, in one study, the intraoperative administration of lidocaine to surgical colic patients was thought to be associated with a reduction in the incidence of POI.[96] In another study of horses undergoing abdominal surgery, the intraoperative administration of lidocaine (0.025 mg/kg/min) combined with CRI of 0.05 mg/kg/min for 24 hours after surgery was considered to have a beneficial effect on intestinal motility.[97] In a study of horses with POI, the administration of lidocaine postoperatively resulted in shorter hospitalization time.[94]

### Effects on Ischemia-Reperfusion Injury

Systemic lidocaine decreases reperfusion injury following ischemia. In a myocardial ischemia model in dogs, lidocaine reduced the size of the myocardial infarct.[98] In an ischemic jejunal model in horses, pretreatment with lidocaine decreased plasma $PGE_2$ metabolite concentration and mucosal cyclooxygenase 2 expression, and ameliorated the effect of flunixin meglumine on promoting mucosal neutrophil infiltration.[99]

### Effects in Endotoxemic Animals

Lidocaine has been investigated for its therapeutic potential in various models of endotoxemia in laboratory animals. In rabbits, lidocaine attenuated the hypotension and metabolic acidosis consequent to the endotoxin administration.[100] In rats, lidocaine attenuated endotoxin-induced changes in leukocyte adhesion to endothelial cells and preserved endothelial integrity, as demonstrated by a decrease in macromolecular leakage.[101]

## METABOLISM AND ELIMINATION OF LIDOCAINE

Metabolism of lidocaine in the horse produces monoethylglycinexylidide and glycinexylidide, which are the pharmacologically active metabolites[81] that are de-ethylation products of lidocaine also produced in the human liver via the cytochrome P450 superfamily of enzymes. Thus, lidocaine may be considered to undergo metabolism via the cytochrome P450 system in horses. Lidocaine and its metabolites are excreted in the urine. Feary and colleagues[102] compared lidocaine kinetics in conscious horses and horses anesthetized with sevoflurane, and concluded that general anesthesia changes lidocaine kinetics. Plasma lidocaine concentrations were increased at all times in the anesthetized group, and this was attributed to a decrease in the volume of distribution and clearance of lidocaine. Lidocaine clearance is greatly dependent on hepatic blood flow,[103] and a decrease in hepatic blood flow, such as may occur during sevoflurane anesthesia, will decrease lidocaine clearance. Additionally, anesthetic drugs metabolized by the cytochrome P450 system may compete for binding sites and delay clearance.

## CONTRAINDICATIONS TO SYSTEMIC ADMINISTRATION OF LIDOCAINE

Because of lidocaine's effects on inflammation and phagocytic cell function, there has been concern that inhibiting these functions might increase the incidence of bacterial infections. It appears, however, that the residual polymorphonuclear cell function is adequate and the bactericidal effect of PMNs from human patients being administered lidocaine infusions is only slightly decreased.[104] Nevertheless, in a study of rats inoculated with *Staphylococcus aureus*, five of six rats treated with systemic lidocaine died, whereas only one of six rats in the control group died.[105] Thus, it may be prudent to avoid the use of systemic lidocaine in patients with gross bacterial contamination. Paradoxically, lidocaine has anti-bacterial effects; however, these effects occur at concentrations greater that what can be safely achieved with systemic administration.[106]

## RECOMMENDATIONS FOR THE USE OF SYSTEMIC LIDOCAINE
### Intraoperative Administration of Lidocaine

Based on currently available data from horses and other species, intraoperative administration of lidocaine is expected to decrease the volatile anesthetic MAC, postoperative pain, the incidence and severity of postoperative ileus, and inflammation.

In the authors' hospital, lidocaine is used with isoflurane, ketamine, and xylazine as part of a multimodal anesthetic regimen. After sedation with xylazine hydrochloride and induction of anesthesia with ketamine and diazepam, a loading dose of lidocaine (3.0 mg/kg over 15 minutes) is given and a CRI of 0.1 mg/kg/min is administered during the first hour. The CRI is decreased to 0.075 and 0.05 mg/kg/min for the second and third hours, respectively. Concurrently, the end-tidal concentration of isoflurane is maintained at 0.4% to 0.6%, and ketamine (2.5 mg/kg/hr) and xylazine (0.25 mg/kg/hr) are infused. The lidocaine infusion is generally stopped approximately 20 minutes before the end of surgery. To delay time to first movement, horses are sedated with romifidine (0.04 mg/kg) and ketamine (0.3 mg/kg) when placed in the recovery box. Problems that can be attributed to lidocaine administration have not been encountered while using this technique in approximately 2,000 horses.

### Lidocaine Administration to Conscious Horses

Systemic lidocaine may be safely used in the conscious horse; however, in this scenario, careful attention must be given to the loading dose and infusion rate. A loading dose of lidocaine (1.3–1.5 mg/kg) is administered over 3 to 5 minutes, and this is followed by a CRI of 0.05 mg/kg/min. Lidocaine can be safely administered at this rate for many hours, and adverse effects, when they occur, are generally due to an unintentional increase in the infusion rate.

## SIGNS AND TREATMENT OF LIDOCAINE TOXICITY

Lidocaine toxicity produces a concentration-dependent spectrum of effects (**Fig. 2**) that are manifested primarily at the central nervous and cardiovascular systems, although cardiac signs of toxicity occur at much greater plasma concentrations.[44]

| Systems | Progression of clinical signs with increasing plasma concentration |
|---|---|
| Central Nervous | Eyelid blinking/ Nystagmus |
| | Muscle twitching |
| | Ataxia |
| | Recumbency |
| | Seizure |
| | Coma |
| Cardiovascular | Hypotension/ Bradycardia |
| | Cardiovascular collapse |

**Fig. 2.** Clinical signs of lidocaine toxicity. The arrow indicates increasing plasma concentrations of lidocaine. These signs may not necessarily occur as a continuum in all horses.

Because of the relatively large volumes of lidocaine required to produce toxicity in an adult horse, toxicity is unlikely to happen under normal circumstances. Treatment of severe lidocaine toxicity may be unrewarding, thus emphasized the importance of vigilance during lidocaine administration.

## CNS Toxicity

Signs of CNS toxicity in conscious horses are initially manifested as eyelid blinking, nystagmus, muscle twitching and ataxia, and the horse may assume sternal recumbency.[107] Some horses have signs of visual dysfunction,[107] which is consistent with reported effects of visual impairment with lidocaine toxicity in human patients.[44] These signs usually resolve fairly quickly once the lidocaine infusion is stopped. However, treatment with a sedative (eg, xylazine, 0.3 mg/kg, IV) or an anticonvulsant (eg, diazepam, 0.05 mg/kg, IV) may be indicated if CNS signs persist beyond a few minutes. In severe overdosing, the aforementioned signs may progress to seizures, unconsciousness, and respiratory arrest. Paradoxically, lidocaine has been shown to suppress seizures at plasma concentrations less than 5.0 μg/mL,[108] and has been used successfully for the treatment of status epilepticus in children.[109]

Treatment of seizures should begin quickly and, in addition to sedatives and anticonvulsants, general anesthesia may be necessary in some cases to control the seizures. Although a GABA agonist, such as thiopental or propofol, may be the ideal agent to induce anesthesia; ketamine combined with a benzodiazepine is probably satisfactory if the horse is heavily sedated (eg, xylazine 1.0 mg/kg, IV) because ketamine significantly prevented lidocaine-induced generalized tonic-clonic seizures in mice.[110] Guaifenesin, a central muscle relaxant, should be beneficial in decreasing the skeletal muscle manifestations of toxicity. Provision of supplemental oxygen is indicated because of the increase in oxygen demands in the brain and muscle; hypoxemia further exacerbates lidocaine toxicity.

## Cardiovascular System Toxicity

Toxicity of the cardiovascular system occurs at plasma lidocaine concentrations much greater than those necessary to cause seizures[44]; thus, cardiovascular depression is less likely to occur during lidocaine administration to horses. In conscious horses, plasma concentrations of lidocaine between 1.85 and 4.53 μg/mL caused statistically significant changes in P-wave duration, P-R interval, R-R interval, and Q-T interval; however, these changes were within the normal reference ranges, and were not deemed to be clinically significant.[107] Nevertheless, lidocaine toxicity can result in hypotension, myocardial depression, and refractory cardiac dysrhythmias. We have observed severe hypotension in an experimental setting where a large dose of lidocaine (5.0 mg/kg IV) was administered over a 5-minute period to ponies anesthetized with halothane. Although hypotension was readily reversed by infusion of dobutamine in those ponies, severe lidocaine-induced cardiovascular depression may, in some cases, be resistant to conventional treatment with anticholinergic drugs and positive inotropes.

## SUMMARY

The antinociceptive effects of systemic lidocaine are well documented in human beings and laboratory animals. There are few studies evaluating the efficacy of systemic lidocaine in horses; however, evidence exists for its anesthetic and antinociceptive effects in this species. Based on findings from the study of human patients, it appears that the best results are obtained when lidocaine is administered in the perioperative period, rather than in the postoperative period only. Administration of lidocaine intraoperatively has the benefit of decreasing volatile anesthetic MAC and the potential to provide postoperative analgesia and decrease the incidence of postoperative ileus.

## REFERENCES

1. Perkins FM, Kehlet H. Chronic pain as an outcome of surgery. A review of predictive factors. Anesthesiology 2000;93(4):1123–33.
2. Jones E, Vinuela-Fernandez I, Eager RA, et al. Neuropathic changes in equine laminitis pain. Pain 2007;132(3):321–31.
3. Sellon DC, Monroe VL, Roberts MC, et al. Pharmacokinetics and adverse effects of butorphanol administered by single intravenous injection or continuous intravenous infusion in horses. Am J Vet Res 2001;62(2):183–9.
4. Boscan P, Van Hoogmoed LM, Farver TB, et al. Evaluation of the effects of the opioid agonist morphine on gastrointestinal tract function in horses. Am J Vet Res 2006;67(6):992–7.
5. Gordon RA. Intravenous novocaine for analgesia in burns (a preliminary report). Can Med Assoc J 1943;49(6):478–81.
6. Gordon RA. Application of intravenous procaine therapy to traumatic surgery. Curr Res Anesth Analg 1950;29(1):54–6.
7. Brittain GJ. Intravenous procaine hydrochloride; post-operative analgesia in 100 cases. Anaesthesia 1949;4(1):30–3.
8. Gilbert CR, Hanson IR, Brown AB, et al. Intravenous use of xylocaine. Curr Res Anesth Analg 1951;30:301–13.
9. Keats AS, D'Alessandro GL, Beecher HK. Controlled study of pain relief by intravenous procaine. J Am Med Assoc 1951;147(18):1761–3.
10. De Clive-Lowe SG, Desmond J, North J. Intravenous lignocaine anaesthesia. Anaesthesia 1958;13(2):138–46.
11. Bartlett EE, Hutserani O. Xylocaine for the relief of postoperative pain. Anesth Analg 1961;40:296–304.
12. Rimback G, Cassuto J, Faxen A, et al. Effect of intra-abdominal bupivacaine instillation on postoperative colonic motility. Gut 1986;27(2):170–5.
13. Rimback G, Cassuto J, Tollesson PO. Treatment of postoperative paralytic ileus by intravenous lidocaine infusion. Anesth Analg 1990;70(4):414–9.
14. Boas RA, Covino BG, Shahnarian A. Analgesic responses to i.v. lignocaine. Br J Anaesth 1982;54(5):501–5.
15. Kastrup J, Petersen P, Dejgard A, et al. Intravenous lidocaine infusion—a new treatment of chronic painful diabetic neuropathy? Pain 1987;28(1):69–75.
16. Chabal C, Russell LC, Burchiel KJ. The effect of intravenous lidocaine, tocainide, and mexiletine on spontaneously active fibers originating in rat sciatic neuromas. Pain 1989;38(3):333–8.
17. Abram SE, Yaksh TL. Systemic lidocaine blocks nerve injury-induced hyperalgesia and nociceptor-driven spinal sensitization in the rat. Anesthesiology 1994;80(2):383–91.
18. Koppert W, Ostermeier N, Sittl R, et al. Low-dose lidocaine reduces secondary hyperalgesia by a central mode of action. Pain 2000;85(1–2):217–24.
19. Dirks J, Fabricius P, Petersen KL, et al. The effect of systemic lidocaine on pain and secondary hyperalgesia associated with the heat/capsaicin sensitization model in healthy volunteers. Anesth Analg 2000;91(4):967–72.

20. Koppert W, Weigand M, Neumann F, et al. Perioperative intravenous lidocaine has preventive effects on postoperative pain and morphine consumption after major abdominal surgery. Anesth Analg 2004;98(4):1050–5.
21. Koppert W, Zeck S, Sittl R, et al. Low-dose lidocaine suppresses experimentally induced hyperalgesia in humans. Anesthesiology 1998;89(6):1345–53.
22. Hollmann MW, Durieux ME. Local anesthetics and the inflammatory response: a new therapeutic indication? Anesthesiology 2000;93(3):858–75.
23. Groudine SB, Fisher HA, Kaufman RP Jr, et al. Intravenous lidocaine speeds the return of bowel function, decreases postoperative pain, and shortens hospital stay in patients undergoing radical retropubic prostatectomy. Anesth Analg 1998;86(2):235–9.
24. Kaba A, Laurent SR, Detroz BJ, et al. Intravenous lidocaine infusion facilitates acute rehabilitation after laparoscopic colectomy. Anesthesiology 2007;106(1): 11–8.
25. Ness TJ. Intravenous lidocaine inhibits visceral nociceptive reflexes and spinal neurons in the rat. Anesthesiology 2000;92(6):1685–91.
26. Cassuto J, Wallin G, Hogstrom S, et al. Inhibition of postoperative pain by continuous low-dose intravenous infusion of lidocaine. Anesth Analg 1985; 64(10):971–4.
27. Cepeda MS, Delgado M, Ponce M, et al. Equivalent outcomes during postoperative patient-controlled intravenous analgesia with lidocaine plus morphine versus morphine alone. Anesth Analg 1996;83(1):102–6.
28. Birch K, Jorgensen J, Chraemmer-Jorgensen B, et al. Effect of i.v. lignocaine on pain and the endocrine metabolic responses after surgery. Br J Anaesth 1987; 59(6):721–4.
29. Brennan TJ, Zahn PK, Pogatzki-Zahn EM. Mechanisms of incisional pain. Anesthesiol Clin North America 2005;23(1):1–20.
30. Strichartz GR. Novel ideas of local anaesthetic actions on various ion channels to ameliorate postoperative pain. Br J Anaesth 2008;101(1):45–7.
31. Woo YC, Park SS, Subieta AR, et al. Changes in tissue pH and temperature after incision indicate acidosis may contribute to postoperative pain. Anesthesiology 2004;101(2):468–75.
32. Kissin I. Vanilloid-induced conduction analgesia: selective, dose-dependent, long-lasting, with a low level of potential neurotoxicity. Anesth Analg 2008; 107(1):271–81.
33. Wood JN, Boorman JP, Okuse K, et al. Voltage-gated sodium channels and pain pathways. J Neurobiol 2004;61(1):55–71.
34. Kenshalo DR Jr, Leonard RB, Chung JM, et al. Facilitation of the response of primate spinothalamic cells to cold and to tactile stimuli by noxious heating of the skin. Pain 1982;12(2):141–52.
35. Hudspith M, Munglani R. A role for presynaptic NMDA receptors in central sensitization in the spinal cord dorsal horn? Br J Anaesth 1998;81(2):294–5.
36. Pogatzki EM, Niemeier JS, Brennan TJ. Persistent secondary hyperalgesia after gastrocnemius incision in the rat. Eur J Pain 2002;6(4):295–305.
37. Crile GW. The kinetic theory of shock and its prevention through anoci-association (shockless operation). Lancet 1913;ii:7–16.
38. Woolf CJ. Evidence for a central component of post-injury pain hypersensitivity. Nature 1983;306(5944):686–8.
39. Tanelian DL, MacIver MB. Analgesic concentrations of lidocaine suppress tonic A-delta and C fiber discharges produced by acute injury. Anesthesiology 1991; 74(5):934–6.

40. Catterall WA. From ionic currents to molecular mechanisms: the structure and function of voltage-gated sodium channels. Neuron 2000;26(1):13–25.
41. Scholz A. Mechanisms of (local) anaesthetics on voltage-gated sodium and other ion channels. Br J Anaesth 2002;89(1):52–61.
42. Alpert LA, Fozzard HA, Hanck DA, et al. Is there a second external lidocaine binding site on mammalian cardiac cells? Am J Physiol 1989;257(1 Pt 2): H79–84.
43. Skarda RT, Tranquilli J. Local anesthetics. In: Tranquilli J, Thurmon JC, Grimm KA, editors. Lumb & Jones' veterinary anesthesia and analgesia. Ames (IA): Blackwell Publishing; 2007. p. 395–418.
44. Barash PG, Cullen BF, Stoelting RK. Handbook of clinical anesthsia. 5th edition. Philadelphia: Lippinkott Williams & Wilkins; 1996.
45. Chernoff DM, Strichartz GR. Kinetics of local anesthetic inhibition of neuronal sodium currents. pH and hydrophobicity dependence. Biophys J 1990;58(1):69–81.
46. Parham SM, Pasieka JL. Effect of pH modification by bicarbonate on pain after subcutaneous lidocaine injection. Can J Surg 1996;39(1):31–5.
47. Tanaka M, Cummins TR, Ishikawa K, et al. SNS Na+ channel expression increases in dorsal root ganglion neurons in the carrageenan inflammatory pain model. Neuroreport 1998;9(6):967–72.
48. Benarroch EE. Sodium channels and pain. Neurology 2007;68(3):233–6.
49. Cox JJ, Reimann F, Nicholas AK, et al. An SCN9A channelopathy causes congenital inability to experience pain. Nature 2006;444(7121):894–8.
50. Nassar MA, Stirling LC, Forlani G, et al. Nociceptor-specific gene deletion reveals a major role for Nav1.7 (PN1) in acute and inflammatory pain. Proc Natl Acad Sci U S A 2004;101(34):12706–11.
51. Waxman SG, Kocsis JD, Black JA. Type III sodium channel mRNA is expressed in embryonic but not adult spinal sensory neurons, and is reexpressed following axotomy. J Neurophysiol 1994;72(1):466–70.
52. Devor M. Neuropathic pain and injured nerve: peripheral mechanisms. Br Med Bull 1991;47(3):619–30.
53. Abdi S, Lee DH, Chung JM. The anti-allodynic effects of amitriptyline, gabapentin, and lidocaine in a rat model of neuropathic pain. Anesth Analg 1998;87(6): 1360–6.
54. Smith FL, Davis RW, Carter R. Influence of voltage-sensitive Ca(++) channel drugs on bupivacaine infiltration anesthesia in mice. Anesthesiology 2001; 95(5):1189–97.
55. Xiong Z, Strichartz GR. Inhibition by local anesthetics of Ca2+ channels in rat anterior pituitary cells. Eur J Pharmacol 1998;363(1):81–90.
56. Hu HJ, Carrasquillo Y, Karim F, et al. The kv4.2 potassium channel subunit is required for pain plasticity. Neuron 2006;50(1):89–100.
57. Brau ME, Vogel W, Hempelmann G. Fundamental properties of local anesthetics: half-maximal blocking concentrations for tonic block of Na+ and K+ channels in peripheral nerve. Anesth Analg 1998;87(4):885–9.
58. Hollmann MW, Strumper D, Herroeder S, et al. Receptors, G proteins, and their interactions. Anesthesiology 2005;103(5):1066–78.
59. Lembo PM, Grazzini E, Groblewski T, et al. Proenkephalin a gene products activate a new family of sensory neuron–specific GPCRs. Nat Neurosci 2002;5(3): 201–9.
60. Hollmann MW, Wieczorek KS, Berger A, et al. Local anesthetic inhibition of G protein-coupled receptor signaling by interference with Galpha(q) protein function. Mol Pharmacol 2001;59(2):294–301.

61. Ferrini F, Salio C, Vergnano AM, et al. Vanilloid receptor-1 (TRPV1)-dependent activation of inhibitory neurotransmission in spinal substantia gelatinosa neurons of mouse. Pain 2007;129(1–2):195–209.
62. Horvath G, Kekesi G, Nagy E, et al. The role of TRPV1 receptors in the antinociceptive effect of anandamide at spinal level. Pain 2008;134(3):277–84.
63. Takeda M, Oshima K, Takahashi M, et al. Systemic administration of lidocaine suppresses the excitability of rat cervical dorsal horn neurons and tooth-pulp-evoked jaw-opening reflex. Eur J Pain 2009;13(9):929–34.
64. Kobayashi K, Fukuoka T, Obata K, et al. Distinct expression of TRPM8, TRPA1, and TRPV1 mRNAs in rat primary afferent neurons with adelta/c-fibers and co-localization with trk receptors. J Comp Neurol 2005;493(4):596–606.
65. Woolf CJ, Salter MW. Neuronal plasticity: increasing the gain in pain. Science 2000;288(5472):1765–9.
66. Liu XJ, Gingrich JR, Vargas-Caballero M, et al. Treatment of inflammatory and neuropathic pain by uncoupling Src from the NMDA receptor complex. Nat Med 2008;14(12):1325–32.
67. Sugimoto M, Uchida I, Mashimo T. Local anaesthetics have different mechanisms and sites of action at the recombinant N-methyl-D-aspartate (NMDA) receptors. Br J Pharmacol 2003;138(5):876–82.
68. Nagy I, Woolf CJ. Lignocaine selectively reduces C fibre-evoked neuronal activity in rat spinal cord in vitro by decreasing N-methyl-D-aspartate and neurokinin receptor-mediated post-synaptic depolarizations; implications for the development of novel centrally acting analgesics. Pain 1996;64(1):59–70.
69. Hahnenkamp K, Durieux ME, Hahnenkamp A, et al. Local anaesthetics inhibit signalling of human NMDA receptors recombinantly expressed in Xenopus laevis oocytes: role of protein kinase C. Br J Anaesth 2006;96(1):77–87.
70. Jaffe RA, Rowe MA. Subanesthetic concentrations of lidocaine selectively inhibit a nociceptive response in the isolated rat spinal cord. Pain 1995;60(2):167–74.
71. Fraser HM, Chapman V, Dickenson AH. Spinal local anaesthetic actions on afferent evoked responses and wind-up of nociceptive neurones in the rat spinal cord: combination with morphine produces marked potentiation of antinociception. Pain 1992;49(1):33–41.
72. Woolf CJ, Wiesenfeld-Hallin Z. The systemic administration of local anaesthetics produces a selective depression of C-afferent fibre evoked activity in the spinal cord. Pain 1985;23(4):361–74.
73. Gold MS, Reichling DB, Shuster MJ, et al. Hyperalgesic agents increase a tetrodotoxin-resistant Na+ current in nociceptors. Proc Natl Acad Sci U S A 1996;93(3):1108–12.
74. Krause KH, Demaurex N, Jaconi M, et al. Ion channels and receptor-mediated Ca2+ influx in neutrophil granulocytes. Blood Cells 1993;19(1):165–73.
75. Huang YH, Tsai PS, Kai YF, et al. Lidocaine inhibition of inducible nitric oxide synthase and cationic amino acid transporter-2 transcription in activated murine macrophages may involve voltage-sensitive Na+ channel. Anesth Analg 2006;102(6):1739–44.
76. Yardeni IZ, Beilin B, Mayburd E, et al. The effect of perioperative intravenous lidocaine on postoperative pain and immune function. Anesth Analg 2009;109(5):1464–9.
77. Legendre P. The glycinergic inhibitory synapse. Cell Mol Life Sci 2001;58(5–6):760–93.
78. Muth-Selbach U, Hermanns H, Stegmann JU, et al. Antinociceptive effects of systemic lidocaine: involvement of the spinal glycinergic system. Eur J Pharmacol 2009;613(1–3):68–73.

79. Li YM, Wingrove DE, Too HP, et al. Local anesthetics inhibit substance P binding and evoked increases in intracellular Ca2+. Anesthesiology 1995;82(1):166–73.

80. Biella G, Lacerenza M, Marchettini P, et al. Diverse modulation by systemic lidocaine of iontophoretic NMDA and quisqualic acid induced excitations on rat dorsal horn neurons. Neurosci Lett 1993;157(2):207–10.

81. Doherty TJ, Frazier DL. Effect of intravenous lidocaine on halothane minimum alveolar concentration in ponies. Equine Vet J 1998;30(4):300–3.

82. Dzikiti TB, Hellebrekers LJ, van Dijk P. Effects of intravenous lidocaine on isoflurane concentration, physiological parameters, metabolic parameters and stress-related hormones in horses undergoing surgery. J Vet Med A Physiol Pathol Clin Med 2003;50(4):190–5.

83. Ringer SK, Kalchofner K, Boller J, et al. A clinical comparison of two anaesthetic protocols using lidocaine or medetomidine in horses. Vet Anaesth Analg 2007; 34(4):257–68.

84. Bubb L, Drissen B, Stafferi F, et al. The isoflurane-sparing effect of intravenous lidocaine administered to horses undergoing exploratory celiotomy [abstract]. In 14th International Veterinary Emergency & Critical Care—Annual Symposium of American College of Veterinary Anesthesiologists. Phoenix (AZ); 2008.

85. Enderle AK, Levionnois OL, Kuhn M, et al. Clinical evaluation of ketamine and lidocaine intravenous infusions to reduce isoflurane requirements in horses under general anaesthesia. Vet Anaesth Analg 2008;35(4):297–305.

86. Lerche P, Muir WW. Co-administration of morphine, lidocaine and ketamine as anesthetic adjuncts in sevoflurane-anesthetized horses [abstract]. In 14th International Veterinary Emergency & Critical Care—Annual Symposium of American College of Veterinary Anesthesiologists. Phoenix (AZ); 2008.

87. Neto PIN, Luna SPL, Steffey EP. Cardiorespiratory and analgesic effects of lidocaine on xylazine, ketamine and guaiphenesin anaesthesia in horses [abstract]. In Association of Veterinary Anaesthetists Autumn conference. Crete (Greece); 2002.

88. Zhang Y, Laster MJ, Eger EI 2nd, et al. Lidocaine, MK-801, and MAC. Anesth Analg 2007;104(5):1098–102.

89. Sinclair M, Valverde A. Short-term anaesthesia with xylazine, diazepam/ketamine for castration in horses under field conditions: use of intravenous lidocaine. Equine Vet J 2009;41(2):149–52.

90. Valverde A, Gunkelt C, Doherty TJ, et al. Effect of a constant rate infusion of lidocaine on the quality of recovery from sevoflurane or isoflurane general anaesthesia in horses. Equine Vet J 2005;37(6):559–64.

91. Murrell JC, White KL, Johnson CB, et al. Investigation of the EEG effects of intravenous lidocaine during halothane anaesthesia in ponies. Vet Anaesth Analg 2005;32(4):212–21.

92. Robertson SA, Sanchez LC, Merritt AM, et al. Effect of systemic lidocaine on visceral and somatic nociception in conscious horses. Equine Vet J 2005; 37(2):122–7.

93. Wallace MS, Laitin S, Licht D, et al. Concentration-effect relations for intravenous lidocaine infusions in human volunteers: effects on acute sensory thresholds and capsaicin-evoked hyperpathia. Anesthesiology 1997;86(6):1262–72.

94. Malone E, Ensink J, Turner T, et al. Intravenous continuous infusion of lidocaine for treatment of equine ileus. Vet Surg 2006;35(1):60–6.

95. Harvey KP, Adair JD, Isho M, et al. Can intravenous lidocaine decrease postsurgical ileus and shorten hospital stay in elective bowel surgery? A pilot study and literature review. Am J Surg 2009;198(2):231–6.

96. Cohen ND, Lester GD, Sanchez LC, et al. Evaluation of risk factors associated with development of postoperative ileus in horses. J Am Vet Med Assoc 2004; 225(7):1070–8.

97. Brianceau P, Chevalier H, Karas A, et al. Intravenous lidocaine and small-intestinal size, abdominal fluid, and outcome after colic surgery in horses. J Vet Intern Med 2002;16(6):736–41.

98. Lesnefsky EJ, VanBenthuysen KM, McMurtry IF, et al. Lidocaine reduces canine infarct size and decreases release of a lipid peroxidation product. J Cardiovasc Pharmacol 1989;13(6):895–901.

99. Cook VL, Jones Shults J, McDowell MR, et al. Anti-inflammatory effects of intravenously administered lidocaine hydrochloride on ischemia-injured jejunum in horses. Am J Vet Res 2009;70(10):1259–68.

100. Taniguchi T, Shibata K, Yamamoto K, et al. Lidocaine attenuates the hypotensive and inflammatory responses to endotoxemia in rabbits. Crit Care Med 1996; 24(4):642–6.

101. Schmidt W, Schmidt H, Bauer H, et al. Influence of lidocaine on endotoxin-induced leukocyte-endothelial cell adhesion and macromolecular leakage in vivo. Anesthesiology 1997;87(3):617–24.

102. Feary DJ, Mama KR, Wagner AE, et al. Influence of general anesthesia on pharmacokinetics of intravenous lidocaine infusion in horses. Am J Vet Res 2005; 66(4):574–80.

103. Engelking LR, Blyden GT, Lofstedt J, et al. Pharmacokinetics of antipyrine, acetaminophen and lidocaine in fed and fasted horses. J Vet Pharmacol Ther 1987; 10(1):73–82.

104. Nakagawara M, Hirokata Y, Yoshitake J. [Effects of anesthetics on the superoxide releasing activity of human polymorphonuclear leukocytes]. Masui 1985; 34(6):754–9 [in Japanese].

105. MacGregor RR, Thorner RE, Wright DM. Lidocaine inhibits granulocyte adherence and prevents granulocyte delivery to inflammatory sites. Blood 1980; 56(2):203–9.

106. Schmidt RM, Rosenkranz HS. Antimicrobial activity of local anesthetics: lidocaine and procaine. J Infect Dis 1970;121(6):597–607.

107. Meyer GA, Lin HC, Hanson RR, et al. Effects of intravenous lidocaine overdose on cardiac electrical activity and blood pressure in the horse. Equine Vet J 2001; 33(5):434–7.

108. DeToledo JC. Lidocaine and seizures. Ther Drug Monit 2000;22(3):320–2.

109. Hamano S, Sugiyama N, Yamashita S, et al. Intravenous lidocaine for status epilepticus during childhood. Dev Med Child Neurol 2006;48(3):220–2.

110. Guler G, Erdogan F, Golgeli A, et al. Ketamine reduces lidocaine-induced seizures in mice. Int J Neurosci 2005;115(8):1239–44.

# Spinal Anesthetics and Analgesics in the Horse

Claudio C. Natalini, DVM, MS, PhD

KEYWORDS

- Spinal analgesia/anesthesia • Horse • Epidural
- Subarachnoid

## IMPORTANCE OF SPINAL ANALGESIA

Spinal and spinal nerve sensory blocks are known to produce anesthesia and analgesia in humans and animals.[1–5] This technique is well established in human medicine but not fully explored in veterinary medicine. Studies on horses have shown the effectiveness and safety of epidural blocks. Types of spinal blocks usually used in horses are the epidural single injection or continuous injection through an epidural catheter and the subarachnoid or intrathecal single injection or continuous injection through a subarachnoid catheter.[6–10]

Spinal analgesia has gained wider acceptance in horses and allows the administration of multiple injections of analgesics and anesthetics for pain control in chronically ill horses and during surgical procedures. In horses, caudal epidural anesthesia is used to desensitize the anus, rectum, perineum, vulva, vagina, urethra, and bladder. The goal is to produce surgical regional anesthesia without losing the motor function of the hind limbs. A combination of a local anesthetic drug with an alpha-2 adrenergic agonist or an opioid is the most popular option as this combination extends the period of action of the epidural anesthesia or analgesia in horses, humans, and small animals. Spinal analgesia and anesthesia have not been used as much in horses as in small animals and humans as an adjunct to general anesthesia. The epidural administration of opioids with or without local anesthetics is commonly performed in dogs and cats before surgery to reduce general anesthetic requirements as well as to provide intraoperative and postoperative pain control. The perioperative use of spinal analgesia in horses is likely to increase in the future as recent studies have shown that the administration of epidural or subarachnoid alpha-2 adrenergic agonists, phencyclidines, opioids, and low-dose local anesthetic produce intense antinociceptive effects.[11–16]

In the past 10 years, there have been many recent advances in spinal techniques in horses, both epidural and subarachnoid, to identify drugs or drug combinations that

Departamento de Farmacologia, Instituto de Ciências Básicas da Saúde, Universidade Federal do Rio Grande do Sul, Rua Sarmento Leite, 500 Sala 202, 90046-902, Porto Alegre RS, Brazil
E-mail address: claudio.natalini@pq.cnpq.br

Vet Clin Equine 26 (2010) 551–564
doi:10.1016/j.cveq.2010.07.005
0749-0739/10/$ – see front matter © 2010 Elsevier Inc. All rights reserved.

have sensory effects without motor nerve paralysis, thus providing pain control without these horses becoming recumbent. Opioids, alpha-2 agonists, dissociative drugs, and others have been investigated. Many of these drugs, which have serious side effects when injected systemically in horses, have been shown to have useful analgesic effects when injected spinally. Morphinelike opioids have the greatest potential for spinal use as they produce long-lasting analgesia without motor effects. Often the doses used spinally are significantly lower than those needed for systemic effects.

## ANATOMY AND PHYSIOLOGY RELATED TO SPINAL INJECTIONS

The spinal cord and meninges of horses generally terminate in the mid sacral region. To access the spinal canal for a subarachnoid injection, the space between the sixth lumbar and the second sacral vertebrae at the midline depression should be located (see section on subarachnoid injection technique). The depth at the lumbosacral joint from the skin to the spinal canal varies from 15 to 20 cm.[17] This limits the usefulness of this site for a single epidural injection although it is the ideal location for a combined spinal-epidural technique.

In the horse, the perineal-inguinal region is innervated by the coccygeal roots of the pudendal and caudal rectal nerve, and by the ventral branches of lumbar nerves L1 to L3. The sacral region is innervated by the caudal cutaneous femoral nerve originating from sacral nerves S1 and S2, and by sacral nerves S1 to S5. The lumbar region is innervated by lumbar nerves L1 to L6. The thoracic area is innervated by thoracic nerves T8 to T18. Studies on spinal analgesic techniques have shown that analgesia is produced up to the thoracic region with epidural or subarachnoid morphine or methadone.[18]

The sacrococcygeal joint may be fused in some horses. An imaginary line joining the 2 hip joints crosses the midline of the sacrococcygeal joint. The spinous process of the first coccygeal bone and, caudally, the first intercoccygeal joint can be palpated in thinner horses. The first intercoccygeal joint is often the first moveable joint in the tail and can be seen and palpated when the tail is raised and lowered. It lies approximately 2.5 to 5 cm (1–2 inches) cranial to the origin of the tail hairs. This joint is at the level of the caudal skin folds that can be seen at each side of the tail when it is raised. Skin, variable amounts of fat, and connective tissue between the dorsal vertebral spinous processes and the interarcuate ligament (ligamentum flavum) overlie the epidural space. The aperture between the 2 coccygeal vertebral arches, the interarcual space, can be relatively small in horses compared with cattle, and sometimes difficult to locate with the needle. The epidural space at this level contains the nerves of the cauda equina, venous sinuses, and epidural fat. The perpendicular (90°) depth from the skin to the first intercoccygeal space is approximately 3.5 to 8 cm.[19] In 1 study in which the needle was angled 10 to 30° to the spinal cord, and the needle tip passed cranially to S5 (sacral vertebra 5), the distance measured from skin to epidural space was 8.5 ± 0.5 cm.[20] The anatomic site for segmental dorsolumbar epidural anesthesia is the T18-L1 space.[21] Difficulties with entering the space and catheter placement in horses have limited the clinical usefulness of this technique.[22]

Nociceptive information is transmitted to supraspinal structures via ascending tracts. Although the neurotransmitters located within the ascending tracts are not known, the activation of supraspinal areas is probably mediated by excitatory amino acids.[23–29] Collateral innervation in the ascending tracts is responsible for simultaneous activation of several brain regions when an ascending nociceptive stimulus is produced.[24] The activation of supraspinal sites is necessary for the perception of pain. The supraspinal sites that process nociceptive information receive several afferent inputs and send out numerous efferents. The activation of systems of descending inhibition has already been described.[29-39] Several studies have shown that multiple areas within the brain contribute to the system of descending inhibition.[28-39] Morphine and morphinelike agents activate systems of descending inhibition similar to endogenous encephalin.[29,36-39]

Painful stimuli are relayed to the spinal cord through A$\delta$ and C fibers. These first-order neurons synapse with secondary neurons in the spinal cord. Release of nociceptive neurotransmitters from these primary afferent fibers activates second-order dorsal horn neurons in the spinal cord. First-order neurons synapse in the dorsal horn of the spinal cord with several different populations of second-order neurons. Nociceptive-specific neurons transmit painful stimuli exclusively and wide dynamic range neurons transmit nonpainful signals. Second-order neurons ascend the spinal cord in multiple tracts relaying painful stimuli to the brain. The quantitatively most important spinothalamic tract ascends the spinal cord in the ventral white matter contralateral to the site of the stimulation.[25-32] The activation of these neurons results in spinal reflex responses as well as activation of ascending tracts, which transmit nociceptive information to supraspinal levels to complete the nociceptive pathway.[29-32] Substance P has been localized to small-diameter primary afferent fibers that terminate in the area of the substantia gelatinosa.[32-34] Other neuropeptides are released from the primary afferent neurons after nociceptive stimulation.[34] Different receptor systems have been localized to the dorsal horn of the spinal cord, and many of these receptor systems may function as specific modulators of nociceptive transmission. Modulation may occur either by inhibiting the release of neurotransmitters from primary afferent fibers or by inhibiting the activation of second-order dorsal horn neurons. Spinal modulation may either be intrinsic or descend from the supraspinal level.[23,29-34,40]

In horses caudal epidural anesthesia is used to desensitize the anus, rectum, perineum, vulva, vagina, urethra, and bladder. The goal is to produce surgical regional anesthesia without losing the motor function of the hind limbs. A combination of a local anesthetic drug with an alpha-2 adrenergic agonist or an opioid is the most popular option as this combination extends the period of action of the epidural anesthesia or analgesia in horses, humans, and small animals. Spinal analgesia and anesthesia has not been used as much in horses as in small animals and humans as an adjunct to general anesthesia. The epidural administration of opioids with or without local anesthetics is commonly performed in dogs and cats before surgery to reduce general anesthetic requirements as well as to provide intraoperative and postoperative pain control. The perioperative use of spinal analgesia in horses is likely to increase in the future as recent studies have shown that the administration of epidural or subarachnoid alpha-2 adrenergic agonists, phencyclidines, opioids, and low-dose local anesthetic produce intense antinociceptive effects.[17-22]

## OPIOID RECEPTORS AND SPINAL ANALGESIA

Opioid receptors such as $\mu$, $\delta$, and $\kappa$ are found in the dorsal horn of the spinal cord, presynaptically and postsynaptically on second-order neurons. Both $\mu$- and $\delta$-opioid agonists inhibit the evoked release of substance P in vivo and other neurotransmitters in vitro, suggesting that opioids inhibit multiple primary afferent neurotransmitters involved in pain transmission. Evidence for a postsynaptic and a presynaptic action of spinal opioids has been reported. Opioid agonists inhibited the firing of the second-order dorsal horn neurons. The intrathecal administration of opioid agonists inhibited the nociceptive behavior produced by intrathecal injection of substance P. These findings provide evidence of a postsynaptic mechanism of action.[29–36]

## ANALGESIC EFFECTS OF EPIDURAL OPIOIDS

Because there are opioid receptors in the substantia gelatinosa of the spinal cord these agents have been used to control acute and chronic pain producing effective and often prolonged analgesia.[36,37] Analgesia that follows epidural placement of opioids reflects diffusion of the drug across the dura mater to gain access to and activate opioid receptors in the spinal cord. Mu opioid receptor activation is primarily responsible for supraspinal and spinal analgesia. Activation of $mu_1$ receptor is speculated to produce analgesia and activation of $mu_2$ receptors is responsible for hypoventilation, bradycardia, and physical dependence.[1,38,39] There is evidence that analgesia results from a regional effect, although systemic absorption occurs and may be responsible for some of the analgesic effects of epidurally administered opioids.[2,3] It has been reported that highly lipophilic opioids such as fentanyl and its derivatives produce analgesia primarily by systemic absorption and there would be no advantage in injecting these agents epidurally.[2,3] Pharmacokinetic studies have found no correlation between analgesia and plasma concentration of opioids and analgesia is present with no morphine detectable in the plasma.[4,5]

There is a relationship between lipid solubility and the onset and duration of analgesia. Onset of analgesia is slower with morphine than with fentanyl, but the duration of analgesia is longer.[2] Epidural administration of equipotent doses in the cat resulted in duration of analgesia of 4 to 20 hours with morphine, 3 to 5 hours with meperidine, and 5 to 12 hours with lofentanil, demonstrating that more hydrophilic agents (morphine) produce a longer analgesic effect than more lipid-soluble opioids (lofentanil).[33] Opioids administered in the epidural space may be taken into epidural fat, undergo systemic absorption, or diffuse across the spinal meninges into the cerebrospinal fluid.[2,3] Doses of morphine of 2, 4, and 8 mg were more effective than 0.5 and 1 mg in humans.[4] In 1 study, 5 mg of epidural morphine was compared with 5 mg methadone and 1 mg hydromorphone, producing 18 hours of analgesic effect in contrast to 7 hours with methadone and 11 hours with hydromorphone. In another study, 4 opioids were compared for control of postoperative pain. Pain relief was longest with morphine, intermediate with methadone and meperidine, and shortest with fentanyl. Morphine also produced more effective analgesia than the other agents.[1–5,36–39] These results suggest that hydrophilic opioids are more effective and the analgesic effects last longer than more lipid-soluble agents.

## SPINAL OPIOIDS IN THE HORSE

Systemic administration of opioids in horses has been described as efficient to provide analgesia although central nervous system (CNS) excitation may occur, which precludes the routine use of these drugs.[41–45] In 1990 the first use of epidural morphine in horses was reported to treat severe somatic pain caused by trauma in the rear limb in a mare.[46] The investigators reported that intractable pain refractory to systemic analgesic administration was successfully controlled with epidural morphine. In 1994, a controlled study proved that 0.05 to 0.1 mg/kg epidural morphine produced segmentally distributed analgesia in horses characterized by sedation and no ataxia; with the higher dose producing a faster onset of analgesia, longer duration, cranial spread, and affecting several dermatomes in more horses than the lower dose. Dorsal nerve branches of the lumbosacral plexus were preferentially affected compared with ventral branches at the 2 doses of morphine given.[47] Recently the combination of morphine and the alpha-2 adrenoceptor agonist detomidine was given epidurally to horses in an amphotericin B–induced synovitis of the left tarsocrural joint model. The investigators concluded that there was a significant decrease in lameness scores after treatment with epidural morphine and detomidine suggesting that the combination produces profound hind-limb analgesia in horses.[48] In another experimentally controlled study, epidural morphine decreased the minimum alveolar concentration (MAC) of halothane in ponies when noxious stimulation was applied to the pelvic limbs but had no effect on MAC when the thoracic limb was stimulated. In the same study, epidural butorphanol produced no change in MAC.[49]

Neuraxial blocks such as spinal and epidural blocks with local anesthetics result in sympathetic block, sensory analgesia, and motor block. Despite these similarities, there are significant physiologic and pharmacologic differences. Spinal anesthesia requires a small mass or volume of drug, virtually devoid of systemic pharmacologic effect to produce profound, reproducible sensory analgesia. In contrast, epidural anesthesia necessitates use of a large mass or volume of local anesthetic that produces pharmacologically active systemic blood levels, which may be associated with side effects and complications.[2] Density is defined as the weight in grams of 1 mL of solution. Density is a major determinant of the distribution, duration, and degree of the clinical block achieved in spinal (subarachnoid) anesthesia with local anesthetics.[1]

Subarachnoidally administered local anesthetics and alpha-2 adrenergic agonists to obtain segmental analgesia in horses have been extensively described.[17,20,21,50–52] Subarachnoid administration of hyperbaric opioids was recently described in the horse.[18] Analgesia obtained after the subarachnoid administration of hyperbaric opioids in horses was considered intense when methadone or morphine was used. The advantage of using hyperbaric opioids subarachnoidally versus epidurally is that the intrathecal route is direct because there is no dura to be penetrated and the drug is deposited close to its site of action, the opioid receptors. Compared with the intrathecal route, epidural administration is complicated by pharmacokinetics of dura mater transfer, epidural fat deposition, and systemic absorption. Some suggestions for techniques and drugs or drug combinations are presented in **Table 1**.

To spinally administer anesthetic and analgesic in a horse, proper technique should be used to prevent trauma and contamination to the vertebral bones and surrounding soft tissue, as well as to the vessel around the vertebral canal, and to the spinal cord.

## EPIDURAL INJECTION AND CATHETERIZATION TECHNIQUE

For epidural injections in adult horses, an 18G 7.5-cm sterile spinal needle with stylet is placed in the first intercoccygeal space in standing horses held in stocks. A regular 20G 3.75-cm hypodermic needle has also been used (**Fig. 1**). The space is located by palpation while manipulating the tail in a dorsoventral direction. The skin over the region is clipped, and surgically prepared. After location of the first intercoccygeal vertebral space, the skin and subcutaneous tissue above the space are desensitized by administration of 3 mL of 2% lidocaine or 2% mepivacaine, using a 16-mm (5/8 inch) 25G needle. Before injection, correct placement of the needle in the epidural space is verified with a drop of sterile water or 0.9% saline in the hub of the needle, which is aspirated when the needle enters the epidural space (hanging drop technique), and negligible resistance to air injection. To ensure that a vein is not inadvertently penetrated, aspiration is performed before injection of the epidural agents. An adhesive clear plastic fenestrated dressing (Bioclusiv transparent dressing, Johnson & Johnson, Arlington, TX, USA) can be placed over the site to prevent contamination. In thick-skinned horses, making a small skin incision with a no. 15 scalpel blade or an 18G needle helps needle

**Table 1**
Drug regimens used for spinal (epidural/intratechal) anesthesia/analgesia and reported volumes and dosages

| Drug | Volume (mL) | Site of Injection | Duration of Effect (Hours) | Comments |
|---|---|---|---|---|
| **Single Drug** | | | | |
| Lidocaine 0.5%–2%[a] | 5–8 | $Co_1$-$Co_2$/L-S | 0.75–1.5 | Epidural/intratechal, rapid onset |
| Mepivacaine 2% | 5–8 | $Co_1$-$Co_2$/L-S | 1.5–3 | Epidural/intratechal, rapid onset |
| Ropivacaine 0.1%–0.5% | 5–10 | $Co_1$-$Co_2$/L-S | 3–8 | Epidural/intratechal, less ataxia |
| Bupivacaine 0.1%–0.5%[a] | 5–8 | $Co_1$-$Co_2$/L-S | 3–8 | Epidural/intratechal, more ataxia |
| Xylazine 0.17 mg/kg[a] | 10 | $Co_1$-$Co_2$/L-S | 1.0–1.5 | Epidural/intratechal, sedation/ataxia |
| Detomidine 20–40 μg/kg | 5–10 | $Co_1$-$Co_2$/L-S | 2–4 | Epidural/intratechal, sedation/ataxia |
| Medetomidine 2–5 μg/kg | 10–30 | $Co_1$-$Co_2$/L-S | 4–6 | Epidural/intratechal, sedation/ataxia |
| Morphine 0.05–0.2 mg/kg[a] | 10–30 | $Co_1$-$Co_2$/L-S | 3–8 | Epidural ONLY, useful for CRI mL/h) via epidural catheter |
| Methadone 0.1 mg/kg | 20 | $Co_1$-$Co_2$ | 3 | Epidural, similar to morphine |
| Tramadol 1 mg/kg | 10–30 | $Co_1$-$Co_2$ | 4–5 | Epidural, similar to morphine |
| Ketamine 0.5–2.0 mg/kg[b] | 10–30 | $Co_1$-$Co_2$ | 0.5–1.25 | Epidural, some ataxia |
| Hydromorphone | 10–30 | $Co_1$-$Co_2$ | 4–5 | Epidural, similar to morphine |
| **Drug Combinations (Balanced Regional Analgesia)** | | | | |
| Lidocaine 2 % + xylazine 0.17 mg/kg | 5–8 | $Co_1$-$Co_2$ | 4–6 | |
| Lidocaine 2 % + morphine 0.1–0.2 mg/kg | 5–8 | $Co_1$-$Co_2$ | 4–6 | |
| Bupivacaine 0.125 % + morphine 0.1–0.2 mg/kg | 10–30 | $Co_1$-$Co_2$/L-S | 8–>12 | Also useful for CRI (0.5–2 mL/h) via epidural catheter |
| Xylazine 0.17 mg/kg + morphine 0.1–0.2 mg/kg | 10–30 | $Co_1$-$Co_2$/L-S | ≥12 | |
| Detomidine 10–30 μg/kg + morphine 0.1–0.2 mg/kg | 5–10 | $Co_1$-$Co_2$/L-S | 24–48 6–8 | Epidural/intratechal moderate pain Epidural/intratechal severe pain |

Use lower doses/volumes of the less concentrated drugs for intratechal injection. Intratechal (subarachnoid) injection potentially increases the risk of infections and inflammation (spinal cord and meninges).

[a] Author's preference for most cases.
[b] May cause injury to the spinal cord.

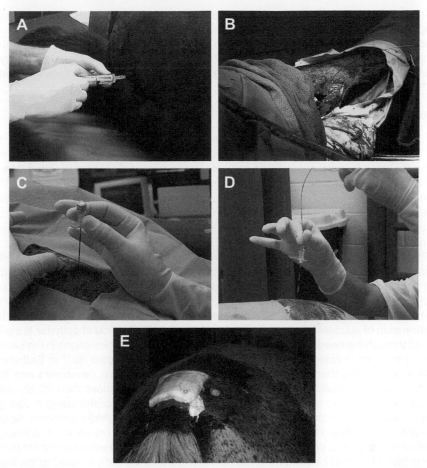

**Fig. 1.** (*A, B*) Single epidural hydromorphone injection as an adjuvant analgesic technique during hind limb wound debridement. (*C–E*) Step by step placement of a 20G radiopaque and closed-tip polyamide epidural catheter into the first intercoccygeal space using an 18G, 8.9-cm (3.5-inch) Tuohy Schliff epidural needle to enter the epidural space (Perifix epidural catheter set, B. Braun Medical, Inc, Bethlehem, PA 18017; product code CE-18T). See text and **Table 1** for more information.

insertion. The spinal needle is introduced perpendicular to the skin with the bevel directed cranially, and pushed down in the median plane until the ligamentum flavum is perforated. Often a popping sensation is detected when the ligament is crossed. If the needle is inserted down to the bony floor of the vertebral canal it should be withdrawn about 0.5 cm to avoid injection into the intervertebral disc.[17–22]

Alternatively, a spinal needle can be inserted at the first intercoccygeal space by placing the needle ventrocranially at an angle of 10 to 30° to the spinal canal. Studies have shown the tip of the needle in the epidural space is generally at the Co1 to S5 vertebral space. The length of needle used should be longer and either an 18G 8.75-cm or 15-cm spinal needle has been recommended.[17,22] This approach to the epidural space can be useful in horses that have developed fibrous tissue over the intercoccygeal space after previous epidural injection.

The amount and volume of anesthetic/analgesic injected depends on the type of drug, the size, and the conformation of the horse. If local anesthetic solution is used, usually less than 10 mL are injected in adult horses to avoid paralysis of the lumbosacral nerves to the hind limbs.[34,54] For single injections of analgesic solutions, total volumes of 10 to 20 mL can be used in adult horses to produce cranial migration of the solution for 6 to 10 vertebral spaces.

## EPIDURAL CATHETERIZATION

For placement of an epidural catheter, the horse should be sedated with 0.5 to 1.0 mg/kg xylazine, administered intravenously. Epidural catheterization is performed using the same technique described earlier for intercoccygeal epidural injection. Many manufacturers produce epidural trays or kits that are suitable for use in the horse.[17–22] An epidural Huber point (Tuohy) needle should be used instead of a spinal needle. This needle design has a slight curve on the end, which aids in directional placement of a catheter and is more blunted at the end making it less likely to sever the catheter than a regular spinal needle.[17,18,22]

The skin should be clipped, surgically prepared, and covered with surgical sterile drapes or clear plastic adhesive drape (Bioclusiv transparent dressing) to avoid catheter contamination. A disposable sterile or reusable 17G or 18G 7.5-cm epidural Tuohy needle (reusable technique needle, Tuohy, thin wall, Becton Dickinson and Company, Franklin Lakes, NJ, USA) is used to penetrate the epidural space. After confirmation of successful epidural puncture, a 19G or 20G epidural catheter is introduced through the needle up to the desired length. Generally for injections in the sacral area, 2 to 4 cm of catheter is advanced cranially from the needle tip.[18,22] Catheters have length marks that are helpful to know how far they have penetrated into the epidural space. Usually the catheter should be inserted no more than 30 cm into the epidural space to avoid catheter kink. The investigators prefer using a spring-wire reinforced catheter, 19G, 91.4 cm (Arrow epidural anesthesia catheter, Arrow International Reading, PA, USA) that facilitates introduction and rarely kinks, although a polyamide or plastic catheter can be used. After the needle is removed and the catheter is placed, it must be secured to the skin using a tape butterfly sutured to the skin. A bacterial filter may be attached to the catheter connector. The site of catheter penetration should be covered with iodine paste and the region covered with sterile dressings and gauze sponges and an adhesive clear plastic dressing. After each drug injection the catheter should be flushed with 0.9% saline. Any presence of blood in the catheter suggests vascular catheterization, which should be ruled out before catheter use. Epidural catheters elicit inflammatory reactions that may become uncomfortable and increase the risk of contamination. Catheter care includes daily inspection and flushing with 0.9% saline or heparinized (10 IU/mL) 0.9% saline and skin cleaning with antiseptic solution.[22]

## SUBARACHNOID INJECTION AND CATHETERIZATION TECHNIQUE

The correct region for subarachnoid catheter placement is determined by palpating the caudal borders of the tuber coxae, the cranial borders of the tuber sacrale, and the midline depression between the sixth lumbar and the second sacral vertebrae (**Fig. 2**). After sedation, the lumbar-sacral vertebral interspace is clipped and the skin surgically prepared and covered with a sterile transparent dressing (**Fig. 2C**). The skin, subcutaneous tissue, and muscle at the lumbar-sacral region, the supraspinous and interspinous ligments are locally anesthetized with 2% lidocaine. A 17G 17.78-cm epidural needle with stylet (**Fig. 2D**) is inserted perpendicularly along the median plane

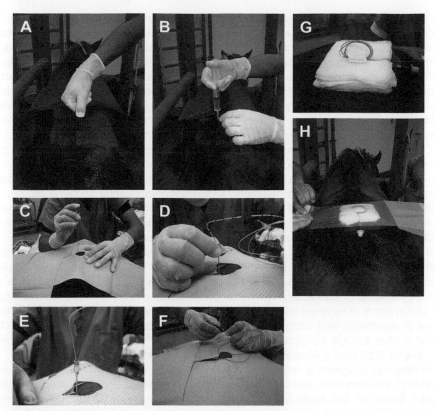

**Fig. 2.** (*A–H*) Step by step placement of a 19G radiopaque 91.4-cm polyurethane, spring-wire reinforced epidural and/or subarachnoid anesthesia catheter at the LS junction. See text and **Table 1** for more information.

of the lumbar-sacral intervertebral space, until the lumbar-sacral subarachnoid space is reached. To confirm successful subarachnoid needle placement, the needle stylet is removed, and a clear cerebrospinal fluid sample should be withdrawn into a syringe. After appropriate placement, the bevel of the needle is directed cephalad and 20 cm of a sterile 19G 91.4-cm polyurethane spring-wire reinforced epidural anesthesia catheter is advanced cranially through the needle into the subarachnoid space. The epidural needle is removed and the catheter is left in place, sutured to the skin and covered with sterile transparent dressing and sterile gauze sponges. After each drug injection the catheter should be flushed with 0.9% saline. Any presence of blood in the catheter suggests vascular catheterization, which should be ruled out before catheter use. As with epidural catheters, subarachnoid catheterization elicits inflammatory reactions that may become uncomfortable and increase the risk of contamination. The catheter is flushed with 1 mL of 10 IU/mL heparinized saline or with nonheparinized saline.[17–22]

## COMPLICATIONS OF SPINAL ANESTHESIA AND ANALGESIA IN HORSES

Systemic absorption of epidurally administered drugs, especially the alpha-2 agonists and lipid-soluble opioids, can lead to sedation (see **Table 1**). Sedation can be manifested as reduced response to external stimuli and by drooping of the head and lower lip. Standard doses of epidural anesthetics may occasionally cause severe ataxia and recumbency in horses (see **Table 1**). This is particularly true for combinations of local anesthetics and alpha-2 agonists or opioids (eg, lidocaine and xylazine).[12] The cause is not always apparent. Spread of local anesthetic too far cranially can paralyze the lumbosacral nerves in pregnant mares or obese horses in which the epidural space is narrowed. Additive effects of combinations of drugs administered epidurally, weakness of the horse from primary disease or exhaustion, or combinations of systemically administered sedatives with analgesic drugs administered epidurally may also contribute. Subarachnoid administration of mu opioids may elicit CNS excitation.

Cranial migration of subarachnoidally administered mu opioid analgesics such as morphine may lead to high concentrations of the opioid in supraspinal structures of the CNS similar to what is seen after intravenous administration, increasing the dopaminergic activity of the substantia nigra, a locomotion-activating center in the CNS, and sympathetic excitation. Recent studies have shown that adding 10% dextrose to mu opioids (morphine, methadone) to produce a hyperbaric solution does not elicit CNS excitation when the solution is administered subarachnoidally in horses.[18]

If motor impairment should occur, if the horse is still standing, it can be supported with a tail-tie until strength in the limbs is regained. If it becomes recumbent then general anesthesia may be necessary to continue surgery or to control the horse if it is very agitated or distressed. Clinical reports described recumbency in horses after caudal epidural anesthesia and lumbosacral epidural anesthesia.[48–54] Recovery after general anesthesia and completion of surgery in 1 horse took approximately 300 minutes after a single injection of 60 µg/kg detomidine[48] and 330 minutes in another horse after 0.22 mg/kg lidocaine with 0.17 mg/kg xylazine.[12]

Inadequate analgesia or anesthesia may occur as a result of improper technique, anatomic abnormalities, and fibrous adhesions from previous epidural injections can cause failure of the technique.[17] Segmental distribution of analgesia has been reported after epidural administration of morphine to horses, in which dorsal dermatomes innervated by lumbosacral nerves had superior analgesia to ventral dermatomes.[19] This would result in inadequate analgesia in ventral areas of the hind limb in some horses. Unilateral blockade with local anesthetics might be caused by the presence of congenital membranes in the epidural space, or adhesions.[17,22] Incorrect epidural catheter placement caused by ventral epidural placement or placement through an intervertebral foramen could also result in unilateral blockace.[17,22]

Neurotoxicity caused by damage to the nerves and spinal cord by epidural solutions is a controversial issue. Reports indicate that clinical doses of local anesthetics used in horses cause no neurotoxicity, whereas in rodents solutions containing the antioxidant sodium bisulphate have produced neuronal damage.[15,17–22,32] The pH of solutions is another possible cause of neuronal injury, although local anesthetics are only mildly acidic.[2] Solutions that contain no preservatives should be used when possible. Large volumes of epidural solutions may cause pain in the spinal canal of horses as a result of compression of sacral and lumbar nerves.[17] Large volumes of subarachnoid solutions may cause pain from spinal cord compression and reflex vertebral venodilation.[2] One study showed no histologic changes in the spinal cord of ponies after administration lidocaine and xylazine epidural.[12]

Sweating is seen in the area affected by lidocaine or xylazine injection.[12] Perineal edema has been observed after xylazine injection. Edematous skin wheals in the perineal area have been seen in some horses after morphine injection, and may be associated with local histamine release.[19] Cardiovascular effects such as bradycardia and second-degree atrioventricular block have occurred after xylazine or detomidine injections.[12,48]

## CLINICAL APPLICATIONS OF SPINAL ANALGESICS

The clinical application of spinal analgesics in horses is recommended for acute and chronic pain control of the rear limbs, perineum, tail, and abdominal wall. Time to effect is influenced by the number of molecules retained in the cerebrospinal fluid and spinal tissue, and by the dissociation kinetics of the drug.[2] Thus, there are differences in onset, spread, and duration that can vary with each drug. Most acute and chronic painful situations involve tissue damage and probably benefit from systemic treatment with concurrent nonsteroidal antiinflammatory drugs.

Segmental analgesia has been reported after epidural morphine administration in horses, which might result in patchy distribution of analgesia in the perineal and lumbosacral areas.[18,19,47] Also, analgesic effects of morphine and hydromorphone, given in the first intercoccygeal space of horses, has been shown to spread cranially as far as the midthoracic region and did not affect the fore limb.[16,53]

Epidural morphine, hydromorphone, and tramadol have been shown to have analgesic effects in horses when used alone. Epidural morphine produces profound analgesia although the long onset of action precludes its use in acute cases without combining it with faster-acting epidural analgesics such as alpha-2 agonists or fentanyl (see **Table 1**). Tramadol has also been combined with fentanyl in horses in severe intractable pain. These combinations usually produce profound analgesic effects that last for 12 to 24 hours.[19] Placement of an epidural catheter allows long-duration pain control in horses.

Subarachnoid hyperbaric morphine and methadone have been shown to produce fast-acting intense analgesic effects. This technique can be recommended for acute pain control because of the faster onset of action compared with epidural administration. Placing a subarachnoid catheter is recommended for chronic pain control when hyperbaric subarachnoid opioids are the treatment of choice. A subarachnoid catheter allows for repeat administration without the hazards of multiple punctures. Care should be taken to prevent contamination of the spinal meninges and the spinal cord. A subarachnoid catheter can be kept in place for several days as long as no signs of infection or spinal cord compression are observed.

For standing surgeries, the lack of motor impairment and profound analgesia produced by epidural morphine, hydromorphone, methadone, and tramadol or subarachnoid hyperbaric morphine and methadone, suggest that these drugs may be combined with low doses of local anesthetics such as lidocaine, mepivacaine, or bupivacaine to produce long-lasting surgical anesthesia/analgesia and prolonged postoperative pain control without ataxia or recumbency (see **Table 1**). Surgical procedures in the perineal and sacral areas could be done using this anesthetic/analgesic technique. Laparoscopic surgery involving the urogenital tract could also be done with an opioid/local anesthetic combination.

## REFERENCES

1. Atweh SF, Kuhar MJ. Autoradiographic localization of opiate receptors in rat brain, I. Spinal cord and lower medulla. Brain Res 1977;124:53–67.
2. Morgan M. The rational use of intrathecal and extradural opioids. Br J Anaesth 1989;63:165–88.
3. Cousins MJ, Mather LE. Intrathecal and epidural administration of opioids. Anesthesiology 1984;61:276–310.
4. Coda BA, Brown MC, Risler L, et al. Equivalent analgesia and side effects during epidural and pharmacokinetically tailored intravenous infusion with matching plasma alfentanil concentration. Anesthesiology 1999;90:98–108.

5. Weddel SJ, Ritter RR. Serum levels following epidural administration of morphine and correlation with relief of postsurgical pain. Anesthesiology 1981;54:210–4.

6. Chopin JB, Wright JD. Complications after the use of a combination of lignocaine and xylazine for epidural anaesthesia in a mare. Aust Vet J 1995;72:354–5.

7. Berti M, Casati A, Fanelli G, et al. 0.2% ropivacaine with or without fentanyl for patient-controlled epidural analgesia after major abdominal surgery: a double-blind study. J Clin Anesth 2000;12:292–7.

8. Bertini L, Mancini S, Di Benedetto P, et al. Postoperative analgesia by combined continuous infusion and patient-controlled epidural analgesia (PCEA) following hip replacement: ropivacaine versus bupivacaine. Acta Anaesthesiol Scand 2001;45:782–5.

9. Badner NH, Reid D, Sullivan P, et al. Continuous epidural infusion of ropivacaine for the prevention of postoperative pain after major orthopaedic surgery: a dose-finding study. Can J Anaesth 1996;43:17–22.

10. Turner G, Blake D, Buckland M, et al. Continuous extradural infusion of ropivacaine for prevention of postoperative pain after major orthopaedic surgery. Br J Anaesth 1996;76:606–10.

11. Tucker GT. Pharmacokinetics of local anaesthetics. Br J Anaesth 1986;58:717–29.

12. Scheling CG, Klein LV. Comparison of carbonate lidocaine and lidocaine hydrochloride for caudal epidural anesthesia in horses. Am J Vet Res 1985;46:1375–7.

13. Grubb TL, Riebold TW, Huber MJ. Comparison of lidocaine, xylazine, and xylazine/lidocaine for caudal epidural analgesia in horses. J Am Vet Med Assoc 1992;20:1187–90.

14. Hendrickson DA, Southwood LL, Lopez MJ, et al. Cranial migration of different volumes of new methylene blue after caudal epidural injection in the horse. Equine Pract 1998;20:12–4.

15. Martin CA, Kerr CL, Pearce SG, et al. Outcome of epidural catheterization for delivery of analgesics in horses: 43 cases (1998–2001). J Am Vet Med Assoc 2003;222(10):1394–8.

16. Natalini CC, Linardi RL. Analgesic effects of epidural administration of hydromorphone in horses. Am J Vet Res 2006;67(1):11–5.

17. Skarda RT. Local and regional anesthetic and analgesic techniques: horses. In: Thurmon JC, Tranquilli WJ, Benson GJ, editors. Lumb and Jones' veterinary anesthesia. 3rd edition. Baltimore (MD): Williams & Wilkins; 1996. p. 448–78.

18. Natalini CC, Linardi RL. Analgesic effects of subarachnoidally administered hyperbaric opioids in horses. Am J Vet Res 2006;67:941–6.

19. Robinson EP, Natalini CC. Epidural anesthesia and analgesia in horses. Vet Clin North Am Equine Pract 2002;18:61–82.

20. Skarda RT, Muir WW. Comparison of antinociceptive, cardiovascular, and respiratory effects, head ptosis, and position of pelvic limbs in mares after caudal epidural administration of xylazine and detomidine hydrochloride solution. Am J Vet Res 1996;57:1338–45.

21. Skarda RT, Muir WW. Continuous caudal epidural and subarachnoid anesthesia in mares: a comparative study. Am J Vet Res 1983;44:2290–8.

22. Skarda RT, Muir WW. Local anesthetic techniques in horses. In: Muir WW, Hubbell JAE, editors. Equine anesthesia: monitoring and emergency therapy. St. Louis (MO): Mosby; 1991. p. 199–246.

23. Jones SL. Anatomy of pain. In: Sinatra RS, Hord AH, Ginsberg B, et al, editors. Acute pain: mechanisms & management. St. Louis (MO): Mosby-Year Book; 1992. p. 8–28.
24. Jensen TS, Yaksh TL. The antinociceptive activity of excitatory amino acids in the rat brainstem: an anatomical and pharmacological analysis. Brain Res 1992;569: 255–67.
25. Harmann PA, Carlton SM, Willis WD. Collaterals of spinothalamic tract cells to the periaqueductal gray: a fluorescence double-labeling study in the rat. Brain Res 1988;441:87–97.
26. Mayer DJ, Price DD. Central nervous system mechanism of analgesia. Pain 1976; 2:379–404.
27. Yaksh TL, Rudy TA. Narcotic analgesics: CNS sites and mechanisms of action as revealed by intracerebral injection techniques. Pain 1978;4:299–359.
28. Kitchell RL. Problems in defining pain and peripheral mechanisms of pain. J Am Vet Med Assoc 1987;191:1195–9.
29. Beitz AJ. Anatomic and chemical organization of descending pain modulation systems. In: Short CE, van Poznak A, editors. Animal pain. New York: Churchill Livingstone; 1992. p. 31–62.
30. Aimone LD. Neurochemistry and modulation of pain. In: Sinatra RS, Hord AH, Ginsberg B, et al, editors. Acute pain: mechanisms & management. St. Louis (MO): Mosby-Year Book; 1992. p. 29–43.
31. Hokfelt T, Kellerth JO, Nilsson G, et al. Experimental immunohistochemical studies on the localization and distribution of substance P in cat primary sensory neurons. Brain Res 1975;100:235–52.
32. Tuchscherer MM, Seybold VS. Immunohistochemical studies of substance P, cholecystokinin-octapeptide, and somatostatin dorsal root ganglia of the rat. Neuroscience 1985;14:593–605.
33. Go VLW, Yaksh TL. Release of substance P from the cat spinal cord. J Physiol 1987;391:141–67.
34. Duggan AW, Morton CR, Zhao ZG, et al. Noxious heating of the skin releases immunoreactive substance P in the substantia gelatinosa of the cat: a study with antibody microprobes. Brain Res 1987;403:345–9.
35. Hamon M, Bourgoin S, LeBars D, et al. In vivo and in vitro release of central neurotransmitters in relation to pain and analgesia. Brain Res 1988;77:431–44.
36. Hutchinson WD, Morton CR, Terenius L, et al. In vivo release in the spinal cord of the cat. Brain Res 1990;532:299–306.
37. Tsou K, Jang CS. Studies on the site of analgesic action of morphine by intracerebral microinjection. Sci Sin 1964;13:1099–109.
38. Fields HL, Basbaum AI. Brainstem control of spinal pain transmission neurons. Annu Rev Physiol 1978;40:217–48.
39. Jensen TS, Yaksh TL. Comparison of the antinociceptive action of mu and delta opioid receptor ligands in the periaqueductal gray matter, medial, and paramedical ventral medulla in the rat as studied by the microinjection technique. Brain Res 1986;372:301–12.
40. Doherty TJ, Geiser DR, Rohrbach BW. Effects of high volume epidural morphine, ketamine and butorphanol on halothane minimum alveolar concentration in ponies. Equine Vet J 1997;29:370–3.
41. Martin R, Salbaing J, Blaise G, et al. Epidural morphine for postoperative pain relief. A dose-response curve. Anesthesiology 1982;56:423–6.
42. Combie J, Dougherty J, Nugent CE, et al. The pharmacology of narcotic analgesics in the horse. IV dose and time response relationships for behavioral

responses to morphine, meperidine, pentazocine, anileridine, methadone, and hydromorphone. J Equine Med Surg 1979;3:377–85.

43. Karmeling SG, DeQuick DJ, Wechman TJ, et al. Dose-related effects of fentanyl on autonomic and behavioral responses in performance horses. Gen Pharmacol 1985;16:253–8.

44. Pascoe PJ, Taylor PM. Effects of dopamine antagonists on alfentanil-induced locomotor activity in horses. Vet Anaesth Analg 2003;30:165–71.

45. Johnson CB, Taylor PM. Effects of alfentanil on the equine electroencephalogram during anesthesia with halothane in oxygen. Res Vet Sci 1997;62:159–63.

46. Tobin T, editor. Drugs and the performance horse. Springfield (IL): Charles C Thomas; 1981.

47. Valverde A, Little CB, Dyson DH. Use of epidural morphine to relieve pain in a horse. Can Vet J 1990;31:211–2.

48. Robinson EP. Preferential dermatomal analgesic effects of epidurally administered morphine in horses. In: Bryden DE, editor. Proceedings, Animal pain, its control. Adelaide and Sydney (Australia): University of Sydney; 1994. p. 417–21.

49. Sysel AM, Pleasant SR, Jacobson JD. Efficacy of an epidural combination of morphine and detomidine in alleviating experimentally induced hindlimb lameness in horses. Vet Surg 1996;25:511–8.

50. Bonica JJ. Pain research and therapy: history, current status, and future goals. In: Short CE, van Poznak A, editors. Animal pain. New York: Churchill Livingstone; 1992. p. 1–30.

51. Skarda RT, Muir WW. Segmental thoracolumbar spinal (subarachnoid) analgesia in conscious horses. Am J Vet Res 1982;34:2121–8.

52. Skarda RT, Muir WW. Caudal analgesia induced by epidural or subarachnoid administration of detomidine hydrochloride solution in mares. Am J Vet Res 1994;55:670–80.

53. Skarda RT, Muir WW. Analgesic, hemodynamic and respiratory effects of caudal epidurally administered ropivacaine hydrochloride solution in mares. Vet Anaesth Analg 2001;28:61–74.

54. Natalini CC, Robinson EP. Evaluation of the analgesic effects of epidurally administered morphine, alfentanil, butorphanol, tramadol, and U50488H in horses. Am J Vet Res 2000;61:1579–86.

# NMDA Receptor Antagonists and Pain: Ketamine

William W. Muir, DVM, PhD

## KEYWORDS

• NMDA receptors • Hypersensitivity • Allodynia • Drug infusion

The transmission and perception of pain-inducing stimuli is dependent on neurotransmitters (eg, glutamate, aspartate) that mediate communication between neurons by binding to 4 distinct types (N-methyl-D-aspartate [NMDA]; α-hydroxy-5-methyl-4-isoxasolepropionic acid [AMPA]; kainite [KA]; metabotropic) of amino acid receptors. These receptors are named for the 4 synthetic activators (agonists) that bind to them. NMDA is a synthetic chemical binding molecule (ligand) that selectively binds to the "slow response" glutamate NMDA receptor (NMDAR). NMDA does bind not to other glutamate receptors (AMPA, KA, metabotropic). NMDARs are important for normal brain function and play a central role in learning, memory, and the development of central nervous system (CNS) hyperactive states.[1] NMDAR activation is essential for the survival of many types of neurons with to little or to much stimulation resulting in cell death. Blockade of NMDARs can enhance analgesia, but when exaggerated can result in memory impairment, excitatory behaviors, dementia, ataxia, and motor incoordination. Although predominantly located in the CNS, NMDARs have been identified in peripheral somatic and visceral sites.[2] Continuous input from polymodal C nociceptive afferent nerve fibers is known to produce progressive increases in the responsiveness ("wind-up") of neurons in the dorsal horn of the spinal cord by activating NMDARs, generating calcium ($Ca^{2+}$) transients that fuel persistent activity after the afferent stimulation has ended ("second" pain). The increase in responsiveness is a form of CNS plasticity that is mediated by NMDA receptors and is responsible for dorsal horn hyperexcitability.[3] Conversely, excessive NMDAR inhibition can kill neurons by reducing the activity of inhibitory interneurons that depend on NMDARs for their activation. The end result of excessive NMDAR blockade is disinhibition of excitatory neurons, pathologically high levels of NMDAR activity, and cell death.

## NMDA RECEPTORS

NMDARs are formed by various combinations of 3 distinct subunits: NR1, NR2, and NR3. The NR1 subunit is essential for the formation of the NMDA ion channel and is

Equine Anesthesia and Analgesia Consulting Services, 338 West 7th Avenue, Columbus, OH 43201, USA
E-mail address: bill.muir@amcny.org

Vet Clin Equine 26 (2010) 565–578
doi:10.1016/j.cveq.2010.07.009
0749-0739/10/$ – see front matter © 2010 Elsevier Inc. All rights reserved.

the major subunit responsible for NMDAR function.[4] There are multiple variants of the NR1 (8 variants) subunit and isoforms of the NR2 (4 isoforms) subunit, but both subunits are required for the formation of functional NMDAR channels.[5] These variants (NR1/NR2 variants) are differentially distributed across multiple cell types. The NR3 subunit is believed to have an inhibitory effect on receptor activity. Differences in the NR2 subunit (2A, 2B, 2C, 2D) in the NR1/NR2 NMDAR channels determine their electrophysiologic properties, sensitivity to magnesium block, and susceptibility and affinity for both agonist and antagonist drugs.[6] NMDARs are ionotropic because they regulate a specific type of cell membrane bound ion channel that is both ligand-gated and voltage-dependent. Normally this ion channel requires coactivation by 2 neurotransmitters, glutamate and glycine, and is specific for but nonselective to sodium and calcium. Ion channel block by extracellular magnesium ($Mg^{2+}$) ions regulates the flow of sodium ($Na^+$) ions and small amounts of calcium ($Ca^{2+}$) ions into the cell, and $K^+$ out of the cell.[7] These activities highlight NMDARs' unique properties: (1) voltage-dependent channel block by endogenous magnesium ($Mg^{2+}$); and (2) high calcium permeability. Intense and sustained activation of NMDARs removes the voltage-dependent $Mg^{2+}$ block facilitating $Ca^{2+}$ influx into the cell.[8] Calcium influx through NMDARs enhances $Ca^{2+}$-sensitive intracellular signaling cascades, which play a critical role in cell membrane excitability, synaptic efficacy, and the recruitment of subliminal inputs. Together these changes contribute to the clinical manifestations of primary hyperalgesia, hypersensitivity in uninjured sites (secondary hyperalgesia), and allodynia. These changes are also responsible for spontaneous pain, and are implicated in the pathogenesis of chronic pain states (**Fig. 1**).

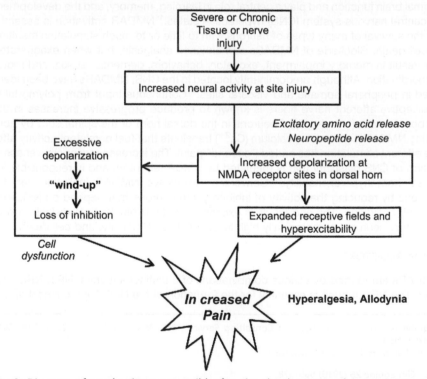

**Fig. 1.** Diagram of mechanisms responsible for the development of hyperalgesia and allodynia.

Of importance, NR1 subunits in the spinal cord are upregulated by nociceptive input, which leads to increased expression of cyclooxygenase-2 (COX-2).[9] Furthermore, NR1 subunits are colocalized with alpha ($\alpha$-2A, $\alpha$-2C) adrenoceptors, and their expression could be one of the mechanisms underlying alpha-2 adrenoceptor analgesia.[10] Experimental studies have also demonstrated that the administration of alpha-2 agonists (eg, clonidine) markedly inhibits the expression, activity, and associated nociceptive behavior associated with NMDAR activation.[10] Furthermore, the combination of NMDA antagonists with opioid agonists or gabapentin significantly increases analgesic activity at spinal, supraspinal, and peripheral levels in addition to decreasing the development of opioid-associated side effects (tolerance, dependence, hypersensitivity).[11,12] Taken together, these studies imply that the administration of nonsteroidal anti-inflammatory drugs (NSAIDs), alpha-2 adrenoceptor agonists, opioids, or gabapentin in conjunction with NMDA antagonists should provide increased therapeutic efficacy for the treatment of severe or chronic pain. Diverse chemicals belonging to various drug families have demonstrated NMDAR antagonistic effects (**Box 1**). To date few, if any, have demonstrated high selectivity for NMDARs. Nevertheless, ketamine has been shown to produce antihyperalgesic effects produced by incision and tissue or nerve damage, and has become popular in equine practice as an anesthetic and more recently as an analgesic for standing surgical procedures and the treatment of laminitis.[13,14] This review focuses on the development of ketamine as an anesthetic and analgesic in horses.

## KETAMINE

Ketamine and xylazine are members of 2 independent families of drugs, used for immobilization, anesthesia, and analgesia in horses. Ketamine is considered a "dissociative anesthetic" providing adequate dosages are administered, and xylazine is a potent sedative, muscle relaxant, and analgesic. Both drugs were admitted to the United States veterinary market in the early 1970s, and were greeted with concern and skepticism due to their "unpredictability" and the frequency of untoward side effects. Both ketamine and xylazine are routine components of the majority of injectable and inhalant anesthetic protocols used in horses. Xylazine's clinical use in horses and cattle was initially reported in 1969.[15] Ketamine was approved for both human and veterinary use in 1970 and, although initially only approved for use in cats, was determined to

| Box 1 |
| --- |
| **Drugs demonstrating NMDAR antagonist effects** |
| Amantadine |
| Memantine |
| Ketamine |
| Phencyclidine |
| Tiletamine |
| Dextromethorphan |
| Dextrorphan |
| Methadone |
| Ethanol |
| Nitrous oxide |

be a suitable short-term anesthetic in horses by several investigators.[16,17] It is important to realize that both drugs (xylazine and ketamine) were approved for veterinary clinical use before their mechanisms of action were understood or appreciated. Suffice it to say, however, that both drugs were considered "safe and effective" providing dosage guidelines were followed and not exceeded. Today xylazine is considered to be an alpha-2 adrenoceptor agonist and is being replaced by newer more selective and more potent alpha-2 adrenoceptor agonists (detomidine, medetomidine, dexmedetomidine, romifidine). Ketamine is considered to be a noncompetitive NMDAR antagonist, although effects on opioids, muscarinic receeptors, and voltage-sensitive calcium channels have been reported.[18] Furthermore, ketamine activates the monoaminergic descending inhibitory system, which may play a key role in ketamine's analgesic effect because blockade of inhibitory mechanisms (disinhibition) facilitates NMDA receptor and associated nociceptive processes.[19,20] Ketamine has evolved to become the most frequently used anesthetic drug in equine veterinary practice, either in conjunction with an alpha-2 adrenoceptor agonist or a centrally acting muscle relaxant (diazepam, midazolam, guaifenesin). Of note, alpha-2 adrenoceptor agonists have recently been demonstrated to significantly reduce an important subunit of the NMDAR that is associated with the development of pain, suggesting that the coadministration of alpha-2 agonists and NMDA antagonists should produce supra-additive (synergistic) effects.[10] It is also important to note that current dosage recommendations for alpha-2 agonists that produce analgesia in the horse are far less than those originally suggested to produce sedation or anesthesia with ketamine.[21]

## Ketamine Pharmacokinetics

Commercial ketamine ([±2-o-chlorophenyl-2(methylamino)cyclohexanone]) is a phenylpiperidine derivative and a racemic mixture of 2 enantiomers, (R)-and (S)-ketamine. It is a dissociative anesthetic, analgesic, and anti-inflammatory drug, and one of a limited number of noncompetitive of NMDAR antagonists (see **Box 1**).[22] The 2 enantiomers (S)- and (R)-ketamine have different binding affinities and potencies: (S)-Ketamine has approximately 4 times greater affinity for the active site of the NMDA receptor.[13] The (S)-enantiomer is less likely to produce psychomimetic and cataleptic side effects including hallucinations, excessive or spontaneous muscle rigidity, involuntary limb movements, excitation, and ataxia.[23] The analgesic and anesthetic potency of (S)-ketamine is 2 to 3 times greater than that of (R)-ketamine. It is conjectured that (R)-ketamine is a sigma opioid agonist, and may be responsible for lowering the seizure threshold observed after ketamine administration.[13] Because (S)-ketamine has greater anesthetic and analgesic effects and fewer side effects than (R)-ketamine, the pure (S)-enantiomer is preferred to the racemic mixture, and is being promoted for clinical use in horses in Europe.[23–26]

Ketamine is metabolized in the liver by the hepatic cytochrome P450 (CYP450) enzyme system.[27,28] Metabolism is enantioselective such that the more pharmacologically active (S)-ketamine is eliminated faster than (R)-ketamine or the racemic mixture.[29,30] Ketamine is initially N-demethylated to (S)- or (R)-norketamine and subsequently hydroxylated to hydroxynorketamine, which is conjugated to water-soluble glucuronide derivatives that are excreted by the kidneys.[31] Of importance is that both (S)- and (R)-norketamine are believed to retain approximately 10% of the anesthetic, analgesic, and anti-inflammatory effects of the parent compound. Current evidence suggests that (R)-ketamine interferes with (S)-ketamine hydroxylation, resulting in faster elimination times and offset of clinical effects when (S)-ketamine is administered alone as compared with when administered as a racemic mixture.[32] Early studies in horses suggested that the elimination half-life of racemic ketamine was approximately 1 hour and that ketamines total body clearance exceeded hepatic blood flow, suggesting that extrahepatic mechanisms in the kidney, lung, or gut participated in ketamine's elimination from the plasma.[33,34] More recent studies investigating the disposition of ketamine enantiomers suggest that ketamine pharmacokinetics are "context sensitive" and differ markedly depending on the dose, mode (bolus vs infusion), and particularly with the duration of administration.[29,35] The range of elimination half-lives for (S)-ketamine (0.3 mg/kg loading dose; 10 µg/kg/min constant rate infusion [CRI]) and S- and (R)-ketamine administered as a racemic mixture (0.6 mg/kg loading dose; 20 µg/kg/min), for example, range from 2.8 to 15.7 minutes and 2.7 to 42.7 minutes, respectively.[29] These values are far less than reported in earlier studies where 2.2 mg/kg racemic ketamine was administered as an intravenous (IV) bolus dose to produce anesthesia.[33,34] Several investigators have suggested that ketamine undergoes "first-pass" metabolism in the lung and liver and that this mechanism explains why arterial plasma concentrations are up to 50% less when compared with venous blood samples.[27,28] In summary, the pharmacokinetic improvements of (S)-ketamine as compared with racemic ketamine, particularly its faster elimination from the plasma, are characterized by a reduced drug load, better control of anesthesia, and improved recovery from anesthesia.[26]

### Clinical Use of Ketmamine in Horses

Ketamine's use as a short-term anesthetic in horses was first described in 1977.[16] Xylazine (1.1 mg/kg, IV) was administered before or simultaneously with ketamine hydrochloride (2.2–6.6 mg/kg, IV). The 2.2 mg/kg IV dose proved to be ideal in providing excellent anesthesia, which was considered to be light anesthesia, and excellent recovery in all horses.[16] Doses of ketamine greater than 4.4 mg/kg, IV (data not presented) were accompanied by an increasing frequency of muscular tremor and rigidity, mydriasis, oculogyric movements, sweating, hypertension, tachycardia, and increased rectal temperature during recovery from anesthesia. Investigators noted that the combination of xylazine and ketamine produced good to excellent short-term (5–10 minutes) anesthesia with stable cardiorespiratory function, provided that xylazine produced good sedation and excessive bolus dosages of ketamine were not administered.[16] The clinical benefits of the xylazine-ketamine drug combination for field anesthesia were subsequently confirmed by several investigators within the next several years.[17,36] Subsequently a clinical trial confirmed that horses that responded poorly to xylazine or did not become sedate either because of inadequate dosing or insufficient

| Table 1 | | |
|---------|---|---|
| **Clinical dosages and use of ketamine in horses** | | |
| **Ketamine: Clinical Uses and Dosages** | | |
| **Route of Administration** | **Clinical Use** | **Dose** |
| Intravenous | Anesthesia | Diazepam, 0.1 mg/kg; |
| Bolus | Standing Analgesia | 2.0–2.2 mg/kg |
| | | 0.3–0.5 mg/kg |
| Infusion (CRI) | Anesthetic Adjunct | 0.5–3.0 mg/kg/h |
| | Standing Analgesia | 0.5–1.5 mg/kg/h |
| Epidural (Note: Not recommended due to tissue toxic effects) | Regional Analgesia | 0.5–2.0 mg/kg |
| Local (neuraxial) block | Local Analgesia | 50–150 mg of a 2 or 3% solution |
| Intraarticular | Articular Analgesia | 0.5 mg/kg |

time (simultaneous administration) failed to become anesthetized.[37] In addition, the benefits of adding diazepam for added muscle relaxation, coadministering reduced (approximately one-half the initial doses) doses of xylazine-ketamine or infusion of a xylazine (0.5 mg/mL)-guaifenesine (50 mg/mL)-ketamine (1.0 mg/mL), 2.75 mL/kg/ h, drug combination to prolong anesthesia were demonstrated (**Table 1**).[38,39] Collectively these studies set the stage for a myriad of drug combination studies wherein ketamine or a closely related congener, tiletamine, combined with zolazepam (Telazol) were administered with various alpha-2 agonists (detomidine, medetomidine, romifidine) to produce or maintain short-term anesthesia.[21,40–43] One study examined the cardiorespiratory and anesthetic effects of a tiletamine/zolazepam-ketamine-detomidine (TZKD) combination in horses.[44] These studies produced directionally similar but more significant changes in cardiorespiratory, acid-base, and blood chemical values compared with xylazine-ketamine drug combination, and generally prolonged the duration of anesthesia but did not improve the quality of recovery from anesthesia, especially when TZKD was administered.[45] Other studies conducted in preconditioned exercising horses administered a combination of xylazine hydrochloride (2.2 mg/kg body weight) and acepromazine maleate (0.04 mg/kg), IV evaluated 4 IV anesthetic regimens: ketamine hydrochloride (2.2 mg/kg); ketamine (2.2 mg/kg) and diazepam (0.1 mg/kg); tiletamine hydrochloride-zolazepam hydrochloride (1 mg/kg); and guaifenesin (50 mg/kg) and thiopental sodium (5 mg/kg) 5 minutes after excersise.[46] These studies demonstrated that the time to lateral recumbency was significantly longer and the quality of recovery was significantly poorer after guaifenesin-thiopental administration than after ketamine-diazepam or tiletamine-zolazepam administration.[46] Furthermore, arterial blood pressure after guaifenesin-thiopental administration was significantly lower than for the ketamine regimens.

Studies originally conducted in halothane-anesthetized horses determined ketamine's ability to reduce inahalant anesthetic requirements.[47] Steady-state plasma concentrations of 0.5, 1.0, 2.0, 4.0, and 8.0 µg/mL were produced in 8 horses by administering IV loading doses and a constant infusion of ketamine. The minimal alveolar concentration (MAC; concentration at which half the horses moved in response to an electrical stimulus) of halothane and plasma ketamine concentration were determined after steady-state concentrations of each ketamine infusion had been reached. Plasma ketamine concentrations greater than 1.0 µg/mL decreased halothane MAC. The MAC reduction was directly related to the square root of the plasma ketamine concentration, reaching a maximum of 37% at a plasma ketamine concentration of $10.8 \pm 2.7$ µg/mL. Heart rate, mean arterial blood pressure, and the rate of increase of right ventricular pressure did not change during the increases in plasma ketamine concentration. Cardiac output increased significantly during ketamine infusions and halothane MAC reduction. These studies were based on an earlier report investigating the pharmacokinetics of IV ketamine in horses, which demonstrated that plasma ketamine concentrations declined biexponentially with a rapid initial distribution phase ($t_{1/2}$: 2.5–3 minutes) followed by a slower elimination phase ($t_{1/2}$: 42–66 minutes).[33,34] Both of these earlier studies suggested that plasma ketamine concentrations of greater than 1.0 µg/mL are required to produce and maintain anesthesia, and provided the background for current experimental and clinical investigations wherein ketamine or various drug combinations containing ketamine have been developed to produce total intravenous anesthetic (TIVA) or as adjunct to inhalant anesthesia.[21,48–53] Recent studies, for example, have compared the anesthetic and cardiorespiratory effects of total IV anesthesia with propofol (P-TIVA) or a ketamine-medetomidine-propofol combination (KMP-TIVA) in horses.[52] The horses received medetomidine (0.005 mg/kg, IV) and anesthesia was induced with midazolam (0.04 mg/kg, IV) and ketamine (2.5 mg/kg, IV). All horses received a loading dose of propofol (0.5 mg/kg, IV), and 6 horses administered P-TIVA (propofol infusion) and 6 horses KMP-TIVA (ketamine [1 mg/kg/h] and medetomidine [0.00125 mg/kg/h]) infusion; the rate of propofol infusion was adjusted to maintain anesthesia.[52] This study concluded that KMP-TIVA and P-TIVA provided clinically acceptable anesthesia and that the infusion of ketamine-medetomidine provided an anesthetic sparing effect on propofol requirements, thereby reducing the potential for the development of cardiorespiratory depression. Similarly, the infusion of guaifenesin, ketamine, and medetomidine in combination with inhalation of sevoflurane versus inhalation of sevoflurane alone and midazolam, ketamine, and medetomidine have been determined in horses.[50,53] Horses were premedicated with xylazine and anesthetized with diazepam and ketamine. Anesthesia was maintained by infusion of guaifenesin, ketamine, and medetomidine and inhalation of sevoflurane (20 horses), or by inhalation of sevoflurane (20 horses).[50] The delivered concentration of sevoflurane was significantly lower, and the quality of transition to inhalation anesthesia and of anesthetic maintenance were significantly better, in horses administered guaifenesin-ketamine-medetomidine infusion than in horses administered sevoflurane alone. Horses that received the guaifenesin-ketamine-medetomidine infusion had better quality transition and maintenance phases of anesthesia, better hemodynamic values, and required fewer attempts to stand after the completion of anesthesia as compared with inhalation of sevoflurane alone.[50] These studies further emphasized the safety and clinical utility of ketamine infusions during TIVA or in conjunction with inhalant anesthesia.

## Ketamine and Analgesia

Today ketamine is gaining increased acceptance as an analgesic that can be used in conjunction with other drugs for standing surgical procedures or to provide multimodal analgesia for acute or chronic pain. In addition, ketamine has been shown to produce local anesthetic and potent anti-inflammatory effects.[54,55] Epidural doses of ketamine (0.5, 1, 2 mg/kg) were evaluated in 6 healthy conscious horses and demonstrated to be effective in producing analgesia of the tail, perineum, and upper hindlimb.[56] Total tail and perineal analgesia times were similar depending on dosage (30 minutes for 0.5 and 1.0 mg/kg and 75 minutes for 2.0 mg/kg). A dose-dependent sedative effect of ketamine was observed, with a peak effect between 15 and 30 minutes post ketamine administration. No cardiopulmonary effects were observed with any dose of ketamine.[56] In other studies horses were randomly chosen and randomly assigned to receive an abaxial sesamoid block of a forelimb with one of the following: saline (0.9% NaCl) solution, 1% ketamine solution, 2% ketamine solution, or 3% ketamine solution.[54] Analgesia to noxious thermal stimulus was assessed by the radiant heat lamp-hoof withdrawal latency reflex (time between lamp illumination and withdrawal of the hoof [HWRL]) test. Hoof withdrawal latency was determined before each nerve block (baseline) and after the nerve block. Local analgesic effects were determined by measuring HWRL at 2 and 5 minutes after injection and then every 5 minutes for a total period of 1 hour. The investigators concluded that abaxial sesamoid block with ketamine produced adequate analgesia in horses, with an onset of action of 2 minutes and a maximal duration of action of 15 minutes.[54] A follow-up study concluded that alkalinization of a 1% ketamine solution produced a more consistent and persistent local analgesia in horses when compared with 1% ketamine alone.[55] Finally, an intra-articular ketamine and tramadol drug combination were demonstrated to be more effective than a ketamine and ropivacaine drug combination on postoperative pain after arthroscopic meniscectomy in humans.[57]

In other studies, infusions of ketamine were investigated on the nociceptive withdrawal reflex (NWR) in both isoflurane-anesthetized and conscious ponies.[58–60] Target plasma concentrationns of 1 μg/mL (S)-ketamine for 120 min during isoflurane anesthesia were produced in Shetland ponies.[60] Quantitative electromyographic assessment of the NWR determined that the peak-to-peak amplitude and the duration of the NWR decreased significantly during ketamine administration and returned slowly toward baseline once the ketamine infusion was discontinued.[60] Similar studies investigating the effects of low-dose racemic ketamine and its (S)-enantiomer were conducted in conscious ponies.[59] Ponies were administered either 0.6 mg/kg racemic ketamine (group RS) or 0.3 mg/kg (S)-ketamine (group S) IV, followed by a CRI of 20 μg/kg/min racemic ketamine (group RS) or 10 μg/kg/min (S)-ketamine (group S) for 59 minutes. The NWR was evoked by transcutaneous electrical stimulation of a peripheral nerve before and 15 and 45 minutes after drug administration, and 15 minutes after the end of the CRI. Electromyographic responses were recorded and analyzed. Minor changes in behavior, heart rate, and mean arterial pressure only occurred within the first 5 to 10 minutes after bolus drug administration in both groups. The investigators concluded that analgesic activity in standing ponies, demonstrated as a depression of the NWR, could only be detected after treatment with racemic ketamine.[59] Finally, several studies have suggested that ketamine could have immunoinhibitory effects, thereby providing a therapeutic benefit to horses suffering from systemic inflammation and endotoxemia.[61] The clinical relevance of these findings to horses with naturally occurring diseases that involve various inflammatory conditions, however, has not been determined.

Ketamine's current clinical usage, although largely confined to anesthetic practices, is gradually expanding to incorporate short- and long-term pain management in conscious horses. Studies in humans suggest that subanesthetic plasma concentrations (<1 μg/mL; range: 0.800–1.200 μg/mL) may produce clinically relevant analgesic effects, and experimental studies in rats suggest that the infusion of subanalgesic (0.030–0.120 μg/mL) doses of ketamine can be administered to improve the analgesic activity of opioids and alpha-2 agonists.[62,63] Studies conducted to determine the pharmacokinetics and pharmacologic effects of ketamine in conscious horses examined infusion rates ranging from 0.4 to 1.6 mg/kg/h for 6 hours in 8 conscious horses.[64] Ketamine was then administered to 6 horses for a total of 12 hours (3 horses at 0.4 mg/kg/h for 6 hours followed by 0.8 mg/kg/h for 6 hours and 3 horses at 0.8 mg/kg/h for 6 hours, followed by 0.4 mg/kg/h for 6 hours). The concentration of ketamine in plasma, heart rate, respiratory rate, blood pressure, physical activity, and analgesia were measured before, during, and following infusion. Analgesic testing was performed with a modified hoof tester applied at a measured force to the withers and radius. Pharmacokinetic data were similar to those reported in earlier studies. Heart rate and mean arterial pressure decreased compared with preinfusion measurements, and an analgesic effect could not be demonstrated during or after infusion.[64] Venous plasma concentrations averaged 0.067, 0.137, and 0.235 μg/mL after ketamine infusions of 0.4 mg/kg/h, 0.8 mg/kg/h, and 1.6 mg/kg/h. One horse administered 1.6 mg/kg/h and a venous plasma concentration of 0.280 μg/mL exhibited increased locomotor activity and exaggerated responses to movement, light, and noise.[64] A separate group of investigators determined the pharmacokinetics and pharmacology of a ketamine infusion, 1.5 mg/kg/h, over 5 hours and 20 minutes following initial drug loading.[31] Cardiopulmonary parameters, arterial blood gases, glucose, lactate, cortisol, insulin, nonesterified fatty acids, and muscle enzyme levels were determined. Respiration and heart rate significantly increased during the early infusion phase. Glucose and cortisol significantly varied both during and after infusion. All other parameters remained within or close to physiologic limits without significant changes from pre-CRI values. The mean venous plasma concentration was was 235 ng/mL (range 118–277 μg/mL) during 1.5 mg/kg/h ketamine infusion.[31] Horses began to demonstrate signs of ketamine effects at approximately 6 hours after beginning the infusion. These studies suggest that ketamine can be safely infused to healthy conscious horses at a rate of 1.5 mg/kg/h for at least 6 h and that signs of ketamine-induced excitability are likely to occur when plasma concentrations exceed 0.280 to 0.300 μg/mL. Greater rates of infusion of 3.6 to 4.8 mg/kg/h could be administered, but for much shorter periods before signs associated with ketamine excess, including increases in respiratory rate, heart rate, arterial blood pressure, and muscle twitching, were produced.[31]

As stated earlier, ketamine is believed to possess analgesic effects when adminis-tered in subanesthetic doses because it is a noncompetitive NMDAR antagonist, an opioid receptor agonist, and an activator of the nomoaminergic descending inhibitory system. It is important that few if any studies have objectively evaluated ketamine's analgesic effects in horses with pain from naturally occurring disease. Furthermore, ket-amine has been demonstrated to produce minimal analgesic effects when adminis-tered alone as the sole analgesic drug postoperatively in humans.[7] Again, similar studies have not been conducted in horses. The reasons for ketamine's poor perfor-mance as a postoperative analgesic in humans remain controversial, but may be related to the principal mechanisms responsible for surgical pain, for example, dependence on activation of AMPA/KA receptors rather than NMDARs. NMDARs only become acti-vated when pain is intense or sustained. Furthermore, most animal models extolling the potential analgesic effects of NMDA antagonists for the treatment of pain are more successful in demonstrating their ability to inhibit hyperexcitability in nociceptive neurons and secondary hyperalgesia (known to be NMDA dependent) without affecting baseline responses to nociceptive stimuli. Do these studies negate the potential benefit of ketamine or other NMDA antagonists for the treament of painful conditions in horses? No, particularly because it is known that CNS sensitization initiated by extensive surgical procedures or degenerative diseases is a key component in the development of chronic pain. These studies highlight, however, that drugs that produce NMDA antagonistic effects are more effective in preventing hyperalgesia and central sensitiza-tion from severe or chronic tissue damage (osteoarthritic laminitis), and are not partic-ularly effective analgesics when pain is produced by mild to moderate acute surgical or accidental events. It is also important, however, that multiple studies conducted in rats wherein subanalgesic doses of ketamine (<0.15 mg/kg/h; <0.040 μg/mL plasma) were administered have demonstrated ketamine's ability to potentiate the analgesic effects of opioids and alpha-2 agonists, and vice versa[10,65–67] Ketamine may also be valuable in preventing or limiting the development of tolerance or side effects associated with opioid administration.[67,68] Collectively these studies provide a reasonable argument for the continued investigation and administration of ketamine as an analgesic in horses. Objectively evaluated, randomized clinical trials remain to be conducted to support and define this practice. In the meantime, these experimental studies suggest that plasma concentrations of ketamine greater than 0.050 μg/mL are likely to poten-tiate the analgesic effects of opioids and alpha-2 agonists, and should help the prevent the development of secondary sensitization and hyperalgesia (pain- or drug-induced).

## OTHER NMDAR ANTAGONISTS

As implied in the introduction, a diverse group of drugs has been identified to produce NMDAR antagonistic effects (see **Box 1**). Other than ketamine, none have been demonstrated to produce analgesic effects in experimental horses or horses with naturally occurring pain. Magnesium sulfate has been suggested for the treatment of postoperative pain from lower limb orthopedic surgery in humans, but most data are inconclusive at best and suspect to experimental design errors.[69] Two antiviral drugs, memantine and amantadine, are purported to produce NMDA antagonistic effects, but neither has been investigated either alone or in combination with other analgesic therapies for the treatment of acute or chronic pain in horses. One study has determined the pharmacokinetics of amantadine in horses and has suggested that administration of 5 mg/kg, IV every 4 h should maintain safe and effective plasma concentrations of amantadine, and the mean bioavailability is between 40% and 60% when an oral dose of 10 to 20 mg/kg is administered.[70] Methadone, a synthetic mu-opioid receptor agonist, is purported to produce analgesic effects similar to morphine in horses and has been demonstrated to produce NMDA antagonistic effects in a spinal neuron pain-related hyperactivity rat model of neuropathic pain.[71,72] Pharmacokinetic studies of the injectable formulation of methadone hydrochloride administered orally in horses, however, do not support its clinical use.[73] No studies, however, have evaluated methadone's effects either alone or in combination with ketamine for the treatment of naturally occurring pain in horses. Randomized, controlled, and blinded experimental and clinical trials with all of the aforementioned drugs are awaited.

## SUMMARY

Similar to other species, NMDARs likely are important in pain processing in horses. Ketamine is a dissociative anesthetic and an NMDA antagonist. Ketamine can be administered by infusion to produce systemic analgesic, anti-inflammatory, and anesthetic effects in horses. Infusion rates ranging from 0.8 to 1.5 mg/kg/h produce venous plasma concentrations (0.130–0.250 µg/mL) that are likely to reduce hyperalgesia and central sensitization and to produce analgesia in horses. Lower infusion rates may enhance the analgesic effects of opioids or be enhanced by the simultaneous administration of alpha-2 agonists or the antisiezue drug gabapentin. (S)-Ketamine may be more potent that (R)-ketamine and is eliminated more rapidly in horses, resulting in better and faster recovery from anesthesia and more control of ketamine infusion, with less potential for side effect. Future investigations should focus on the potential clinical utility of ketamine's local analgesic effects and the clinical efficacy of ketamine administration to horses suffering from painful diseases.

## REFERENCES

1. Petrenko AB, Yamakura T, Baba H, et al. The role of N-methyl-D-Aspartate (NMDA) receptors in pain: a review. Anesth Analg 2003;97:1108–16.
2. Carlton SM, Hargett GL, Coggeshall RE. Localization and activation of glutamate receptors in unmyelinated and myelinated axons of rat glabrous skin. Neurosci Lett 1995;197:25–8.
3. Latremoliere A, Woolf CJ. Central sensitization: a generator of pain hypersensitivity by central neural plasticity. J Pain 2009;10(9):895–926.
4. Mori H, Mishina M. Structure and function of the NMDA receptor channel. Neuropharmacology 1995;34:1219–37.
5. Laube B, Hirai H, Sturgess M, et al. Molecular determinants of agonist discrimination by NMDA receptor subunits: analysis of the glutamate binding site on the NR2B subunit. Neuron 1997;18:493–503.
6. Yamakura T, Shimoji K. Subunit-and site-specific pharmacology of the NMDA receptor channel. Prog Neurobiol 1999;59:279–98.

7. DeKock MF. The clinical role of NMDA receptor antagonists for the treatment of postoperative pain. Best Pract Res Clin Anaesthesiol 2007;21:85–98.
8. Costigan M, Woolf CJ. Pain: molecular mechanisms. J Pain 2000;1(Suppl 3): 35–44.
9. Cheng HT, Suzuki M, Hegarty DM, et al. Inflammatory pain-induced signaling events following a conditional deletion of the N-methyl-D-aspartate receptor in spinal cord dorsal horn. Neuroscience 2008;155(3):948–58.
10. Roh D, Seo H, Yoon S, et al. Activation of spinal a-2 adrenoceptors, but not u-opioid receptors, reduces the intrathecal n-methyl-D-aspartate-induced increase in spinal NR1 subunit phosphorylation and nociceptive behaviors in the rat. Anesth Analg 2010;110:622–9.
11. Subramaniam K, Subramaniam B, Steinbrook RA. Ketamine as adjuvant analgesic to opioids: a quantitative and qualitative systematic review. Anesth Analg 2004;99:482–95.
12. Cheng J, Cheng C, Yang J, et al. The antiallodynic action target of intrathecal gabapentin: Ca2+ channels, KATP channels or N-methyl-D-aspartate acid receptors. Anesth Analg 2006;102:182–7.
13. Visser E, Schug SA. The role of ketamine in pain management. Biomed Pharmacother 2006;60:341–8.
14. Jones E, Vinuela-Fernandz I, Eager RA, et al. Neuropathic changes in equine laminitis pain. Pain 2007;132:321–31.
15. Clarke KW, Hall LW. "Xylazine"–a new sedative for horses and cattle. Vet Rec 1969;85(19):512–7.
16. Muir WW, Skarda RT, Milne DW. Evaluation of xylazine and ketamine hydrochloride for anesthesia in horses. Am J Vet Res 1977;38(2):195–201.
17. Butera TS, Moore JN, Garner HE, et al. Diazepam/xylazine/ketamine combination for short-term anesthesia in the horse. Vet Med Small Anim Clin 1978;73(4):495–6.
18. Kawamata T, Omote H, Sonoda H, et al. Analgesic mechanisms of ketamine in the presence and absence of peripheral inflammation. Anesthesiology 2000;93:520–8.
19. Koizuka S, Obata H, Sasaki M, et al. Systemic ketamine inhibits hypersensitivity after surgery via descending inhibitory pathways in rats. Can J Anaesth 2005;52: 498–505.
20. Costigan M, Scholz J, Woolf CJ. Neuropathic pain: a maladaptive response of the nervous system to damage. Annu Rev Neurosci 2009;32:1–32.
21. Yamashita K, Muir WW. Intravenous anesthetic and analgesic adjunct to inhalation anesthesia. In: Muir WW, Hubbell JA, editors. Equine anesthesia: monitoring and emergency therapy. 2nd edition. St Louis (MO): Saunders Elsevier; 2009. p. 261–72.
22. Mazar J, Rogachev B, Shked G, et al. Involvement of adenosine in the anti-inflammatory action of ketamine. Anesthesiology 2005;102:1174–81.
23. Filzek U, Fischer U, Ferguson J. Intravenous anaesthesia in horses: racemic ketamine versus S-(+)-ketamine. Pferdeheilkunde 2003;19:501–6.
24. Rossetti RB, Gaido Cortopassi SR, Intelizano T, et al. Comparison of ketamine and S(+)-ketamine, with romifidine and diazepam, for total intravenous anesthesia in horses. Vet Anaesth Analg 2008;35:30–7.
25. Larenza MP, Knobloch M, Landoni MF, et al. Stereoselective pharmacokinetics of ketamine and norketamine after racemic ketamine or S-ketamine administration in Shetland ponies sedated with xylazine. Vet J 2008;177(3):432–5.
26. Larenza MP, Ringer SK, Kutter AP, et al. Evaluation of anesthesia recovery quality after low-dose racemic or S-ketamine infusions during anesthesia with isoflurane in horses. Am J Vet Res 2009;70(6):710–8.

27. Schmitz A, Portier CJ, Thormann W, et al. Stereoselective biotransformation of ketamine in equine liver and lung microsomes. J Vet Pharmacol Ther 2008; 31(5):446–55.

28. Capponi L, Schmitz A, Thormann W, et al. In vitro evaluation of differences in phase 1 metabolism of ketamine and other analgesics among humans, horses, and dogs. Am J Vet Res 2009;70(6):777–86.

29. Larenza MP, Peterbauer C, Landoni MF, et al. Stereoselective pharmacokinetics of ketamine and norketamine after constant rate infusion of a subanesthetic dose of racemic ketamine or S-ketamine in Shetland ponies. Am J Vet Res 2009;70(7):831–9.

30. Larenza MP, Landoni MF, Levionnois OL, et al. Stereoselective pharmacokinetics of ketamine and norketamine after racemic ketamine or S-ketamine administration during isoflurane anaesthesia in Shetland ponies. Br J Anaesth 2007;98(2): 204–12.

31. Lankveld DP, Driessen B, Soma LR, et al. Pharmacodynamic effects and pharmacokinetic profile of a long-term continuous rate infusion of racemic ketamine in healthy conscious horses. J Vet Pharmacol Ther 2006;29(6):477–88.

32. Ihmsen H, Geisslinger G, Schuttler J. Sterioselective pharmacokinetics of ketamine: R(-)-ketmaine inhibits the elimination of S(+)-ketmaine. Clin Pharmacol Ther 2001;70:431–8.

33. Kaka JS, Klavano PA, Hayton WL. Pharmacokinetics of ketmaine in the horse. Am J Vet Res 1979;50:978–81.

34. Waterman AE, Robertson SA, Lane JG. The pharmacokinetics of intravenously administered ketamine in the horse. Res Vet Sci 1987;42:161–6.

35. White M, de Graaff P, Renshof B, et al. Pharmacokinetics of S(+) ketamine derived from target controlled infusion. Br J Anaesth 2006;96:330–4.

36. Parsons LE, Walmsley JP. Field use of an acetylpromazine, methadone, ketamine combination for anaesthesia in the horse and donkey. Vet Rec 1982;111(17):395.

37. Trim CM, Adams JG, Hovda LR. Failure of ketamine to induce anesthesia in two horses. J Am Vet Med Assoc 1987;190(2):201–2.

38. Muir WW, Skarda RT, Sheehan W. Evaluation of xylazine, guaifenesin, and ketamine hydrochloride for restraint in horses. Am J Vet Res 1978;39(8):1274–8.

39. Greene SA, Thurmon JC, Tranquilli WJ, et al. Cardiopulmonary effects of continuous intravenous infusion of guaifenesin, ketamine, and xylazine in ponies. Am J Vet Res 1986;47(11):2364–7.

40. Clarke KW, Taylor PM, Watkins SB. Detomidine/ketamine anaesthesia in the horse. Acta Vet Scand Suppl 1986;82:167–79.

41. Kaegi B. [Anesthesia by injection of xylazine, ketamine and the benzodiazepine derivative climazolam and the use of the benzodiazepine antagonist Ro 15–3505]. Schweiz Arch Tierheilkd 1990;132(5):251–7 [in German].

42. McCarty JE, Trim CM, Ferguson D. Prolongation of anesthesia with xylazine, ketamine, and guaifenesin in horses: 64 cases (1986–1989). J Am Vet Med Assoc 1990;197(12):1646–50.

43. Wan PY, Trim CM, Mueller PO. Xylazine-ketamine and detomidine-tiletamine-zolazepam anesthesia in horses. Vet Surg 1992;21(4):312–8.

44. Muir WW 3rd, Gadawski JE, Grosenbaugh DA. Cardiorespiratory effects of a tiletamine/zolazepam-ketamine-detomidine combination in horses. Am J Vet Res 1999;60(6):770–4.

45. Muir WW 3rd, Lerche P, Robertson JT, et al. Comparison of four drug combinations for total intravenous anesthesia of horses undergoing surgical removal of an abdominal testis. J Am Vet Med Assoc 2000;217(6):869–73.

46. Hubbell JA, Hinchcliff KW, Schmall LM, et al. Anesthetic, cardiorespiratory, and metabolic effects of four intravenous anesthetic regimens induced in horses immediately after maximal exercise. Am J Vet Res 2000;61(12):1545–52.

47. Muir WW 3rd, Sams R. Effects of ketamine infusion on halothane minimal alveolar concentration in horses. Am J Vet Res 1992;53(10):1802–6.

48. Clarke KW, Song DY, Alibhai HI, et al. Cardiopulmonary effects of desflurane in ponies, after induction of anaesthesia with xylazine and ketamine. Vet Rec 1996;139(8):180–5.

49. Yamashita K, Satoh M, Umikawa A, et al. Combination of continuous intravenous infusion using a mixture of guaifenesin-ketamine-medetomidine and sevoflurane anesthesia in horses. J Vet Med Sci 2000;62(3):229–35.

50. Yamashita K, Muir WW 3rd, Tsubakishita S, et al. Infusion of guaifenesin, ketamine, and medetomidine in combination with inhalation of sevoflurane versus inhalation of sevoflurane alone for anesthesia of horses. J Am Vet Med Assoc 2002;221(8):1150–5.

51. Umar MA, Yamashita K, Kushiro T, et al. Evaluation of total intravenous anesthesia with propofol or ketamine-medetomidine-propofol combination in horses. J Am Vet Med Assoc 2006;228(8):1221–7.

52. Umar MA, Yamashita K, Kushiro T, et al. Evaluation of cardiovascular effects of total intravenous anesthesia with propofol or a combination of ketamine-medetomidine-propofol in horses. Am J Vet Res 2007;68(2):121–7.

53. Yamashita K, Wijayathilaka TP, Kushiro T, et al. Anesthetic and cardiopulmonary effects of total intravenous anesthesia using a midazolam, ketamine and medetomidine drug combination in horses. J Vet Med Sci 2007;69(1):7–13.

54. López-Sanromán FJ, Cruz JM, Santos M, et al. Evaluation of the local analgesic effect of ketamine in the palmar digital nerve block at the base of the proximal sesamoid (abaxial sesamoid block) in horses. Am J Vet Res 2003;64(4):475–8.

55. López-Sanromán J, Cruz J, Santos M, et al. Effect of alkalinization on the local analgesic efficacy of ketamine in the abaxial sesamoid nerve block in horses. J Vet Pharmacol Ther 2003;26(4):265–9.

56. Gómez de Segura IA, De Rossi R, Santos M, et al. Epidural injection of ketamine for perineal analgesia in the horse. Vet Surg 1998;27(4):384–91.

57. Altunkaya AH, Bayar A, Turan IO, et al. The effect of intraarticular combinations of tramadol and ropivacaine with ketamine on postoperative pain after arthroscopic meniscectomy. Arch Orthop Trauma Surg 2010;130:307–12.

58. Levionnois OL, Menge M, Thormann W, et al. Effect of ketamine on the limb withdrawal reflex evoked by transcutaneous electrical stimulation in ponies anaesthetised with isoflurane. Vet J 2009. [Epub ahead of print].

59. Peterbauer C, Larenza PM, Knobloch M, et al. Effects of a low dose infusion of racemic and S-ketamine on the nociceptive withdrawal reflex in standing ponies. Vet Anaesth Analg 2008;35(5):414–23.

60. Knobloch M, Portier CJ, Levionnois OL, et al. Antinociceptive effects, metabolism and disposition of ketamine in ponies under target-controlled drug infusion. Toxicol Appl Pharmacol 2006;216(3):373–86.

61. Lankveld DP, Bull S, Van Dijk P, et al. Ketamine inhibits LPS-induced tumour necrosis factor-alpha and interleukin-6 in an equine macrophage cell line. Vet Res 2005;36.257–62.

62. Grant IS, Nimmo WS, Clements JA. Pharmacokinetics and analgesic effects of IM and oral ketamine. Br J Anaesth 1981;53:805–10.

63. Himmelseher S, Durieux ME. Ketamine for perioperative pain management. Anesthesiology 2005;102(1):211–20.

64. Fielding CL, Brumbaugh GW, Matthews NS, et al. Pharmacokinetics and clinical effects of a subanesthetic continuous rate infusion of ketamine in awake horses. Am J Vet Res 2006;67(9):1484–90.

65. Shulte H, Sollevi A, Segerdahl M. The synergistic effect of combined treatment of systemic ketamine and morphine on experimentally induced windup-like pain in humans. Anesth Analg 2004;98:1574–80.

66. Zhang GH, Min SS, Seol GH, et al. Inhibition of the N-methyl-D-aspartate receptor unmasks the antinociception of endogenous opioids in the periphery. Pain 2009; 143:233–7.

67. Lauline J, Maurette P, Corcuff J, et al. The role of ketamine in preventing fentanyl-induced hyperalgesia and subsequent acute morphine tolerance. Anesth Analg 2002;94:1263–9.

68. Inturrisi CE. The role of N-methyl-D-aspartate (NMDA) receptors in pain and morphine tolerance. Minerva Anestesiol 1994;60:401–3.

69. Dabbagh A, Elyasi H, Razavi SS, et al. Intravenous magnesium sulfate for postoperative pain in patients undergoing lower limb orthopedic surgery. Acta Anaesthesiol Scand 2009;53:1088–91.

70. Rees WA, Harkins JD, Woods WE, et al. Amantadine and equine influenza: pharmacology, pharmacokinetics and neurologicalneurologic effects in the horse. Equine Vet J 1997;29(2):104–10.

71. Pippi NL, Lumb WV. Objective tests of analgesic drugs in ponies. Am J Vet Res 1979;40(8):1082–6.

72. Sotgiu ML, Valente M, Storchi R, et al. Cooperative N-methyl-D-aspartate (NMDA) receptor antagonism and mu-opioid receptor agonism mediate the methadone inhibition of the spinal neuron pain-related hyperactivity in a rat model of neuropathic pain. Pharmacol Res 2009;60(4):284–90.

73. Linardi RL, Stokes AM, Barker SA, et al. Pharmacokinetics of the injectable formulation of methadone hydrochloride administered orally in horses. J Vet Pharmacol Ther 2009;32(5):492–7.

# The Role of Manual Therapies in Equine Pain Management

Kevin K. Haussler, DVM, DC, PhD

**KEYWORDS**

- Manual therapy • Touch • Stretching • Massage • Mobilization
- Manipulation • Pain

*Beyond all doubt the use of the human hand, as a method of reducing human suffering, is the oldest remedy known to man; historically no date can be given for its adaptation.*

*John Mennell, MD*

The use of touch, massage, or manipulation of painful articulations or tense muscles is arguably one of the oldest and most universally accepted forms of therapy to relieve pain and suffering.[1] Firmly grasping an acutely injured thumb after a misdirected hammer blow or rubbing a sore muscle or stiff joint after a long-day's work are simple and often effective methods of providing short-term pain relief in humans. Similarly, animals lick, scratch, or rub wounds or areas of irritation on themselves or their offspring in an apparent attempt to reduce pain and suffering. Horses are known to respond favorably to grooming, to stretch, roll on their backs, and rub up against objects, presumably because these activities provide some sense of comfort. Over time, both lay and licensed practitioners have developed a spectrum of manual methods to provide varying levels of pain relief to both humans and animals. However, most organized medicine often remains skeptical of any purported effects of massage or other forms of manual therapy, and routinely ostracizes practitioners that apply these techniques.[2] In the last few decades, considerable advances have been made in conducting investigations into plausible mechanisms of action and scientific reviews of the clinical efficacy of manual therapy in pain management.

All forms of manual therapy involve the application of the hands to the body, with a diagnostic or therapeutic intent.[3] Abdominal and rectal palpation, soft tissue and bony palpation of musculoskeletal structures, or moving a joint through its expected range of motion are considered essential diagnostic techniques used routinely in veterinary medicine (**Fig. 1**). Touch therapies, massage, physical therapy, osteopathy,

Gail Holmes Equine Orthopaedic Research Center, Department of Clinical Sciences, College of Veterinary Medicine and Biomedical Sciences, Colorado State University, 300 West Drake Road, Fort Collins, CO 80523, USA

*E-mail address:* Kevin.Haussler@ColoState.edu

Vet Clin Equine 26 (2010) 579–601
doi:10.1016/j.cveq.2010.07.006
0749-0739/10/$ – see front matter © 2010 Elsevier Inc. All rights reserved.

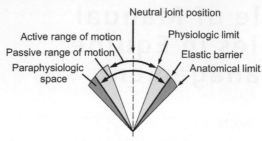

**Fig. 1.** Joint mechanics as it relates to active and passive joint range of motion. The physiologic limit demarcates active versus passive joint range of motion. The paraphysiologic space is defined by the elastic barrier and the anatomic limit of the articulation. Inducing motion beyond the anatomic limit of the joint induces tissue damage and results in joint subluxation or luxation.

and chiropractic are techniques that have been developed for treatment of musculoskeletal disorders in humans and transferred for use in horses. Each treatment method has a unique origin and different proposed biomechanical or physiologic effects; however, all forms of manual therapy are characterized by applying variable gradations of manual force and degrees of soft tissue or articular displacement (**Fig. 2**).[4] The goal of all manual therapies is to influence reparative or healing processes within the neuromusculoskeletal system, which often includes pain relief.

The therapeutic effects of manual therapies may be generalized to the entire body by inducing relaxation or altering behavior; regional effects may include alterations in pain perception or neuromuscular control; or effects may be localized to specific tissues and cellular responses.[3] The challenge for practitioners is in selecting the most appropriate and effective form of manual therapy to produce the desired physiologic effect within an individual patient, such as increasing joint range of motion, reducing pain, or promoting general body relaxation. Anecdotally, all forms of manual therapy have varying reported levels of effectiveness in humans and horses. Unfortunately, most claims are not supported by high levels of evidence from randomized, controlled trials or systematic reviews of the literature. The purpose of this article is provide a brief description and overview of the scientific literature on the efficacy,

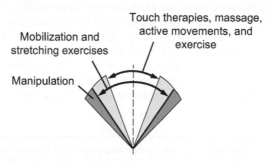

**Fig. 2.** Joint mechanics as it relates to the site of action of various manual therapies. Touch therapies and massage do not typically induce joint motion, whereas all forms of exercise occur within the active range of joint motion. Passive stretching and joint mobilization occur within the passive range of joint motion. Joint manipulation, characterized by a high-velocity, low-amplitude thrust, occurs outside of the limits of passive joint motion; within the paraphysiologic space.

safety, and mechanisms of action of the different manual therapy techniques commonly applied to horses, with a specific focus on their role in acute and chronic pain management.

## ANTINOCICEPTIVE EFFECTS OF MANUAL THERAPIES

Pain represents a series of complex molecular, cellular, physiologic, physical, and behavioral attributes and interactions.[5] Nociception involves the processes of transduction (at the sensory nerve ends), transmission (via peripheral sensory nerves), modulation (within the spinal cord), projection (via ascending pain pathways), and pain perception (within the thalamus and cerebral cortex).[6] The exact mechanisms by which manual therapies relieve pain are unknown; however, the various forms of manual therapy may influence the nociceptive processes at each of these levels. The problem, in part, is in defining and objectively measuring the primary cause of musculoskeletal pain.[1] Transduction may be altered by local biochemical changes induced by massage that modulates local blood flow and oxygenation of tissues.[7] Pinching the skin at the site of an injection is a form of a manually induced counterirritant or afferent stimulation that acts to reduce the perception of pain associated with percutaneous injections. The transmission of nociceptive signals may be altered by mechanical and neurophysiologic mechanisms associated with spinal manipulation, which influence primary afferent neurons from paraspinal tissues, the motor control system, and pain processing.[8,9] Modulations of spinal pathways act to inhibit central sensitization and influence referred pain. Peripheral and central sensitization are characterized by increased sensitivity of local tissues and the spinal cord to noxious and innocuous stimuli, which causes an increase in pain perception. Spinal manipulation is theorized to produce an inhibitory effect mediated by induced stretching of spinal mechanoreceptors that reduce central sensitization of the segmental dorsal horn neurons.[8,10] Neuronal and synaptic plasticity of spinal neurons may also be influenced by manual therapies.[11] The gate-control theory predicts that massaging a particular area stimulates large diameter nerve fibers, which have an inhibitory input within the spinal cord.[7] Projection of nociceptive signals may be altered by descending pain inhibitory systems projecting from the brain to the spinal cord, which can be activated by spinal manipulation via sympathoexcitatory effects.[12] Manual therapies may also increase pain thresholds through the release of endorphins and serotonin and modulate activity within subcortical nuclei that influence mood and pain perception.[7] Pain perception may be influenced through physical and mental relaxation.[7] Placebo or psychological effects also play a role in human pain; however the magnitude of these effects within the veterinarian-client-patient relationship is unknown.[13]

Manual therapy is considered to produce physiologic effects within local tissues, on sensory and motor components of the nervous system, and at a psychological or behavioral level.[3] It is likely that specific manual therapy techniques are inherently more effective than others in addressing each of these local, regional, or systemic components.[14] The challenge is in choosing the most appropriate form of manual therapy or combination of techniques that will be efficacious for an individual patient with specific musculoskeletal disabilities (**Table 1**). If soft tissue restriction and pain are identified as the primary components of a musculoskeletal injury, then massage, stretching, and soft tissue mobilization techniques are indicated for increasing tissue extensibility (**Fig. 3**).[15] However, if the musculoskeletal dysfunction is localized to articular structures, then stretching, joint mobilization, and manipulation are the most indicated manual therapy techniques for restoring joint range of motion and reducing pain.[16]

**Table 1**
**Potential indications for application of various equine manual therapy techniques**

| Manual Therapy Technique | Indications |
| --- | --- |
| Touch therapies | Pain |
| Massage | Muscle hypertonicity, soft tissue restriction, pain |
| Stretching | Soft tissue restriction, joint stiffness |
| Soft tissue mobilization | Soft tissue restriction, pain |
| Joint mobilization | Joint stiffness, pain |
| Joint manipulation | Joint stiffness, pain, muscle hypertonicity |

Local tissue effects produced by manual therapy techniques relate to direct mechanical stimulation of skin, fascia, muscles, tendons, ligaments, and joint capsules.[17] Direct mechanical loading of tissues can alter tissue healing, the physical properties of tissues (eg, elongation), and local tissue fluid dynamics associated with extracellular or intravascular fluids. Normal tissue repair and remodeling relies on mechanical stimulation of cells and tissues to restore optimal structural and functional properties, such as tensile strength and flexibility. Nonspecific back pain is most likely related to a functional impairment and not a structural disorder; therefore, many back problems may be related to muscle or joint dysfunction with secondary soft tissue irritation and pain generation.[18] Soft tissue contractures and adhesions are unwanted effects associated with musculoskeletal injuries and postsurgical immobilization.[19] Stretching exercises or direct mechanical mobilization of the affected tissue can be used to elongate contracted or fibrotic connective tissues to improve soft tissue extensibility and increase joint range of motion.[15] Tissue viability is highly dependent on its vascular and lymphatic supply, which is often compromised as a result of mechanical disruption or ischemia. Soft tissue or joint mobilization may facilitate flow to and from the affected tissues, help to reduce pain and edema, and decrease joint effusion.[20] Joint manipulation can improve restricted joint mobility and may reduce the harmful effects associated with joint immobilization and joint capsule contractures. Limb and joint mobilization can also have direct mechanical effects on nerve roots and the dura mater, which may have clinical application in the treatment of perineural adhesions and edema.[21]

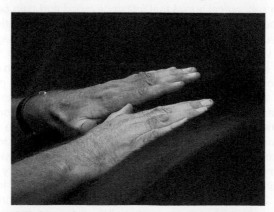

**Fig. 3.** Soft tissue mobilization of the skin overlying the trunk. The skin and superficial fascia is mobilized in cranial-caudal and medial-lateral directions to assess or treat any soft tissue restrictions in movement.

Joint mobilization and manipulation are believed to produce different physiologic effects; however, the evidence in humans is mixed. Manipulation has been shown to immediately reduce spontaneous myoelectrical activity and paraspinal muscle spindles, whereas mobilization has not.[22,23] For neck pain in humans, manipulation produces significant reductions in pain and disability, compared with mobilization.[24] However, both joint mobilization and manipulation increase cervical range of motion to a similar degree.[25] Other studies report that neither manipulation nor mobilization are beneficial or significantly different for mechanical neck disorders.[26] For acute low back pain in humans, there is moderate evidence that spinal manipulation provides more short-term pain relief than does mobilization.[16] It has been theorized that spinal manipulation preferentially influences a sensory bed, which, in terms of anatomic location and function, is different from the sensory bed influenced by spinal mobilization techniques.[27] Manipulation may particularly stimulate receptors within deep intervertebral muscles, whereas mobilization techniques most likely affect more superficial axial muscles. In horses, spinal manipulation increased the dorsoventral displacement of the trunk and applied force, which indicate increased spinal flexibility and increased tolerance to pressure in the thoracolumbar region of the equine vertebral column, compared with mobilization alone.[28,29] The literature suggests that any stimulus that activates high-threshold receptors within the periarticular tissues has the potential to initiate unique neurologic reflexes associated with joint manipulation.[30,31]

Tissue manipulation has the additional effect of stimulating regional or systemic changes in neurologic signaling related to pain processing and motor control.[32] Manual therapy can provide effective management of pain and neuromuscular deficits associated with musculoskeletal injuries, alterations in postural control, and locomotory issues related to antalgic or compensatory gait.[3] In response to chronic pain or stiffness, new movement patterns are developed by the nervous system and adopted in an attempt to reduce pain or discomfort. Long after the initial injury has healed, adaptive or secondary movement patterns may continue to persist, which predispose adjacent articulations or muscles to injury.[18] Activation of proprioceptors, nociceptors, and components of the muscle spindles provide afferent stimuli that have direct and widespread influences on components of the peripheral and central nervous systems that directly regulate muscle tone and movement patterns.[18] The various forms of manual therapy are believed to affect different aspects of joint function via diverse mechanical and neurologic mechanisms.[4] Alterations in articular neurophysiology from mechanical or chemical injuries can affect both mechanoreceptor and nociceptor function via increased joint capsule tension and nerve ending hypersensitivity.[33] Mechanoreceptor stimulation induces reflex paraspinal musculature hypertonicity and altered local and systemic neurologic reflexes. Nociceptor stimulation results in a lowered pain threshold, sustained afferent stimulation (ie, facilitation), reflex paraspinal musculature hypertonicity, and abnormal neurologic reflexes. Touch and light massage preferentially stimulate superficial proprioceptors, whereas any technique that involves deep tissue massage, stretching, muscle contraction, or joint movement has the potential to stimulate deep proprioceptors.[3] Massage, stretching, and joint mobilization are also considered to affect more superficial epaxial muscles, such as the longissimus muscle, and to have a multisegmental effect. In contrast, manipulation preferentially stimulates mechanoreceptors within deep multifidi muscles and has a more segmental focus.[27] Joint manipulation can affect mechanoreceptors (ie, Golgi tendon organ and muscle spindles) to induce reflex inhibition of pain and muscle relaxation and to correct abnormal movement patterns.[8] Because of somatovisceral innervation, mobilization and manipulation within the trunk has possible influences on the autonomic system and visceral functions; however, the clinical significance and repeatability of these effects are largely unknown.[34,35]

The effects of touch or massage on psychological issues such as behavior or emotion are often dismissed as an insignificant component of the overall healing process in patients.[3] Promoting general body relaxation and reducing anxiety may be significant components of pain management protocols.[36] Behaviors related to pain, depression, or fear are associated with patterned somatic responses, which may be manifest as generalized changes in muscle tone, autonomic activity, or altered pain tolerance. Other psychological factors associated with manual therapies include placebo effects and patient satisfaction. Unfortunately, the role of placebo effects in horses and their owners is currently unknown.

## THERAPEUTIC TOUCH

The physical act of touching another human being or an animal can induce physiologic responses and is often considered therapeutic.[37] Interacting with animals during animal-assisted therapy sessions has been shown to reduce blood pressure and cholesterol, decrease anxiety, improve a person's sense of well-being, and cause a significant reduction in pain levels in humans.[38,39] Similarly, petting a horse or a dog can cause physiologic changes within the animal itself.[40] In humans, therapeutic touch is used by nurses to nurture premature infants, for supportive care in cancer or terminally ill patients, and for support of the bereaved.[41] Recognized touch therapy techniques in humans include Healing Touch, Therapeutic Touch and Reiki.[42] These techniques are considered a form of energy-based therapy in which practitioners move their hands over the body but do not contact the patient or use a gentle touch over certain areas of the body with the goal of facilitating physical, emotional, mental, and spiritual health. Human patients often use touch therapies for relaxation, stress reduction, and symptom relief. Mechanical devices or squeeze machines have also been developed to induce deep pressure or full-body compression, which induce calming behaviors in both autistic human patients and animals.[43,44] Reviews of controlled studies in humans evaluating effectiveness of touch therapies show promising results for pain relief, but further rigorous studies are needed to define clinical applications and mechanisms of action.[42,45] Trials conducted by more experienced practitioners appeared to yield greater effects in pain reduction.

In horses, touch therapies have been primarily developed and promoted by Linda Tellington-Jones in a collection of techniques named the Tellington Touch Equine Awareness Method (TTEAM) or Tellington TTouch.[46] Anecdotally, therapeutic touch is considered to improve behavior, performance, and well-being of horses and enhance the relationship between horse and rider, but no controlled studies exist to support these claims. Similar touch therapy techniques have been used in foals at birth to assess the effects of touch or imprint training on behavioral reactions during selected handling procedures.[47] Conditioned foals were significantly less resistant to touching the front and hind limbs and picking up the hind feet at 3 months of age. Well-designed and controlled studies are needed to determine the effectiveness of touch theories in managing behavior and musculoskeletal pain in horses.

## MASSAGE THERAPY

Massage therapy is defined as the manipulation of the skin, muscle, or superficial soft tissues either manually (eg, rubbing, kneading, or tapping) or with an instrument or mechanical device (eg, mechanical vibration) for therapeutic purposes (**Fig. 4**). Massage techniques do not typically cause movement or changes in articular

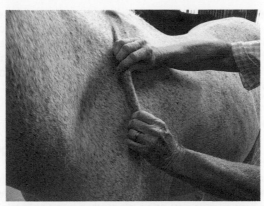

**Fig. 4.** Mobilization of the skin overlying the lateral scapular region using a skin-rolling technique to assess the quality and quantity of soft tissue mobilization in the region.

positioning and include many named methods such as Swedish massage, Rolfing, myofascial release, trigger point therapy, lymphatic drainage, and acupressure.[7] The manual techniques used in massage include effleurage, pétrissage, friction, kneading, or hacking, and often vary in the depth or speed of the applied pressure and in the specific tissues or regions of interest.[48] Massage is indicated for a wide variety of conditions in which pain relief, reduction of swelling, or mobilization of adhesive tissues are desired.[49] Massage is generally recognized as a safe intervention with minimal adverse effects. However, deep friction, compression, or ischemic compression have been reported to produce temporary postmassage soreness or ecchymosis in humans.[50] Massage is contraindicated for acute injuries, open wounds, and skin infections.[48]

Clinically, massage and soft tissue mobilization are believed to increase blood flow, promote relaxation, reduce muscle hypertonicity, increase tissue extensibility, reduce pain, and speed return to normal function; however, few controlled studies exist to support these claims.[7,51] There are many anecdotal reports of the beneficial effects of massage on human athletic performance; however, strong evidence in the form of controlled studies does not exist for the effects of massage on preventing injuries, recovery from exercise, or enhancing performance.[52] Systematic reviews suggest that massage may be beneficial for patients with subacute and chronic nonspecific low back pain in humans, especially when combined with exercises and education programs.[53,54] There is moderate evidence that acupressure may be more effective than Swedish massage for chronic low back pain.[7] Massage is also a popular adjunct to cancer palliation and systematic reviews suggest that massage can alleviate a wide range of cancer-associated symptoms in humans: pain, nausea, anxiety, depression, anger, stress, and fatigue.[55,56] Unfortunately, the methodological quality of most massage studies is poor, which prevents definitive conclusions and recommendations.[57] More research is needed to determine which type of massage is indicted for similar clinical presentations within patients, such as higher baseline pain scores, muscle spasms, or stress and anxiety.[7]

In horses, massage therapy has been shown to be effective for reducing stress-related behavior[40] and lowering mechanical nociceptive thresholds within the thoracolumbar region.[58] A noncontrolled, clinical trial using 8 horses measured increased stride lengths at the walk and trot before and after massage, but changes were not significant because of the small sample size.[59] Manual lymph drainage has been described for use in the management of lymphedema in horses; however, no controlled studies exist evaluating its effectiveness.[60] In a clinical trial in dogs, massage was significantly more effective in increasing lymph flow than passive flexion and extension of the forelimb or electrical stimulation of the forelimb musculature.[61] More high-quality, objective, outcome-based evidence is needed to support the use of massage therapy in horses.[62,63]

## PASSIVE STRETCHING EXERCISES

Passive stretching consists of applying forces to a limb or body segment to lengthen muscles or connective tissues beyond their normal resting lengths, with the intent of increasing joint range of motion and promoting flexibility.[64] Passive joint range of motion or stretching exercises differ neurophysiologically from active joint motion or exercise, which requires muscle activation, strength, and coordination. Active stretching involves using the patient's own movements to induce a stretch, whereas passive stretches are applied to relaxed muscles or connective tissues during passive soft tissue or joint mobilization. In horses, active stretches of the neck and trunk are often induced with baited (ie, carrot) stretches with the goal in increasing flexion, extension, or lateral bending of the axial skeleton (**Fig. 5**).[65] Asking horses to produce active stretching of specific articulations is often difficult; therefore, passive stretches are most commonly prescribed in horses (**Fig. 6**).[66] Distraction or traction refers to applying manual or mechanical forces to induce separation of adjacent joint surfaces, which causes stretching of the joint capsule, reduced intraarticular pressure, and is often used to reduce joint luxations (**Fig. 7**).

Stretching exercises vary according to the direction, velocity, amplitude, and duration of the applied force or induced movement. However, it is difficult to identify which combination of positions, techniques, and durations of stretching are the most effective

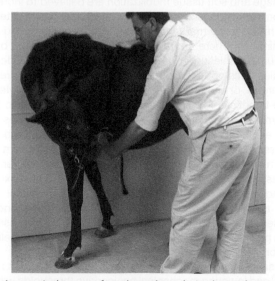

**Fig. 5.** Induced active cervical range of motion using a baited stretch. Note that the horse is positioned up against a wall to prevent lateral movement of the trunk as the hay is positioned at the girth region to induce left lateral bending of the cervical region. Active range of motion helps to identify left-to-right asymmetries in joint range of motion.

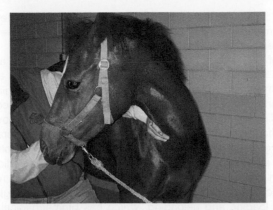

**Fig. 6.** Induced passive right lateral bending of the lower cervical region. The intervertebral articulation of interest (eg, C5–C6) is stabilized with one hand as the head and neck of the horse is brought into lateral bending. Gentle joint mobilization at the end range of motion helps to localize and lateralize signs of pain, joint stiffness, and muscle hypertonicity to specific cervical intervertebral articulations.

to induce increased joint range of motion and reduced pain within a specified articulation.[67] Stretching should be performed slowly to maximize tissue elongation due to creep and stress relaxation within fibrotic or shortened periarticular soft tissues.[15] Sustained low-load stretching is more effective than rapid high-load stretching for altering viscoelastic properties within soft tissues.[68] Rapid stretching may exceed the tissue's mechanical properties and produce additional trauma within injured tissues.[69] The force applied during stretching exercises should be tailored to specific phases of tissue repair.[15] During the acute inflammatory phase, stretching should be mostly avoided because of the increased risk of tissue injury. During the regenerative and remodeling phases of healing, tissues progressively regain tensile strength and applied manual forces can be gradually increased. The amount of force applied during passive stretching is largely based on the patient's response and signs of pain. Musculoskeletal injuries are often characterized by multiple tissue involvement, each of which has a different

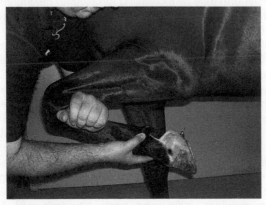

**Fig. 7.** Passive distraction of the carpus. The distal limb is passively flexed over the doctor's forearm to induce a distractive force to the carpal articulations and associated joint capsules.

healing rate and unique mechanical response to stretching. Therefore, effective stretching programs are best tailored to address specific soft tissue injuries and not only focused on restoring joint motion.

The duration of the applied stretch is dependent on the force applied, affected tissue shape and size, the amount of damage or fibrosis present, and the stage of tissue healing.[15] In humans, the recommended duration for stretching the musculotendinous unit varies from 6 to 60 seconds.[69] Stretching for 30 seconds has been shown to be significantly more effective than 15-second stretches; however, structural and functional differences within each affected tissue makes general recommendations for stretching a particular articulation or limb difficult to establish.[70] The mode of loading during an applied stretch varies from continuous to cyclic. Continuous or static loading can be uncomfortable for some patients and is not recommended.[15] Cyclic or rhythmical stretching is more comfortable and physiologic as it provides periods of tissue loading and unloading, which has biomechanical and neurologic benefits. Cyclic loading also has cumulative effects on soft tissues as a result of incremental elongation and stress relaxation within each stretch cycle; however, these effects are maximized approximately within the first 4 cycles of loading.[69] Therefore, recommendations for optimal passive stretching include applying 4 to 5 repetitions of slow low-load forces held at the end range of motion of the affected tissues, with each stretch applied and released in 30-second cycles, without inducing pain. If performed inappropriately, stretches may cause or aggravate injuries.[71] Therefore, thorough patient evaluation and formulation of a proper stretching program are required before implementing any stretching exercises.

Stretching soft tissues is believed to increase joint range of motion, enhance flexibility, improve coordination and motor control, increase blood flow to muscles, and helps to prevent injuries.[72] Systematic reviews of the human literature suggest that stretching may have beneficial effects on increasing joint range of motion, reducing pain, and preventing work-related musculoskeletal disorders.[71,73] There is strong evidence that stretching and strengthening exercises are effective for reducing pain, improving function, and producing favorable long-term global effects in human patients with subacute and chronic mechanical neck disorders.[74] Randomized studies suggest that regular stretching increases joint range of motion (average of 8°) for more than 1 day after cessation of stretching and that the effects of stretching are possibly greater in muscle groups with limited extensibility.[75] Regular stretching has been shown to improve performance by increasing force, jump height, and speed.[76] Other reviews of the literature report that there is not sufficient evidence to endorse or discontinue routine stretching before or after exercise to prevent injury among competitive or recreational human athletes.[77–79] Because of the relatively low methodological quality of most studies, further research is needed to determine the proper role of stretching in human sports. Stretching combined with strengthening provides the largest improvement in nonspecific chronic neck or low back pain in humans.[80,81]

In horses, passive stretching exercises of the limbs and axial skeleton have anecdotal effects of increasing stride length and joint range of motion and improving overall comfort (Fig. 8).[66] In a noncontrolled study, passive thoracic limb stretching lowered wither height as a result of possible relaxation of the fibromuscular thoracic girdle.[82] However, a randomized controlled trial in riding school horses evaluating the effect of 2 different 8-week passive stretching programs reported no significant changes in stride length at the trot but had a detrimental effect of decreasing joint range of motion within the shoulder, stifle, and hock articulations.[83] The investigators concluded that daily stretching may be too intensive in normal horses and may actually cause negative biomechanical effects. Additional studies on the effects of different

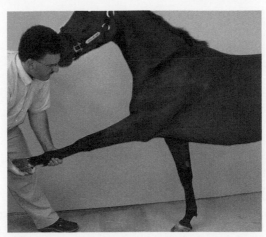

**Fig. 8.** Induced passive thoracic limb protraction. At the end range of motion, the horse is asked to actively extend the thoracic limb into the doctor's hands in an effort to stimulate neuromuscular reflexes and improve active protraction of the limb.

stretching techniques and frequency for specific disease processes using objective outcome measures need to be completed before any further claims of performance enhancement or pain reduction in horses can be made.

## SOFT TISSUE AND JOINT MOBILIZATION

Mobilization is defined as manually or mechanically induced movement of articulations or soft tissues for therapeutic purposes. Soft tissue mobilization focuses on restoring movement to the skin, connective tissue, ligaments, tendons, and muscles with the goal of modulating pain, reducing inflammation, improving tissue repair, increasing extensibility, and improving function.[51] Neural mobilization techniques have been developed to induce movement within specific spinal or peripheral nerves and the dura mater with the intent of reducing neural adhesions and edema.[21,32] Joint mobilization is characterized as nonimpulsive repetitive joint movements induced within the passive range of joint motion with the purpose of restoring normal and symmetric joint range of motion, to stretch connective tissues, and to reduce pain (**Fig. 9**).[84] Biomechanical characteristics of joint mobilization include low velocity movements, low peak forces, and large displacements. Mobilization is typically applied with oscillatory forces within or at the limits of physiologic joint range of motion without imparting a thrust or impulse. Mobilization is also performed within the patient's ability to resist the applied motion and therefore requires cooperation and relaxation of the patient. Joint mobilization is usually applied in a graded manner, with each grade increasing the range of joint movement. Grade 1 and 2 mobilizations are characterized by slow oscillations within the first 25% to 50% of the available joint motion, with the goal of reducing pain. Grade 3 and 4 mobilizations involve slow oscillations at or near the end of available joint motion, which are used to increase joint range of motion. Some soft tissue and joint mobilization techniques may include a hold and stretch at the end range of motion.

Soft tissue and joint mobilization is used to assess the quality and quantity of joint range of motion and as a primary means of treating musculoskeletal disorders. Adjunctive physical therapy techniques include therapeutic exercises and rehabilitation of

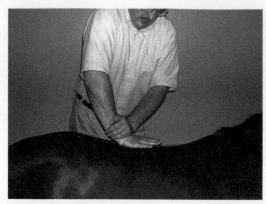

**Fig. 9.** Spinal mobilization at the thoracolumbar junction. A ventral force is applied rhythmically to assess the quality and quantity of passive joint range of motion and the joint endfeel (ie, anatomic limit of the articulation) in extension at sequential intervertebral levels.

neuromotor control, where manual forces are used to induce passive stretching, weight shifting or activation of spinal reflexes, which help to increase flexibility, stimulate proprioception and strengthen core musculature.[32,65] There is strong evidence that a multimodal approach of cervical mobilization, manipulation, and exercise are effective for reducing pain, improving function, and producing favorable long-term global effects in human patients with subacute and chronic mechanical neck disorders.[74] Active range of motion exercises may be more effective for acute pain reduction in human patients with whiplash-associated disorders.[85] There is mediate evidence in humans that mobilization and manipulation produce similar effects on pain, function, and patient satisfaction at intermediate-term follow-up.[86] Peripheral nerve and nerve root mobilization techniques and exercises are also used for the postoperative rehabilitation of low back pain.[87]

Few formal studies exist to support the use of active soft tissue, joint, or spinal mobilization techniques in horses.[28] Most mobilization studies in horses involve a period of induced joint immobilization by a fixture or cast followed by allowing the horse to spontaneously weight bear and locomote on the affected limb, without evaluation of specific soft tissue or joint mobilization techniques.[19] Spinal mobilization has been shown to be effective at increasing spinal flexibility in ridden horses without clinical signs of back pain.[29] Spinal manipulation, characterized by high-velocity, low-amplitude thrusts, produced immediate and larger increases in displacement within treatment sessions; whereas the effects of spinal mobilization had a delayed effect of increasing displacement, which suggests 2 possibly different mechanisms of action for spinal mobilization and manipulation.[88] Spinal mobilization is generally considered a more conservative or low-force technique applied in acute pain conditions; whereas manipulation is theoretically considered a more specific and forceful type of manual therapy that has shown more beneficial effects for chronic neck or back pain in humans.[16]

## MANIPULATION

Joint manipulation is characterized by the application of a high-velocity, low-amplitude thrust or impulse that moves a joint or vertebral segment beyond its physiologic range of motion, without exceeding the anatomic limit of the articulation.[89] Differences in the magnitude and rate of loading associated with mobilization versus manipulation are likely to produce variable therapeutic effects because of the viscoelastic nature of the soft tissues surrounding the vertebral column.[88,90] Spinal manipulation involves the application of controlled thrust or impulse to articular structures within the axial skeleton with the intent of reducing pain and muscle hypertonicity and increasing joint range of motion.[91]

Both the chiropractic and osteopathic professions use high-velocity, low-amplitude thrusts to induce therapeutic effects in articular structures, muscle function, and neurologic reflexes with the goal of increasing joint range of motion and reducing pain.[4,92] Most human chiropractic patients seek care because of headaches or spinal pain; more than 70% have neck or lower back pain.[93] Human research has demonstrated reductions in pain and muscle hypertonicity and increased joint range of motion after chiropractic treatment.[16,25,94] In humans, osteopathic care significantly reduces low back pain and effects can persist for at least 3 months.[95] Few studies have assessed the efficacy of preventative spinal manipulation for managing chronic low back pain.[96] The therapeutic dose of joint manipulation is varied by the number of vertebrae or articulations treated, the amount of force applied, and the frequency and duration of treatment. Unfortunately, there is not good scientific evidence on which to base optimal dosage recommendations for continued care, therefore therapeutic trials are often used on an individual basis.[97] There is low quality evidence that cervical manipulation alone compared with a control may provide short-term pain relief following 1 to 4 treatment sessions, and that 9 to 12 sessions were superior to 3 treatments for pain and disability in patients with cervicogenic headache.[86] High-dose manipulation is superior to low-dose manipulation for chronic low back pain in the short-term.[98]

In horses, anecdotal evidence and clinical experience suggest that manipulation is an effective adjunctive modality for the conservative treatment of select musculoskeletal-related disorders.[99] However, therapeutic trials of spinal manipulation are often used because there is limited formal research available about the effectiveness of osteopathic or chiropractic techniques in equine practice. Equine osteopathic evaluation and treatment procedures have been described in textbooks and case reports, but no formal hypothesis-driven research exists.[92,100,101] Human osteopathic techniques also include highly controversial methods associated with mobilizing cranial bones and abdominal viscera, which have questionable application to horses.[92,102] The focus of recent equine chiropractic research has been on assessing the clinical effects of spinal manipulation on pain relief, improving flexibility, reducing muscle hypertonicity, and restoring spinal motion symmetry. Obvious criticism has been directed at the physical ability to even induce movement in the horse's back. Pilot work has shown that manually applied forces associated with chiropractic techniques are able to produced substantial segmental spinal motion.[103] Two randomized, controlled clinical trials using pressure algometry to assess mechanical nociceptive thresholds in the thoracolumbar region of horses have shown that both manual and instrument-assisted spinal manipulation can reduce back pain (or increase mechanical nociceptive thresholds).[58,104] Additional studies have assessed the effects of equine chiropractic techniques on increasing passive spinal mobility (ie, flexibility)[28,29] and reducing longissimus muscle tone.[105] The effect of manipulation on asymmetrical spinal movement patterns in horses with documented back pain suggest that chiropractic treatment elicits slight but significant changes in thoracolumbar and pelvic kinematics and that some of these changes are likely to be beneficial.[106,107]

## MANUAL-ASSISTED TECHNIQUES

In humans, the application of manual forces can be combined with a wide diversity of therapeutic or medical techniques to produce varying effects. Hand-held spring-loaded or electromechanical devices can be used to apply single or multiple impulses to articulations or tissues in a series of techniques named manually assisted, mechanical force procedures. It has been reported that approximately 40 N of force is required to activate mechanical and neurologic responses associated with spinal manipulation.[108] Manual impulses applied to the human cervical and lumbar spine range from 40 to 400 N and occur for 30 to 150 milliseconds. Similar amplitudes of force have been measured with instrument-assisted manipulations (ie, 72 N to 230 N); however, the impulse occurs for a much smaller time (ie, 0.1–5.0 milliseconds). It is hypothesized that the velocity of the applied force may be more important than the amplitude of the applied force.[108] Randomized studies have shown similar effectiveness using either manual or instrument-assisted treatment techniques.[109,110] Using a stick and mallet or similar percussive device to apply sharp mechanical forces to dorsal spinous processes has been reported in horses to reduce back pain and increase spinal range of motion, but controlled studies are lacking.[106] Theoretically, there is an increased risk for injury using instrument-assisted techniques or hammers to treat horses because of the possibility of applying excessive forces by inexperienced or lay practitioners with little or no knowledge of spinal or joint biomechanics.

Joint mobilization and manipulation can be combined with sedation or general anesthesia, which provides increased relaxation and analgesia for evaluation of subtle joint motion restrictions or treatment of joint contractures and spinal pain, without the influence of conscious pain or protective muscle guarding.[111] Manipulation under anesthesia generally consists of 4 stages: sedation, mobilization/stretching/traction, manipulation, and aftercare of active rehabilitation and additional manual therapy.[112] Indications for manipulation under anesthesia in humans include pain that will not allow conscious manipulation, conditions that do not respond to conscious spinal manipulation within 4 to 8 weeks, chronic joint or soft tissue fibrosis, acute myofascial rigidity and painful inhibition, severe joint dysfunction, refractory contained disc herniation, and multiple recurrences of a condition.[113] The risks of manipulation under sedation or general anesthesia include the inability of patients to provide verbal feedback on pain or to resist overzealous manipulation because intrinsic guarding mechanisms associated with voluntary muscle contraction are absent, which can produce an increased risk of iatrogenic injuries.[113] There is currently insufficient evidence to make any recommendations regarding the use of manipulation under anesthesia for chronic low back pain in humans.[112]

Spinal manipulation under sedation and anesthesia has been used in horses to address reduced joint mobility; however, controlled studies are lacking.[101,114,115] In a case series of 86 horses, 88% of horses maintained improved ranges of pain-free joint motion after cervical mobilization and sustained stretching at the end range of motion while under anesthesia.[114] Similar indications and risks associated with the mobilization or manipulation under anesthesia in humans are expected in horses. No significant adverse effects were reported with cervical mobilization under general anesthesia in horses.[114] Well-designed controlled studies are needed to further investigate the safety and effectiveness of these techniques in equine practice.

Manipulation combined with epidural analgesia or epidural medications consists of segmental anesthesia with simultaneous epidural corticosteroid injection and spinal manipulation.[111] In humans, epidural anesthesia is less costly and is associated with fewer risks than general anesthesia, patients are able to cooperate during treatment, and epidural corticosteroids reduce inflammation and reduce fibrosis and adhesions, compared with manipulation under anesthesia alone. One possible indication for using this technique in horses is severe or compensatory spinal pain or stiffness associated with chronic limb lameness.

Joint mobilization or manipulation combined with intraarticular injection of either local anesthetic or corticosteroids has also been reported to reduce pain and inflammation associated with osteoarthritis and is believed to more effectively restore joint mobility.[111] Indications in humans include recalcitrant joint pain that prevents mobilization or rehabilitation of the affected region. In horses, one possible indication includes cervical facet osteoarthritis, where acute pain and inflammation can be initially controlled with intraarticular facet injections; however, recurrent stiffness and disability are common. Intraarticular injections combined with a series of spinal manipulations, stretching, and strengthening exercises provides the opportunity to increase pain-free cervical mobility and reduce long-term morbidly or recurrence. Controlled clinical trials are needed to assess other possible clinical indications and effectiveness of manipulation combined with intraarticular injections in horses.

## INDICATIONS FOR MANUAL THERAPIES

Most of the current knowledge about equine manual therapies has been borrowed from human techniques, theories, and research, and applied to horses. Therapeutic trials are often used because of limited knowledge about the effectiveness for specific disease conditions or the duration of action of select manual therapies in horses. The indications for joint mobilization and manipulation are similar and include restricted joint range of motion, muscle spasms, pain, fibrosis, or contracted soft tissues.[84] The principal indications for spinal manipulation are neck or back pain, localized or regional joint stiffness, poor performance, and altered gait that is not associated with overt lameness. A thorough diagnostic workup is required to identify soft tissue and osseous disorders, neurologic disorders, or other lameness conditions that may not be responsive to manual therapy. Clinical signs that indicate a primary spinal disorder include localized musculoskeletal pain, muscle hypertonicity, and restricted joint motion. This triad of clinical signs can also be found in a variety of lower limb disorders; however, they are most evident in horses with neck or back problems. Clinical signs that indicate chronic or secondary spinal disorders include regional or diffuse pain, generalized stiffness, and widespread muscle hypertonicity. In these cases, further diagnostic evaluation or imaging should be done to identify the primary cause of lameness or poor performance. Manual therapy may help in the management of muscular, articular, and neurologic components of select musculoskeletal injuries in performance horses. Musculoskeletal conditions that are chronic or recurring, not readily diagnosed, or are not responding to conventional veterinary care may be indicators that manual therapy evaluation and treatment is needed. Manual therapy is usually more effective in the early clinical stages of disease processes versus end-stage disease when reparative processes have been exhausted. Joint manipulation is usually contraindicated in the acute stages of soft tissue injury; however, mobilization is safer than manipulation and has been shown to have short-term benefits for acute neck or back pain in humans.[116] Manipulation is probably more effective than mobilization for chronic neck or back pain and has the potential to help restore normal joint motion, thus limiting the risk of reinjury.[18]

Contraindications for mobilization and manipulation are often based on clinical judgment and are related to the technique applied and skill or experience of the practitioner.[84] Few absolute contraindications exist for joint mobilization if techniques are applied appropriately. Manual therapy is not a cure-all for all joint or back problems and is generally contraindicated in the presence of fractures, acute inflammatory or infectious joint disease, osteomyelitis, joint ankylosis, bleeding disorders, progressive neurologic signs, and primary or metastatic tumors.[84] Joint mobilization and manipulation cannot reverse severe degenerative processes or overt pathology. Acute episodes of osteoarthritis, impinged dorsal spinous processes, and severe articular instability, such as joint subluxation or luxation, are often contraindications for manipulation. Inadequate physical or spinal examinations and poorly developed manipulative skills are also contraindications for applying manual therapy.[113] All horses with neurologic diseases should be evaluated fully to assess the potential risks or benefits of joint mobilization or manipulation. Cervical vertebral myelopathy occurs because of both structural and functional disorders.[117] Static compression caused by vertebral malformation and dynamic lesions caused by vertebral segment hypermobility are contraindications for cervical manipulation; however, adjacent regions of hypomobile vertebrae may benefit from mobilization or manipulation to help restore joint motion and reduce biomechanical stresses in the affected vertebral segments. Life-threatening injuries or diseases requiring immediate medical or surgical care need to be ruled out and treated by conventional veterinary medicine before any routine manual therapy is initiated. However, manual techniques may contribute to the rehabilitation of most postsurgical cases or severe musculoskeletal injuries by helping to restore normal joint motion and function. Horses that have concurrent hock pain (eg, osteoarthritis) and a stiff, painful thoracolumbar or lumbosacral vertebral region are best managed by addressing all areas of musculoskeletal dysfunction. A multidisciplinary approach entails combined medical treatment of the hock osteoarthritis and manual therapy evaluation and treatment of the back problem.

In humans, adverse effects or risks of complications associated with joint mobilization are minimal. Mobilization is considered safer than manipulation.[116] Some investigators suggest that given the higher risk of adverse reactions and lack of demonstrated effectiveness of manipulation over mobilization, then manual therapists should consider conservative mobilization, especially in human patients with severe neck pain.[118] In humans, most adverse events associated with spinal manipulation are benign and self-limiting.[119] Potential mild adverse effects from properly applied manipulations include transient stiffness or worsening of the condition after treatment. Data from prospective studies suggest that minor, transient adverse events occur in approximately half of all patients during a course of spinal manipulative therapy.[120,121] However, these mild adverse effects do not cause patients to stop seeking manipulative care. Mild adverse effects usually last less than 1 to 2 days and resolve without concurrent medical intervention. Severe complications following spinal manipulation are typically uncommon and estimates of the incidence range from 1 in 200,000 to 1 per 100 million manipulations in humans.[116,122,123] The most common serious adverse events in humans are vertebrobasilar accidents, disk herniation, and cauda equina syndrome.[120] However, there is no evidence of increased risk of vertebrobasilar artery stroke associated with chiropractic care compared with primary medical care.[124] Even though the complication rate of spinal manipulation is small, the potential for adverse outcomes must be considered because of the possibility of permanent impairment or death.[116] The benefits of chiropractic care in humans seem to outweigh the potential risks.[125] The risk of adverse effects associated with joint mobilization or spinal manipulation is unknown in horses. The apparent safety of spinal manipulation, especially compared with other medically accepted treatments for neck or low back pain in humans, should stimulate its use in the conservative treatment of spinal-related problems.[123,126] If an exacerbation of musculoskeletal dysfunction or lameness is noted after spinal manipulation, then a thorough re-examination and appropriate medical treatment should be pursued. If the condition does not improve with conservative care, referral for more extensive diagnostic evaluation or more aggressive medical treatment is recommended.

## FUTURE STUDIES

Further research is needed to assess the effectiveness of specific manual therapy recommendations or combined treatments for pain management and select lameness conditions. Currently there is no validated equine model for studying the effects of manual therapies that would allow characterization of the anatomic, biomechanical, neurophysiologic, pathophysiologic, cellular, or biochemical changes associated with soft tissue and joint mobilization or high-velocity thrusts. Further understanding of the local and systemic effects of mobilization and manipulation on pain reduction and tissue healing is also needed. Additional studies are needed to determine the duration of the clinical effects of manual therapies and the multimodal use of mobilization or manipulation and analgesics or other pain management strategies. Controlled trials using different forms of spinal manipulation (eg, manual thrusts vs instrument-assisted thrusts vs manipulation under anesthesia) need to be done to determine which method is most effective for addressing specific disease processes. Studies are needed to identify which pain or patient characteristics are likely to benefit from the various forms of manual therapy, either individually or in combination. New methods of objectively measuring musculoskeletal dysfunction and further studies into the pathophysiology of chronic pain syndromes are needed to help assess the effectiveness of manual therapies on reducing morbidity and improving overall performance in equine athletes.

## SUMMARY

A thorough knowledge of equine anatomy, soft tissue and joint biomechanics, musculoskeletal pathology, tissue-healing processes, and pain mechanisms is required to understand the basic principles and application of the various forms of manual therapies for pain management. There is a notable lack of evidence for using touch, massage, stretching exercises, and joint mobilization techniques in horses. However, spinal manipulation has been shown in several studies to be effective for reducing pain, improving flexibility, reducing muscle tone, and improving symmetry of spinal kinematics in horses. Because of potential misuse and safety issues, mobilization and manipulative therapies should be provided only by specially trained veterinarians or licensed human manual therapists.

## REFERENCES

1. Haldeman S, Hooper PD. Mobilization, manipulation, massage and exercise for the relief of musculoskeletal pain. In: Wall PD, Melzack R, editors. Textbook of pain. 4th edition. New York: Churchill Livingstone; 1999. p. 1399–418.
2. Ramey D, Ernst E. Common misconceptions about alternative medicine. In: Ramey D, editor. Consumer's guide to alternative therapies in the horse. Foster City (CA): Howell Book House; 1999. p. 35–42.
3. Lederman E. Fundamentals of manual therapy: physiology, neurology and psychology. St. Louis (MO): Churchill Livingstone; 1997.
4. Bergmann TF. High-velocity low-amplitude manipulative techniques. In: Haldeman S, editor. Principles and practice of chiropractic. 3rd edition. New York: McGraw-Hill; 2005. p. 755–66.
5. Taylor PM, Pascoe PJ, Marna KR. Diagnosing and treating pain in the horse. Where are we today? Vet Clin North Am Equine Pract 2002;18(1):1–19, v.
6. Muir W. Recognizing and treating pain in horses. In: Reed SM, Bayly WM, Sellon DC, editors. Equine internal medicine. 2nd edition. St. Louis (MO): Saunders; 2004. p. 1529–41.

7. Imamura M, Furlan AD, Dryden T, et al. Evidence-informed management of chronic low back pain with massage. Spine J 2008;8(1):121–33.

8. Pickar JG. Neurophysiological effects of spinal manipulation. Spine J 2002;2(5):357–71.

9. Colloca CJ, Keller TS, Gunzburg R. Neuromechanical characterization of in vivo lumbar spinal manipulation. Part II. Neurophysiological response. J Manipulative Physiol Ther 2003;26(9):579–91.

10. Vernon H. Qualitative review of studies of manipulation-induced hypoalgesia. J Manipulative Physiol Ther 2000;23(2):134–8.

11. Boal RW, Gillette RG. Central neuronal plasticity, low back pain and spinal manipulative therapy. J Manipulative Physiol Ther 2004;27:314–26.

12. Wright A. Hypoalgesia post-manipulative therapy: a review of a potential neurophysiological mechanism. Man Ther 1995;1(1):11–6.

13. Wall PD. The placebo and the placebo response. In: Wall PD, Melzack R, editors. Textbook of pain. 4th edition. New York: Churchill Livingstone; 1999. p. 1419–30.

14. Triano J. The theoretical basis for spinal manipulation. In: Haldeman S, editor. Principles and practice of chiropractic. 3rd edition. New York: McGraw-Hill; 2005. p. 361–81.

15. Lederman E. The biomechanical response. Fundamentals of manual therapy: physiology, neurology and psychology. St. Louis (MO): Churchill Livingstone; 1997. p. 23–37.

16. Bronfort G, Haas M, Evans RL, et al. Efficacy of spinal manipulation and mobilization for low back pain and neck pain: a systematic review and best evidence synthesis. Spine J 2004;4(3):335–56.

17. Threlkeld AJ. The effects of manual therapy on connective tissue. Phys Ther 1992;72(12):893–902.

18. Liebenson C. Rehabilitation of the spine. 1st edition. Baltimore (MD): Williams & Wilkins; 1996.

19. van Harreveld PD, Lillich JD, Kawcak CE, et al. Clinical evaluation of the effects of immobilization followed by remobilization and exercise on the metacarpophalangeal joint in horses. Am J Vet Res 2002;63(2):282–8.

20. Lederman E. Changes in tissue fluid dynamics. In: Lederman E, editor. Fundamentals of manual therapy: physiology, neurology and psychology. St. Louis (MO): Churchill Livingstone; 1997. p. 39–54.

21. Gruenenfelder FI, Boos A, Mouwen M, et al. Evaluation of the anatomic effect of physical therapy exercises for mobilization of lumbar spinal nerves and the dura mater in dogs. Am J Vet Res 2006;67(10):1773–9.

22. Leach RA. Segmental dysfunction hypothesis. The chiropractic theories: principles and clinical applications. 3rd edition. Baltimore (MD): Williams & Wilkins; 1994. p. 43–54.

23. Pickar JG, Sung PS, Kang YM, et al. Response of lumbar paraspinal muscles spindles is greater to spinal manipulative loading compared with slower loading under length control. Spine J 2007;7(5):583–95.

24. Cleland JA, Glynn P, Whitman JM, et al. Short-term effects of thrust versus non-thrust mobilization/manipulation directed at the thoracic spine in patients with neck pain: a randomized clinical trial. Phys Ther 2007;87(4):431–40.

25. Cassidy JD, Lopes AA, Yong-Hing K. The immediate effect of manipulation versus mobilization on pain and range of motion in the cervical spine: a randomized controlled trial. J Manipulative Physiol Ther 1992;15(9):570–5.

26. Gross AR, Hoving JL, Haines TA, et al. A Cochrane review of manipulation and mobilization for mechanical neck disorders. Spine (Phla Pa 1976) 2004;29(14):1541–8.

27. Bolton PS, Budgell BS. Spinal manipulation and spinal mobilization influence different axial sensory beds. Med Hypotheses 2006;66(2):258–62.
28. Haussler KK, Hill AE, Puttlitz CM, et al. Effects of vertebral mobilization and manipulation on kinematics of the thoracolumbar region. Am J Vet Res 2007; 68(5):508–16.
29. Haussler KK, Martin CE, Hill AE. Efficacy of spinal manipulation and mobilization on trunk flexibility and stiffness in horses: a randomized clinical trial. Equine Vet J Suppl, in press.
30. Triano JJ. Studies on the biomechanical effect of a spinal adjustment. J Manipulative Physiol Ther 1992;15(1):71–5.
31. Dishman JD, Burke J. Spinal reflex excitability changes after cervical and lumbar spinal manipulation: a comparative study. Spine J 2003;3(3):204–12.
32. Goff LM. Manual therapy of the horse – a contemporary perspective. J Equine Vet Sci 2009;29(11):799–808.
33. Cameron MH. Physical agents in rehabilitation. Philadelphia: WB Saunders; 1999.
34. Schmid A, Brunner F, Wright A, et al. Paradigm shift in manual therapy? Evidence for a central nervous system component in the response to passive cervical joint mobilisation. Man Ther 2008;13(5):387–96.
35. Nansel D, Szlazak M. Somatic dysfunction and the phenomenon of visceral disease simulation: a probable explanation for the apparent effectiveness of somatic therapy in patients presumed to be suffering from true visceral disease. J Manipulative Physiol Ther 1995;18(6):379–97.
36. Moyer CA, Rounds J, Hannum JW. A meta-analysis of massage therapy research. Psychol Bull 2004;130(1):3–18.
37. Coppa D. The internal process of therapeutic touch. J Holist Nurs 2008;26(1): 17–24.
38. Friedmann E, Son H. The human-companion animal bond: how humans benefit. Vet Clin North Am Small Anim Pract 2009;39(2):293–326.
39. Braun C, Stangler T, Narveson J, et al. Animal-assisted therapy as a pain relief intervention for children. Complement Ther Clin Pract 2009;15(2):105–9.
40. McBride SD, Hemmings A, Robinson K. A preliminary study on the effect of massage to reduce stress in the horse. J Equine Vet Sci 2004;24(2):76–82.
41. Monroe CM. The effects of therapeutic touch on pain. J Holist Nurs 2009;27(2): 85–92.
42. So PS, Jiang Y, Qin Y. Touch therapies for pain relief in adults. Cochrane Database Syst Rev 2008;(4):CD006535.
43. Edelson SM, Edelson MG, Kerr DC, et al. Behavioral and physiological effects of deep pressure on children with autism: a pilot study evaluating the efficacy of Grandin's Hug Machine. Am J Occup Ther 1999;53(2):145–52.
44. Grandin T. Calming effects of deep touch pressure in patients with autistic disorder, college students, and animals. J Child Adolesc Psychopharmacol 1992;2(1):63–72.
45. Bardia A, Barton DL, Prokop LJ, et al. Efficacy of complementary and alternative medicine therapies in relieving cancer pain: a systematic review. J Clin Oncol 2006;24(34):5457–64.
46. Tellington-Jones L, Lieberman B. The ultimate horse behavior and training book. North Pomfret (VT): Trafalgar Square Books; 2006.
47. Spier SJ, Berger Pusterla J, Villarroel A, et al. Outcome of tactile conditioning of neonates, or "imprint training" on selected handling measures in foals. Vet J 2004;168(3):252–8.

48. Scott M, Swenson LA. Evaluating the benefits of equine massage therapy: a review of the evidence and current practices. J Equine Vet Sci 2009;29(9): 687–97.

49. Frey Law LA, Evans S, Knudtson J, et al. Massage reduces pain perception and hyperalgesia in experimental muscle pain: a randomized, controlled trial. J Pain 2008;9(8):714–21.

50. Cherkin DC, Eisenberg D, Sherman KJ, et al. Randomized trial comparing traditional Chinese medical acupuncture, therapeutic massage, and self-care education for chronic low back pain. Arch Intern Med 2001;161(8):1081–8.

51. Bromiley MW. Massage techniques for horse and rider. Wiltshire (UK): The Crowood Press; 2002.

52. Hemmings BJ. Physiological, psychological and performance effects of massage in sport: a review of the literature. Phys Ther Sport 2001;2:165–70.

53. Furlan AD, Imamura M, Dryden T, et al. Massage for low-back pain. Cochrane Database Syst Rev 2008;(4):CD001929.

54. Ernst E. Massage therapy for low back pain: a systematic review. J Pain Symptom Manage 1999;17(1):65–9.

55. Ernst E. Massage therapy for cancer palliation and supportive care: a systematic review of randomised clinical trials. Support Care Cancer 2009;17(4):333–7.

56. Wilkinson S, Barnes K, Storey L. Massage for symptom relief in patients with cancer: systematic review. J Adv Nurs 2008;63(5):430–9.

57. Ernst E. Manual therapies for pain control: chiropractic and massage. Clin J Pain 2004;20(1):8–12.

58. Sullivan KA, Hill AE, Haussler KK. The effects of chiropractic, massage and phenylbutazone on spinal mechanical nociceptive thresholds in horses without clinical signs. Equine Vet J 2008;40(1):14–20.

59. Wilson J. The effects of sports massage on athletic performance and general function. Massage Therapy J 2002;90–100, Summer.

60. Fedele C, Berens von Rautenfeld D. Manual lymph drainage for equine lymphoedema-treatment strategy and therapist training. Equine Vet Educ 2007; 19(1):26–31, February.

61. Ladd MP, Kottke FJ, Blanchard RS. Studies of the effect of massage on the flow of lymph from the foreleg of the dog. Arch Phys Med 1952;604–12, October.

62. Ramey DW, Tiidus PM. Massage therapy in horses: assessing its effectiveness from empirical data in humans and animals. Compendium 2002;24(5):418–23.

63. Buchner HH, Schildboeck U. Physiotherapy applied to the horse: a review. Equine Vet J 2006;38(6):574–80.

64. Blignault K. Stretch exercises for your horse. London: JA Allen; 2003.

65. Stubbs NC, Clayton HM. Activate your horse's core: unmounted exercises for dynamic mobility, strength and balance. Mason (MI): Sport Horse Publications; 2008.

66. Frick A. Fitness in motion: keeping your equine's zone at peak performance. Guilford (CT): The Lyons Press; 2007.

67. Decoster LC, Cleland J, Altieri C, et al. The effects of hamstring stretching on range of motion: a systematic literature review. J Orthop Sports Phys Ther 2005;35(6):377–87.

68. Light KE, Nuzik S, Personius W, et al. Low-load prolonged stretch vs. high-load brief stretch in treating knee contractures. Phys Ther 1984;64(3):330–3.

69. Taylor DC, Dalton JD Jr, Seaber AV, et al. Viscoelastic properties of muscle-tendon units. The biomechanical effects of stretching. Am J Sports Med 1990; 18(3):300–9.

70. Bandy WD, Irion JM. The effect of time on static stretch on the flexibility of the hamstring muscles. Phys Ther 1994;74(9):845–50.
71. da Costa BR, Vieira ER. Stretching to reduce work-related musculoskeletal disorders: a systematic review. J Rehabil Med 2008;40(5):321–8.
72. Frick A. Stretching exercises for horses: are they effective? J Equine Vet Sci 2010;30(1):50–9.
73. Radford JA, Burns J, Buchbinder R, et al. Does stretching increase ankle dorsi-flexion range of motion? A systematic review. Br J Sports Med 2006;40(10): 870–5 [discussion: 875].
74. Gross AR, Goldsmith C, Hoving JL, et al. Conservative management of mechan-ical neck disorders: a systematic review. J Rheumatol 2007;34(5):1083–102.
75. Harvey L, Herbert R, Crosbie J. Does stretching induce lasting increases in joint ROM? A systematic review. Physiother Res Int 2002;7(1):1–13.
76. Shrier I. Does stretching improve performance? A systematic and critical review of the literature. Clin J Sport Med 2004;14(5):267–73.
77. Thacker SB, Gilchrist J, Stroup DF, et al. The impact of stretching on sports injury risk: a systematic review of the literature. Med Sci Sports Exerc 2004; 36(3):371–8.
78. Herbert RD, Gabriel M. Effects of stretching before and after exercising on muscle soreness and risk of injury: systematic review. Br Med J 2002; 325(7362):468.
79. Small K, Mc Naughton L, Matthews M. A systematic review into the efficacy of static stretching as part of a warm-up for the prevention of exercise-related injury. Res Sports Med 2008;16(3):213–31.
80. Hayden JA, van Tulder MW, Tomlinson G. Systematic review: strategies for using exercise therapy to improve outcomes in chronic low back pain. Ann Intern Med 2005;142(9):776–85.
81. Kay TM, Gross A, Goldsmith C, et al. Exercises for mechanical neck disorders. Cochrane Database Syst Rev 2005;(3):CD004250.
82. Giovagnoli G, Plebani G, Daubon JC. Withers height variations after muscle stretching. Proceedings Conference on Equine Sports Medicine and Science. Oslo, Norway, CESMAS, 2004. p. 172–6.
83. Rose NS, Northrop AJ, Brigden CV, et al. Effects of a stretching regime on stride length and range of motion in equine trot. Vet J 2009;181(1):53–5.
84. Scaringe J, Kawaoka C. Mobilization techniques. In: Haldeman S, editor. Princi-ples and practice of chiropractic. 3rd edition. New York: McGraw-Hill; 2005. p. 767–85.
85. McKinney LA. Early mobilisation and outcome in acute sprains of the neck. Br Med J 1989;299(6706):1006–8.
86. Gross A, Miller J, D'Sylva J, et al. Manipulation or mobilisation for neck pain. Co-chrane Database Syst Rev 2010;(1):CD004249.
87. Ellis RF, Hing WA. Neural mobilization: a systematic review of randomized controlled trials with an analysis of therapeutic efficacy. J Man Manip Ther 2008;16(1):8–22.
88. Keller TS, Colloca CJ, Gunzburg R. Neuromechanical characterization of in vivo lumbar spinal manipulation. Part I. Vertebral motion. J Manipulative Physiol Ther 2003;26(9):567–78.
89. Gatterman MI. What's in a word. In: Gatterman MI, editor. Foundations of chiro-practic. St. Louis (MO): Mosby-Year Book; 1995. p. 5–17.
90. Harms MC, Bader DL. Variability of forces applied by experienced therapists during spinal mobilization. Clin Biomech (Bristol, Avon) 1997;12(6):393–9.

91. Haussler KK. Chiropractic evaluation and management. Vet Clin North Am Equine Pract 1999;15(1):195–209.
92. Verschooten F. Osteopathy in locomotion problems of the horse: a critical evaluation. Vlaams Diergeneeskd Tijdschr 1992;61:116–20.
93. Coulter ID, Hurwitz EL, Adams AH, et al. Patients using chiropractors in North America: who are they, and why are they in chiropractic care? Spine (Phila Pa 1976) 2002;27(3):291–6 [discussion: 297–8].
94. Nansel DD, Waldorf T, Cooperstein R. Effect of cervical spinal adjustments on lumbar paraspinal muscle tone: evidence for facilitation of intersegmental tonic neck reflexes. J Manipulative Physiol Ther 1993;16(2):91–5.
95. Licciardone JC, Brimhall AK, King LN. Osteopathic manipulative treatment for low back pain: a systematic review and meta-analysis of randomized controlled trials. BMC Musculoskelet Disord 2005;6:43.
96. Descarreaux M, Blouin JS, Drolet M, et al. Efficacy of preventive spinal manipulation for chronic low-back pain and related disabilities: a preliminary study. J Manipulative Physiol Ther 2004;27(8):509–14.
97. Bronfort G, Haas M, Evans R. The clinical effectiveness of spinal manipulation for musculoskeletal conditions. In: Haldeman S, editor. Principles and practice of chiropractic. 3rd edition. New York: McGraw-Hill; 2005. p. 147–66.
98. Haas M, Groupp E, Kraemer DF. Dose-response for chiropractic care of chronic low back pain. Spine J 2004;4(5):574–83.
99. Herrod-Taylor EE. A technique for manipulation of the spine in horses. Vet Rec 1967;81:437–9.
100. Evrard P. Introduction aux techniques ostéopathiques struturelles appliquées au cheval. Thy-Le-Château: Olivier éditeur; 2002.
101. Pusey A, Colles C, Brooks J. Osteopathic treatment of horses – a retrospective study. Br Osteo J 1995;16:30–2.
102. Parsons J, Marcer N. Osteopathy: models for diagnosis, treatment and practice. Philadelphia: Churchill Livingstone; 2006.
103. Haussler KK, Bertram JEA, Gellman K. In-vivo segmental kinematics of the thoracolumbar spinal region in horses and effects of chiropractic manipulations. Proc Am Assoc Equine Practitioners 1999;45:327–9.
104. Haussler KK, Erb HN. Pressure algometry: objective assessment of back pain and effects of chiropractic treatment. Proc Am Assoc Equine Practitioners 2003;49:66–70.
105. Wakeling JM, Barnett K, Price S, et al. Effects of manipulative therapy on the longissimus dorsi in the equine back. Equine Comp Exerc Physiol 2006;3(3): 153–60.
106. Faber MJ, van Weeren PR, Schepers M, et al. Long-term follow-up of manipulative treatment in a horse with back problems. J Vet Med A Physiol Pathol Clin Med 2003;50(5):241–5.
107. Gómez Alvarez CB, L'Ami JJ, Moffat D, et al. Effect of chiropractic manipulations on the kinematics of back and limbs in horses with clinically diagnosed back problems. Equine Vet J 2008;40(2):153–9.
108. Fuhr AW, Menke JM. Status of activator methods chiropractic technique, theory, and practice. J Manipulative Physiol Ther 2005;28(2):e1–20.
109. Shearar KA, Colloca CJ, White HL. A randomized clinical trial of manual versus mechanical force manipulation in the treatment of sacroiliac joint syndrome. J Manipulative Physiol Ther 2005;28(7):493–501.
110. Wood TG, Colloca CJ, Matthews R. A pilot randomized clinical trial on the relative effect of instrumental (MFMA) versus manual (HVLA) manipulation in the

treatment of cervical spine dysfunction. J Manipulative Physiol Ther 2001;24(4): 260–71.

111. Kohlbeck FJ, Haldeman S. Medication-assisted spinal manipulation. Spine J 2002;2(4):288–302.

112. Dagenais S, Mayer J, Wooley JR, et al. Evidence-informed management of chronic low back pain with medicine-assisted manipulation. Spine J 2008; 8(1):142–9.

113. West DT, Mathews RS, Miller MR, et al. Effective management of spinal pain in one hundred seventy-seven patients evaluated for manipulation under anesthesia. J Manipulative Physiol Ther 1999;22(5):299–308.

114. Ahern TJ. Cervical vertebral mobilization under anesthetic (CVMUA): a physical therapy for the treatment of cervico-spinal pain and stiffness. J Equine Vet Sci 1994;14(10):540–5.

115. Brooks J, Colles C, Pusey A. The role of osteopathy in the treatment of the horse. In: Rossdale P, Green R, editors. Guardians of the horse II. Newmarket (UK): Romney Publications; 2001. p. 40–9.

116. Hurwitz EL, Aker PD, Adams AH, et al. Manipulation and mobilization of the cervical spine. A systematic review of the literature. Spine (Phila Pa 1976) 1996;21(15):1746–59 [discussion: 1759–60].

117. Levine JM, Adam E, MacKay RJ, et al. Confirmed and presumptive cervical vertebral compressive myelopathy in older horses: a retrospective study (1992–2004). J Vet Intern Med 2007;21(4):812–9.

118. Hurwitz EL, Morgenstern H, Vassilaki M, et al. Frequency and clinical predictors of adverse reactions to chiropractic care in the UCLA neck pain study. Spine (Phila Pa 1976) 2005;30(13):1477–84.

119. Rubinstein SM. Adverse events following chiropractic care for subjects with neck or low-back pain: do the benefits outweigh the risks? J Manipulative Physiol Ther 2008;31(6):461–4.

120. Stevinson C, Ernst E. Risks associated with spinal manipulation. Am J Med 2002;112(7):566–71.

121. Senstad O, Leboeuf-Yde C, Borchgrevink C. Frequency and characteristics of side effects of spinal manipulative therapy. Spine (Phila Pa 1976) 1997;22(4): 435–40 [discussion: 440–1].

122. Thiel HW, Bolton JE, Docherty S, et al. Safety of chiropractic manipulation of the cervical spine: a prospective national survey. Spine (Phila Pa 1976) 2007; 32(21):2375–8 [discussion: 2379].

123. Oliphant D. Safety of spinal manipulation in the treatment of lumbar disk herniations: a systematic review and risk assessment. J Manipulative Physiol Ther 2004;27(3):197–210.

124. Cassidy JD, Boyle E, Cote P, et al. Risk of vertebrobasilar stroke and chiropractic care: results of a population-based case-control and case-crossover study. Spine (Phila Pa 1976) 2008;33(Suppl 4):S176–83.

125. Rubinstein SM, Leboeuf-Yde C, Knol DL, et al. The benefits outweigh the risks for patients undergoing chiropractic care for neck pain: a prospective, multicenter, cohort study. J Manipulative Physiol Ther 2007;30(6):408–18.

126. Dabbs V, Lauretti WJ. A risk assessment of cervical manipulation vs. NSAIDs for the treatment of neck pain. J Manipulative Physiol Ther 1995;18(8):530–6.

# Treatment of Visceral Pain in Horses

Sheilah A. Robertson, BVMS, PhD, MRCVS[a],*,
L. Chris Sanchez, DVM, PhD[b]

**KEYWORDS**

- Colic • Visceral pain • Analgesia • Opioids
- Nonsteroidal anti-inflammatory agents • Lidocaine

Visceral pain can be defined as pain originating in any internal organ and is often subdivided to include the organs contained within each major body cavity, which are the thorax, abdomen, and pelvis (**Table 1**). Using this categorization, pain arising from the bladder would be a form of pelvic visceral pain. The term "colic" should be clearly defined because it is often misused. "Colic" is not a diagnosis; it is a clinical sign resulting from visceral pain within the abdomen. Mair and colleagues[1] state that there are approximately 100 conditions that result in abdominal pain in the horse, but the most common sources are the small and large intestine, hence the term "colic" most typically refers to gastrointestinal pain. Visceral pain may be acute, chronic, or recurrent in fashion, and some individuals may experience a combination of these manifestations. The cause of visceral pain may be organic (identifiable structural change in an organ) or dysfunctional (an abnormal change in organ function without identifiable pathologic changes).[2] Irritable bowel syndrome (IBS) in humans is an example of a dysfunctional disease that may affect up to 25% of the population[2]; whether similar syndromes exist in horses is less clear, but is considered plausible.[3,4] Ischemia, inflammation, muscle contraction (spasm) or distension may be the primary underlying cause of pain, and identifying which of these is responsible for the patient's discomfort is important for directing therapy. Considering the number of internal organs, it is not surprising that visceral pain is common in horses; however, it presents a challenge to the clinician because it can be difficult to make a definitive diagnosis. Ideally treatment is aimed at addressing the underlying pathology, but is often symptomatic with a primary focus on relieving pain; the latter is the focus of this article. Although treatment options for visceral pain have expanded in recent years, they remain suboptimal. In horses, the small and large intestines are the most prevalent

[a] Section of Anesthesia and Pain Management, Department of Large Animal Clinical Sciences, College of Veterinary Medicine, University of Florida, PO Box 100136, Gainesville, FL 32610-0136, USA
[b] Department of Large Animal Clinical Sciences, College of Veterinary Medicine, University of Florida, PO Box 100136, Gainesville, FL 32610-0136, USA
* Corresponding author.
*E-mail address:* robertsons@ufl.edu

Vet Clin Equine 26 (2010) 603–617
doi:10.1016/j.cveq.2010.08.002
0749-0739/10/$ – see front matter © 2010 Elsevier Inc. All rights reserved.

**Table 1**
**Origin and examples of visceral pain in the horse**

| Origin | Example: Acute | Example: Chronic |
|---|---|---|
| Thorax<br>  • Lung<br>  • Pleura<br>  • Esophagus<br>  • Heart | • Pleuropneumonia<br>• Choke<br>• Trauma<br>• Pericarditis | • Pleural abscessation<br>• Neoplasia<br>• Pericarditis |
| Abdomen<br>  • Stomach<br>  • Small intestine<br>  • Large intestine<br>    Cecum<br>    Large colon<br>    Small colon<br>  • Spleen<br>  • Liver<br>  • Pancreas<br>  • Kidneys<br>  • Ureters<br>  • Ovaries<br>  • Uterus | • Most causes of acute colic<br>• Pancreatitis<br>• Nephrolithiasis<br>• Uterine artery hematoma, rupture<br>• Metritis<br>• Cholelithiasis<br>• Uterine torsion | • Inflammatory bowel diseases<br>• Enterolithiasis<br>• Chronic diarrhea<br>• Nephrolithiasis<br>• Neoplasia<br>• Cholelithiasis |
| Pelvis<br>  • Bladder<br>  • Testicles<br>  • Rectum<br>  • Anus<br>  • Vagina | • Cystitis<br>• Urolithiasis<br>• Testicular torsion<br>• Rectal tear<br>• Foaling trauma<br>• Necrotic vaginitis | • Cystitis<br>• Urolithiasis<br>• Neoplasia |

source of visceral pain, and this type of pain has received the most research and clinical attention. The pleura, kidneys, and stomach are, however, well recognized sources of pain and resultant suffering in equine patients. Horses of all ages, breeds, and sex may present with visceral pain, and examples are given in **Table 1**.

## INCIDENCE AND IMPACT OF VISCERAL PAIN

Gastrointestinal and musculoskeletal diseases are two of the most clinically and economically important medical problems facing horses and their owners. In the National Animal Health Monitoring Systems (NAHMS) equine study conducted by the United States Department of Agriculture (USDA) in 2005, "colic" affected 2.4% of horses on a yearly basis (http://www.aphis.usda.gov/vs/ceah/ncahs/nahms/equine/equine98/economics.PDF). The economic impact of this was estimated to be $115 million per year in the equivalent study published in 1998 (http://www.aphis.usda.gov/vs/ceah/ncahs/nahms/equine/equine05/equine05reportpart1.pdf). These figures represent overall costs to the industry due to loss of use, hospitalization, veterinary care, and mortality.

## VISCERAL PAIN ASSESSMENT

When assessing pain in animals and nonverbal human beings, one must remember that the assessment is always based on observations and interpretation of what is seen. Thus, when addressing an animal's status, one must be aware of inherent differences based on species, age, sex, genetics, environment, and source and duration of the pain. Most published studies on visceral pain in horses, whether they are research or clinically based, are confined to abdominal causes and more specifically the intestinal tract.

## Research Models

For research models of pain in animals, Gebhart and Ness[5] proposed the following necessary criteria: the subject must be conscious, the experimental stimulus mimics a natural stimulus, the stimulus is minimally invasive and ethically acceptable, the stimulus is controllable, reproducible, and quantifiable, and the responses are reliable and quantifiable. Most models of visceral pain in horses and other species involve acute distension of a portion of the gastrointestinal tract. Because many naturally occurring conditions causing abdominal visceral pain involve distension, such models have provided clinically meaningful information regarding analgesic medications for use in the horse. These models have involved cecal,[6,7] duodenal,[8–10] and colorectal[11,12] distension. The primary advantage of the cecal and duodenal distension models is that both the stimulus (distension) and associated behaviors (pawing, flank watching, and so forth) mimic the clinical syndrome of "colic." With colorectal distension, the associated response is not as clear and results may be more closely associated with the "urge to defecate" response in humans, and therefore not truly nociceptive in nature.[11] The major disadvantage of the cecal and duodenal models is the need for visceral cannulation, which is not necessary for colorectal distension; however, as is discussed later, the response to analgesic agents is not uniform throughout the intestinal tract.

## Pain Assessment Tools

To claim that one has treated pain effectively implies that one can recognize it and measure or quantify it. Objective measures such as vital signs and plasma cortisol concentration circumvent the subjective nature of assessment; however, vital signs that might be predicted to be useful are affected not only by pain but a variety of other factors including hydration status, perfusion, sepsis and/or endotoxemia, fear, anxiety, and sedative or analgesic drugs. Pain-scoring tools must therefore be primarily based on behavioral indicators,[13] in combination with the judicious use of vital signs such as heart rate.[14]

To be useful, a pain-scoring system should meet the following criteria: it should include clearly defined assessment criteria, be suitable for all observers, be simple and quick to use, be sensitive, have identified strengths and weaknesses, and be validated. Possible deficiencies include bias and inter- and intraobserver variability. A lack of agreement between observers is one of the flaws of simple scoring systems such as the visual analog scale (VAS). When critically assessing scoring systems, the investigator should control for signalment (age, breed, sex), observer (veterinarian, student, owner/trainer), type and source of pain, and other effects (eg, food withdrawal and anesthesia). In a review of behavioral assessments of pain in equidae, Ashley and colleagues[13] point out that although some nonspecific "pain behaviors" are reported, specific behaviors can be identified and these differ depending on the cause of pain; for example, abdominal versus limb and hoof or dental pain. Vocalization (groaning), rolling, kicking at the abdomen, flank watching, and stretching are overt behaviors associated with abdominal pain[13]; however, other indicators can be easily overlooked. Pritchett and colleagues[14] recorded physiologic and behavioral variables in horses that underwent exploratory laparotomy for a variety of surgically correctable intestinal lesions, and compared these with control horses (no anesthesia, no surgery) and horses anesthetized for nonpainful procedures. Horses were videotaped and detailed "time budgets" were calculated. Observers used a numerical rating scale (NRS) of behavior, which included head position, ear position, location in the stall, activity, lifting of the feet, and response to food. After surgery, horses spent significant periods of time doing nothing (resting) and had higher NRS scores compared with the other 2 groups, but displayed very few overt pain behaviors such as rolling, kicking, and pawing. In clinical practice these animals will often be overlooked and not given analgesics. Thus, this or similar scoring systems can be used to guide pain management in horses with abdominal pain, with the aim being to restore normal behaviors and activity levels (Table 2) and not simply to avoid overt pain behaviors.

## TREATMENT OPTIONS
### Approaches to Treatment of Visceral Pain

When identifiable, treatment is focused on correcting the underlying pathology; however, in many cases a definitive diagnosis may not be made or may take time to reach. It has been argued that pain management should be withheld until the cause of the pain has been identified because masking it will confound any ongoing diagnostic tests. However, this approach must be weighed against the dangers that painful horses pose to personnel working on them, the imposition of additional "procedural pain," for example, abdominocentesis and thoracocentesis, and, clearly, the welfare of the horse.

**Table 2**
**Numerical rating scale for scoring abdominal pain in horses**

| Behavior Category | 1 | 2 | 3 | 4 |
|---|---|---|---|---|
| Overt pain behaviors[a,b] | None | | Occasional | Continuous |
| Head position[b] | Above withers | | At withers | Below withers |
| Ear position[b] | Forward, frequently moving | | Slightly back, infrequent movement | |
| Location in stall[b] | At the exit, watching | In the center, watching exit | In the center, watching walls | At the middle or back, facing away from exit |
| Spontaneous locomotion[b] | Moving freely | Occasional steps | | No movement |
| Response to door opening[c] | Moves toward door | Looks at door | | No response |
| Response to approach[c] | Moves toward the person, with ears forward | Looks at person, with ears forward | Moves away from the person | Does not move, ears back |
| Foot lifting | Lifts feet easily if asked | Can lift feet if encouraged | | Unwilling to lift feet |
| Response to offered food[c] | Reaches for food | Looks at food | | No interest in food |

[a] Overt pain behaviors include pawing, sweating, flank watching, flehmen, rolling, lying down and standing up repeatedly, groaning.
[b] Combine all these scores to obtain a posture score.
[c] Combine these scores to obtain a socialization score.
   *Data from* Pritchett LC, Ulibarri C, Robertson MC, et al. Identification of potential physiologic and behavioral indicators of post-operative pain in horses after exploratory celiotomy for colic. Appl Anim Behav Sci 2003;80:31–43.

Pain itself can result in ileus, which has many negative consequences (reflux, fluid and electrolyte losses) and adds to the overall pain burden of the patient. In addition, it is now well understood that the longer pain goes untreated, the greater the risk of long-term sensitization and hyperalgesia that result from an unmitigated afferent barrage of noxious stimuli into the central nervous system.[15] Thus, pain control emerges as the single most important therapeutic factor when treating visceral pain in horses.

## Surgery

Whereas many painful visceral conditions can be treated medically, conditions such as strangulating and nonstrangulating bowel obstructions and removal of renal, cystic, or ureteral calculi require surgical intervention, and pleuritis typically requires thoraco-centesis at a minimum, possibly with thoracoscopy or rib resection. If surgical therapy is not a practical or financial option for a given individual with such a condition, eutha-nasia may represent the most practical and humane method of analgesia. If surgical therapy is elected, analgesia is an important component of perioperative management.

## SYSTEMIC PHARMACOLOGIC THERAPY

There are a limited number of analgesics available to treat severe pain in horses. At present, the most commonly used analgesic medications include the $\alpha_2$-adrenergic agonists, nonsteroidal anti-inflammatory drugs (NSAIDs), and opioids. Because many of these do not always produce the desired results or are associated with adverse effects, other more novel analgesic drugs are currently under investigation for use in the horse, and are also discussed here. In the horse, most available informa-tion pertaining to visceral pain is restricted to the gastrointestinal tract. However, the drugs discussed in this article are likely to have similar effects on visceral pain arising from other organs. The commonly used drugs and their suggested doses are outlined in **Table 3**.

## $\alpha_2$-Adrenergic Drugs

Major disadvantages of all the $\alpha_2$-adrenergic agonists for prolonged analgesic therapy include the immediate and profound decrease in gastrointestinal motility that occurs after their administration and the relatively short duration of analgesia provided.[16–19] Fewer undesirable side effects are seen when butorphanol is administered as a constant rate infusion instead of boluses; whether this approach would be beneficial when using $\alpha_2$-adrenergic drugs to treat horses with abdominal pain has not been thoroughly explored.

### Specific $\alpha_2$-adrenergic drugs

**Xylazine** Xylazine is very commonly used to provide sedation and analgesia for both diagnostic procedures and treatment of visceral pain in horses. Xylazine provides excellent visceral analgesia of short duration; up to 90 minutes in some models.[7,20,21] Adverse effects associated with its administration include the aforementioned nega-tive effects on motility combined with hypertension and bradycardia followed by hypo-tension.[17,22–24] Due to the relatively short duration of its effects, xylazine, either alone or in conjunction with butorphanol, is an excellent choice for sedation and analgesia during the initial evaluation of horses presenting for colic. Dosages from 150 to 250 mg for an average 450 to 550 kg adult horse typically facilitate passage of a nasogas-tric tube and rectal palpation.

**Detomidine** Detomidine is commonly used in horses to provide sedation for diag-nostic procedures and to alleviate abdominal pain.[25] Its use results in a characteristic

**Table 3**
Commonly used visceral analgesic medications

| Class of Drug | Drug | Dosage (mg/kg) | Route | Dosing Interval (h) | Comments |
|---|---|---|---|---|---|
| NSAIDs | Flunixin | 0.25–1.1 | IV, PO | 8–24 | Avoid max. dose >2×/d |
| | Ketoprofen | 2.2 | IV | 24 | |
| | Phenylbutazone | 2.2–4.4 | IV, PO | 12–24 | Avoid extravascular injection |
| $\alpha_2$-Agonists | Xylazine | 0.2–1.1 | IV, IM | prn | Sedation typically outlasts analgesia |
| | Detomidine | 0.005–0.04 | IV, IM | prn | Sedation typically outlasts analgesia |
| | Medetomidine | 0.004–0.01 | IV | prn | |
| Opioids | Butorphanol bolus | 0.02–0.1 | IV, IM | 3–4 | Can increase locomotion if used as sole agent in adults |
| | Butorphanol infusion | 18 µg/kg bolus over 15 min then 13–23 µg/kg/h | IV | CRI | Typically not used longer than 12–24 h |
| | Morphine | 0.12–0.66 | IV | | Combine with $\alpha_2$-agonist |
| Other | Lidocaine (2%, 20 mg/mL) | 1.3 mg/kg bolus over 10–15 min then 3 mg/kg/h (75 mL/h for 500 kg) | IV | CRI | Main adverse effects are neurologic and associated with rapid administration or accumulation |
| | N-Butylscopolammonium bromide | 0.3 mg/kg | Slow IV | Once | Causes transient tachycardia |
| | Ketamine | 0.4–1.2 mg/kg/h | IV | CRI | Hyperexcitability possible at higher dosages |

Please note that these are suggested dosages and routes only. The dose, route, and frequency of administration should be considered individually for each case. Special consideration should be given to the current medical status, organ function, and concurrently administered medications.

*Abbreviations:* CRI, continuous rate infusion; IM, intramuscular; IV, intravenous; PO, by mouth; prn, "as needed."

dose-dependent head drop, ataxia, and decrease in heart rate, respiratory rate, and gastrointestinal motility.[26,27] In an experimental model of cecal distension, detomidine was effective in alleviating the associated pain.[28] In a duodenal distension model, a marked and immediate decrease in duodenal contractions occurred after 10 and 20 μg/kg (intravenously), but analgesia was both dose and location dependent; 10 μg/kg provided no visceral antinociception whereas 20 μg/kg provided 15 minutes of antinociception. The effects on colorectal distension were different, with 10 μg/kg and 20 μg/kg increasing colorectal distension threshold for 15 and 165 minutes, respectively.[16] Elfenbein and colleagues[16] measured the plasma concentration that correlated with visceral analgesia, which provides the pharmacokinetic data necessary to design infusion rates for future study. These investigators also demonstrated that the plasma concentration required for analgesia was in the order of 10 times that required for sedation, which emphasizes that sedation does not equal analgesia, especially with the $\alpha_2$-agonists.

**Medetomidine/dexmedetomidine** Medetomidine and dexmedetomidine are not licensed for use in the horse and are considerably more expensive than xylazine, detomidine, and romifidine. Medetomidine infusions have been used successfully as part of a balanced anesthetic protocol.[29] Medetomidine combined with morphine (both given as infusions) provided suitable conditions for standing laparoscopy in horses[30] and is discussed later in the section Multimodal Approaches to Therapy. Commercially, medetomidine has now been replaced by dexmedetomidine, and to the authors' knowledge this drug has not been evaluated in horses for its visceral analgesic properties in a research or clinical setting.

### Nonsteroidal Anti-Inflammatory Drugs

NSAIDs have well-documented visceral analgesic and anti-inflammatory properties, but adverse effects including gastric and colonic ulceration, impairment of jejuna, epithelial restitution following ischemic injury, and renal tubular necrosis are reported.[21,31–33] Despite this fact, flunixin meglumine remains likely the most important and commonly used medication available for the treatment of visceral pain in horses. As such, many horses with abdominal pain will recover completely with one administration of 1 mg/kg flunixin via the intravenous, intramuscular, or oral route. The positive and negative effects of this class of drugs are discussed in detail elsewhere in this issue and thus are not further discussed here.

### Opioids

Opioids have not been widely used to treat clinical pain in horses in comparison with other species including humans. Reasons for this include the apparent narrow margin between analgesia and excitation or arousal, and difficulty in demonstrating a consistent and quantifiable analgesic action.[34] In pain-free horses, opioid administration has resulted in adverse effects, predominantly excitement, whereas clinical reports of opioid use in painful animals are more encouraging. Opioid receptor–binding studies demonstrate distinct differences in the distribution and density of opioid receptors within the central nervous system between horses and other species, but the clinical significance of these data is still unclear.[35,36]

#### Specific opioids
**Butorphanol** Butorphanol is a κ (OP2) agonist and competitive μ (OP3) antagonist, which is labeled for use in horses. When administered by bolus injection, butorphanol provides a moderate degree of somatic and a slightly greater degree of visceral analgesia in the horse; however, it also causes decreased gastrointestinal

motility.[17,21,37,38] Adverse effects such as ataxia, decreased defecation, and borborygmi after a single intravenous injection are less apparent when it is given as a continuous infusion.[39] No antinociceptive properties were measurable when an infusion was used in a research model of visceral distension.[10] The effect of butorphanol on gastrointestinal motility appears to vary with the segment of the gastrointestinal tract, dosage, and method of administration. Bolus administration of butorphanol did not significantly alter antroduodenal motility in one study[40] but resulted in delayed gastric emptying in another.[18] When administered as a constant rate infusion, butorphanol did not significantly alter duodenal motility.[10] In clinical patients undergoing exploratory laparotomy for colic, butorphanol infusion (13 μg/kg/h for 24 hours) did delay passage of feces following surgery. However, overall there were clear advantages to its use in this manner[39]: pain scores were significantly decreased in the immediate postoperative period; horses lost significantly less weight, had improved recovery characteristics, and on average were discharged 3 days earlier than control horses (flunixin meglumine only).[39] These benefits translated to an overall cost savings of approximately $1000.

**Morphine** The use of morphine in horses is controversial. When used at doses of 0.1 to 0.2 mg/kg intravenously or as an infusion (0.1 mg/kg/h) in horses undergoing surgery, no undesirable effects were reported and it significantly improved the quality of recovery, presumably because of its analgesic effects or perhaps its sedative effects in a clinical setting.[41–43] Morphine provided pain relief in a cecal distension model but inhibited colonic motility.[6] The role of systemically administered morphine for the alleviation of abdominal pain is currently unclear; as with the $\alpha_2$-agonists, short-term use may be effective and beneficial, but long-term use (several days) may result in ileus. As with butorphanol, infusions may reduce the unwanted side effects, and deserve further study.

The biggest concerns regarding the use of morphine are its effects on gastrointestinal motility and therefore the potential increased risk of colic. A dose of 0.5 mg/kg intravenously every 12 hours for 6 days to normal horses resulted in decreased defecation frequency, fecal moisture content, and gastrointestinal sounds.[44] Those effects were mostly mitigated by the concurrent administration of $N$-methylnaltrexone, an opioid antagonist that does not cross the blood-brain barrier.[45]

In a study of 496 horses that underwent orthopedic surgery, 14 developed colic; the use of morphine was associated with a fourfold increased risk of colic compared with the use of no opioids or butorphanol.[46] In another study of 533 horses that underwent anesthesia but not surgery or nonabdominal surgery, 3.6% of horses developed colic within 7 days of anesthesia; significantly more horses were in the surgery group, but the use of morphine was not associated with an increased risk.[47]

**Fentanyl** In conscious research horses, fentanyl failed to produce significant visceral or somatic antinociception at serum concentrations above the nociceptive threshold in other species.[9] At high plasma concentrations (>5 ng/mL), some but not all horses became agitated. Also, very high (13.31 ng/mL) serum concentrations of fentanyl are necessary to achieve minimal (18%) isoflurane minimum alveolar concentration reduction in horses.[48] The use of transdermal fentanyl patches was initially met with enthusiasm, but uptake of fentanyl from a transdermal patch is highly variable in horses.[49,50] This information, combined with the disappointing results of intravenous infusions and cost, limit the utility of fentanyl for treatment of visceral pain in horses.

**Tramadol** Tramadol is an analogue of codeine and although not a controlled substance, some of its analgesic properties are related to its opioid properties.

Tramadol has a short half-life, low oral bioavailability (~3%), and the active metabolite M1 is a minor metabolite that may limit its usefulness in horses relative to other species.[51] No opioid-related excitement was reported but somatic analgesia could not be demonstrated with tramadol administration at doses ranging from 0.1 to 1.6 mg/kg intravenously.[52] Epidural administration of tramadol (1.0 mg/kg) resulted in significant antinociception at lumbar and thoracic dermatomes within 3 hours of administration, which lasted for 5 hours,[53] but it is currently unknown whether this would translate to visceral analgesia. Thus, the role of tramadol for the alleviation of pain in horses remains to be determined.

### Sodium Channel Blockers

Lidocaine is an aminoamide local anesthetic that prevents propagation of action potentials by binding to voltage-gated sodium channels. Lidocaine, administered as an intravenous infusion, is commonly used in horses for its potential analgesic, prokinetic, and anti-inflammatory properties.[8,54–58] Variable doses of intravenous lidocaine are reported; loading doses vary from 1.3 to 5.0 mg/kg and infusion rates vary from 25 to 100 μg/kg/min. Clinical signs of toxicity in conscious horses include skeletal muscle tremors, altered visual function, anxiety, ataxia, collapse, and electrocardiographic changes, which can occur at serum concentrations between 1.65 and 4.53 μg/mL (mean 3.24 ± 0.74 [SD] μg/mL).[59] It is noteworthy that the neurologic manifestations of toxicosis may be masked by general anesthesia.

Using electroencephalographic changes as an objective measure of nociception in anesthetized ponies, intravenous lidocaine infusion (5 mg/kg loading dose, 100 μg/kg/min infusion) obtunded the response to castration, lending support to the role of lidocaine as a visceral analgesic.[60]

Lidocaine administration following exploratory laparotomy has been associated with reduced small intestinal size and peritoneal fluid accumulation,[57] and improved survival.[61] In one hospital setting, the intraoperative use of lidocaine was thought to reduce the incidence of postoperative ileus by approximately 50%[62] and in a multicenter study of horses with enteritis or postoperative ileus, lidocaine infusion decreased the volume and duration of reflux compared with saline-treated controls.[56] Following experimentally induced small intestinal ischemia, lidocaine improved mucosal healing by an unknown mechanism that may be related to the decreased production of inflammatory cytokines.[63]

Because treatment of horses with gastrointestinal disease may need to be prolonged, it is important to understand how the duration of infusion affects the disposition of lidocaine and also how the pharmacokinetics might be altered by disease or general anesthesia, so that appropriate changes in the infusion rate can be made to avoid toxicosis. The target steady-state concentration of lidocaine for the treatment of ileus is thought to be between 1.0 and 2.0 μg/mL (mean 0.98 μg/mL).[64] In healthy horses, steady-state serum concentrations slightly below this suggested that targets were reached 3 hours after starting a continuous rate infusion at 50 μg/kg/min (no bolus), and did not accumulate over a 96-hour study period.[65] However, in a clinical setting accumulation can be demonstrated.[66] Cetiofur sodium and flunixin meglumine decrease the protein binding of lidocaine, therefore lower infusion rates of lidocaine should be used in horses receiving highly protein bound drugs.[66] Plasma concentrations may also be affected by liver disease or by changes in liver blood flow that occur under general anesthesia. A bolus dose of 1.3 mg/kg followed by an infusion of 50 μg/kg/min results in higher serum concentrations in anesthetized as compared with awake horses,[67] and in the former these were within the range reported to be toxic in conscious horses.[59]

### Lidocaine: other applications

Many horses that present with abdominal pain will undergo a rectal palpation. Intra-rectal lidocaine (15 mL, 2% solution) increases rectal wall compliance and facilitates rectal palpation, and likely decreases the risk of rectal tears.[11] The pain associated with other diagnostic procedures such as thoracocentesis and abdominocentesis can be decreased by local infiltration with lidocaine or another local anesthetic.

In mares undergoing laparoscopic ovariectomy, the addition of 10 mL of 2% lidocaine injected into the mesovarium to a protocol of intravenous xylazine and butor-phanol and epidural detomidine resulted in fewer pain responses compared with intra-ovarian injection of saline.[68]

## N-Methyl-D-Aspartate Antagonists

Ketamine, an N-methyl-D-aspartate (NMDA) receptor antagonist commonly used for dissociative anesthesia, may have a very important role to play in the prevention of central hypersensitivity,[15] and has somatic antinociceptive properties when adminis-tered as a constant rate infusion at subanesthetic doses in both anesthetized and conscious horses.[69,70] Subanesthetic doses of ketamine decreased overall gastroin-testinal transit time in comparison with saline control,[71] in contrast to studies in dogs.[72] The ability for ketamine to produce visceral analgesia in horses is currently unknown. Ketamine also has well-documented anti-inflammatory properties in several species; it reduced the production of tumor necrosis factor $\alpha$, interleukin (IL)-6, and IL-8 in human blood and in dogs in response to endotoxin stimulation.[73,74]

## Antispasmodic Medications

N-Butylscopolammonium bromide (NBB) has both anticholinergic and antispasmodic properties, and is labeled for the treatment of spasmodic colic. In an experimental model of cecal balloon distension, NBB had an analgesic effect in 6 of 8 ponies.[75] In another similar trial, NBB had a brief analgesic effect as well as a transient negative effect on cecal contractions.[76] In horses, administration of NBB produced visceral antinociception, as indicated by a significantly increased colorectal distension threshold and a small but nonsignificant increase in duodenal distension threshold.[10] The administration of NBB also decreases rectal tone for facilitation of a rectal exam-ination.[77] In all reports the duration of effect is of short duration (15–20 minutes).

## NONPHARMACOLOGIC THERAPY

Despite anecdotal reports in individual horses, the benefits of acupuncture for the relief of abdominal pain in horses have not been substantiated by large clinical trials or in a research model of duodenal distension.[78] This is clearly an area in need of further research.

## MULTIMODAL APPROACH TO THERAPY

Severe pain may be refractory to single analgesic therapy and may require a multi-modal approach to pain management, employing drugs with different mechanisms of action. Despite the potential for improved analgesia, for example in a small clinical study of horses with pain that was refractory to NSAID therapy alone, the addition of the fentanyl transdermal therapeutic system appeared to be effective based on subjective evaluation.[79] However, others have warned that the use of such combina-tions may also increase the potential for adverse effects, especially alterations in gastrointestinal motility or behavior.[17]

As previously discussed, infusions of drugs often result in fewer adverse effects. An infusion of medetomidine (5 µg/kg/h) combined with morphine (30 µg/kg/h) provided reliable sedation and stable cardiorespiratory function during standing laparoscopy surgery.[30] Only a few drug combinations and doses have been studied to date, but this concept should be further explored to find the most effective protocols to treat severe, especially chronic, visceral pain in horses.

## FUTURE DIRECTIONS
### New Approaches to Treatment

There is much work to be done to develop effective treatment protocols that do not have significant adverse effects for horses with visceral pain. The rigorous use of pain-scoring systems will produce more reliable information from clinical studies. The role of infusions and combinations of drugs looks promising. Because of the high prevalence of visceral pain in humans and the need for more effective treatments, this is an area of intense research. New targets include transient receptor channels, and purinergic and adenosine receptors,[80–82] which may also apply to horses.

## SUMMARY

Overall, although much work has focused on the evaluation and treatment of visceral pain in horses, the basic tenets of treatment involve identification of the source and cause of pain and alleviation of that cause, if possible. Pharmacologic therapy typically involves unimodal therapy with an NSAID (phenylbutazone, firocoxib, or most commonly, flunixin meglumine) as a starting point for mild cases. For more severe or prolonged causes of pain, a combination of an $\alpha_2$-adrenergic agonist (xylazine, detomidine) with an opioid (typically butorphanol) as single or repeated bolus injection allows for facilitation of diagnostic procedures or short-term (<24 hours) therapy. For protracted cases, constant rate infusion of lidocaine, with or without addition of butorphanol or ketamine, can provide visceral analgesia with the potential for a decreased incidence of adverse effects.

## REFERENCES

1. Mair T, Divers T, Ducharme N. Etiology, risk factors, and pathophysiology of colic. In: Mair T, Divers T, Ducharme N, editors. Manual of equine gastroenterology. London: WB Saunders; 2002. p. 101–6.
2. Giamberardino MA. Visceral pain. International association for the study of pain; Clinical Updates 2005;XIII(6):1–6.
3. Hunter JO. Do horses suffer from irritable bowel syndrome? Equine Vet J 2009; 41(9):836–40.
4. Hudson NP, Merritt AM. Equine gastrointestinal motility research: where we are and where we need to go. Equine Vet J 2008;40(4):422–8.
5. Gebhart GF, Ness TJ. Central mechanisms of visceral pain. Can J Physiol Pharmacol 1991;69(5):627–34.
6. Kohn CW, Muir WW 3rd. Selected aspects of the clinical pharmacology of visceral analgesics and gut motility modifying drugs in the horse. J Vet Intern Med 1988;2(2):85–91.
7. Muir WW, Robertson JT. Visceral analgesia: effects of xylazine, butorphanol, meperidine, and pentazocine in horses. Am J Vet Res 1985;46(10):2081–4.
8. Robertson SA, Sanchez LC, Merritt AM, et al. Effect of systemic lidocaine on visceral and somatic nociception in conscious horses. Equine Vet J 2005; 37(2):122–7.

9. Sanchez LC, Robertson SA, Maxwell LK, et al. Effect of fentanyl on visceral and somatic nociception in conscious horses. J Vet Intern Med 2007;21(5): 1067–75.

10. Sanchez LC, Elfenbein JR, Robertson SA. Effect of acepromazine, butorphanol, or N-butylscopolammonium bromide on visceral and somatic nociception and duodenal motility in conscious horses. Am J Vet Res 2008;69(5):579–85.

11. Sanchez LC, Merritt AM. Colorectal distention in the horse: visceral sensitivity, rectal compliance and effect of i.v. xylazine or intrarectal lidocaine. Equine Vet J 2005;37(1):70–4.

12. Skarda RT, Muir WW 3rd. Comparison of electroacupuncture and butorphanol on respiratory and cardiovascular effects and rectal pain threshold after controlled rectal distention in mares. Am J Vet Res 2003;64(2):137–44.

13. Ashley FH, Waterman-Pearson AE, Whay HR. Behavioural assessment of pain in horses and donkeys: application to clinical practice and future studies. Equine Vet J 2005;37(6):565–75.

14. Pritchett LC, Ulibarri C, Robertson MC, et al. Identification of potential physiological and behavioral indicators of post-operative pain in horses after exploratory celiotomy for colic. Appl Anim Behav Sci 2003;80:31–43.

15. Pozzi A, Muir WW, Traverso F. Prevention of central sensitization and pain by N-methyl-D-aspartate receptor antagonists. J Am Vet Med Assoc 2006;228(1):53–60.

16. Elfenbein JR, Sanchez LC, Robertson SA, et al. Effect of detomidine on visceral and somatic nociception and duodenal motility in conscious adult horses. Vet Anaesth Analg 2009;36(2):162–72.

17. Merritt AM, Burrow JA, Hartless CS. Effect of xylazine, detomidine, and a combination of xylazine and butorphanol on equine duodenal motility. Am J Vet Res 1998;59(5):619–23.

18. Doherty TJ, Andrews FM, Provenza MK, et al. The effect of sedation on gastric emptying of a liquid marker in ponies. Vet Surg 1999;28(5):375–9.

19. Freeman SL, England GC. Effect of romifidine on gastrointestinal motility, assessed by transrectal ultrasonography. Equine Vet J 2001;33(6):570–6.

20. Brunson DB, Majors LJ. Comparative analgesia of xylazine, xylazine/morphine, xylazine/butorphanol, and xylazine/nalbuphine in the horse, using dental dolorimetry. Am J Vet Res 1987;48(7):1087–91.

21. Kalpravidh M, Lumb WV, Wright M, et al. Effects of butorphanol, flunixin, levorphanol, morphine, and xylazine in ponies. Am J Vet Res 1984;45(2):217–23.

22. Clark ES, Thompson SA, Becht JL, et al. Effects of xylazine on cecal mechanical activity and cecal blood flow in healthy horses. Am J Vet Res 1988;49(5):720–3.

23. Lester GD, Merritt AM, Neuwirth L, et al. Effect of alpha 2-adrenergic, cholinergic, and nonsteroidal anti-inflammatory drugs on myoelectric activity of ileum, cecum, and right ventral colon and on cecal emptying of radiolabeled markers in clinically normal ponies. Am J Vet Res 1998;59(3):320–7.

24. Sutton DG, Preston T, Christley RM, et al. The effects of xylazine, detomidine, acepromazine and butorphanol on equine solid phase gastric emptying rate. Equine Vet J 2002;34(5):486–92.

25. Clarke KW, Taylor PM. Detomidine: a new sedative for horses. Equine Vet J 1986; 18(5):366–70.

26. Wilson DV, Bohart GV, Evans AT, et al. Retrospective analysis of detomidine infusion for standing chemical restraint in 51 horses. Vet Anaesth Analg 2002;29:54–7.

27. Freeman SL, England GC. Investigation of romifidine and detomidine for the clinical sedation of horses. Vet Rec 2000;147(18):507–11.

28. Lowe JE, Hilfiger J. Analgesic and sedative effects of detomidine compared to xylazine in a colic model using i.v. and i.m. routes of administration. Acta Vet Scand Suppl 1986;82:85–95.

29. Ringer SK, Kalchofner K, Boller J, et al. A clinical comparison of two anaesthetic protocols using lidocaine or medetomidine in horses. Vet Anaesth Analg 2007; 34(4):257–68.

30. Solano AM, Valverde A, Desrochers A, et al. Behavioural and cardiorespiratory effects of a constant rate infusion of medetomidine and morphine for sedation during standing laparoscopy in horses. Equine Vet J 2009;41(2):153–9.

31. MacAllister CG, Morgan SJ, Borne AT, et al. Comparison of adverse effects of phenylbutazone, flunixin meglumine, and ketoprofen in horses. J Am Vet Med Assoc 1993;202(1):71–7.

32. Tomlinson JE, Blikslager AT. Effects of cyclooxygenase inhibitors flunixin and deracoxib on permeability of ischaemic-injured equine jejunum. Equine Vet J 2005; 37(1):75–80.

33. Cook VL, Meyer CT, Campbell NB, et al. Effect of firocoxib or flunixin meglumine on recovery of ischemic-injured equine jejunum. Am J Vet Res 2009;70(8): 992–1000.

34. Bennett RC, Steffey EP. Use of opioids for pain and anesthetic management in horses. Vet Clin North Am Equine Pract 2002;18(1):47–60.

35. Hellyer PW, Bai L, Supon J, et al. Comparison of opioid and alpha-2 adrenergic receptor binding in horse and dog brain using radioligand autoradiography. Vet Anaesth Analg 2003;30(3):172–82.

36. Thomasy SM, Moeller BC, Stanley SD. Comparison of opioid receptor binding in horse, guinea pig, and rat cerebral cortex and cerebellum. Vet Anaesth Analg 2007;34(5):351–8.

37. Kalpravidh M, Lumb WV, Wright M, et al. Analgesic effects of butorphanol in horses: dose-response studies. Am J Vet Res 1984;45(2):211–6.

38. Sellon DC, Monroe VL, Roberts MC, et al. Pharmacokinetics and adverse effects of butorphanol administered by single intravenous injection or continuous intravenous infusion in horses. Am J Vet Res 2001;62(2):183–9.

39. Sellon DC, Roberts MC, Blikslager AT, et al. Effects of continuous rate intravenous infusion of butorphanol on physiologic and outcome variables in horses after celiotomy. J Vet Intern Med 2004;18(4):555–63.

40. Merritt AM, Campbell-Thompson ML, Lowrey S. Effect of butorphanol on equine antroduodenal motility. Equine Vet J Suppl 1989;7:21–3.

41. Mircica E, Clutton RE, Kyles KW, et al. Problems associated with perioperative morphine in horses: a retrospective case analysis. Vet Anaesth Analg 2003; 30(3):147 55.

42. Love EJ, Lane JG, Murison PJ. Morphine administration in horses anaesthetized for upper respiratory tract surgery. Vet Anaesth Analg 2006;33(3):179–88.

43. Clark L, Clutton RE, Blissitt KJ, et al. The effects of morphine on the recovery of horses from halothane anaesthesia. Vet Anaesth Analg 2008; 35(1):22–9.

44. Boscan P, Van Hoogmoed LM, Farver TB, et al. Evaluation of the effects of the opioid agonist morphine on gastrointestinal tract function in horses. Am J Vet Res 2006;67(6):992–7.

45. Boscan P, Van Hoogmoed LM, Pypendop BH, et al. Pharmacokinetics of the opioid antagonist N-methylnaltrexone and evaluation of its effects on gastrointestinal tract function in horses treated or not treated with morphine. Am J Vet Res 2006;67(6):998–1004.

46. Senior JM, Pinchbeck GL, Dugdale AH, et al. Retrospective study of the risk factors and prevalence of colic in horses after orthopaedic surgery. Vet Rec 2004;155(11):321–5.

47. Andersen MS, Clark L, Dyson SJ, et al. Risk factors for colic in horses after general anaesthesia for MRI or nonabdominal surgery: absence of evidence of effect from perianaesthetic morphine. Equine Vet J 2006;38(4):368–74.

48. Thomasy SM, Steffey EP, Mama KR, et al. The effects of i.v. fentanyl administration on the minimum alveolar concentration of isoflurane in horses. Br J Anaesth 2006;97(2):232–7.

49. Orsini JA, Moate PJ, Kuersten K, et al. Pharmacokinetics of fentanyl delivered transdermally in healthy adult horses—variability among horses and its clinical implications. J Vet Pharmacol Ther 2006;29(6):539–46.

50. Mills PC, Cross SE. Regional differences in transdermal penetration of fentanyl through equine skin. Res Vet Sci 2007;82(2):252–6.

51. Shilo Y, Britzi M, Eytan B, et al. Pharmacokinetics of tramadol in horses after intravenous, intramuscular and oral administration. J Vet Pharmacol Ther 2008; 31(1):60–5.

52. Dhanjal JK, Wilson DV, Hughs CG, et al. Effects of intravenous tramadol in horses. Paper presented at: ACVA Annual Meeting. New Orleans (LA), September 27, 2007.

53. Natalini CC, Robinson EP. Evaluation of the analgesic effects of epidurally administered morphine, alfentanil, butorphanol, tramadol, and U50488H in horses. Am J Vet Res 2000;61(12):1579–86.

54. Van Hoogmoed LM, Nieto JE, Snyder JR, et al. Survey of prokinetic use in horses with gastrointestinal injury. Vet Surg 2004;33(3):279–85.

55. Milligan M, Beard W, Kukanich B, et al. The effect of lidocaine on postoperative jejunal motility in normal horses. Vet Surg 2007;36(3):214–20.

56. Malone E, Ensink J, Turner T, et al. Intravenous continuous infusion of lidocaine for treatment of equine ileus. Vet Surg 2006;35(1):60–6.

57. Brianceau P, Chevalier H, Karas A, et al. Intravenous lidocaine and small-intestinal size, abdominal fluid, and outcome after colic surgery in horses. J Vet Intern Med 2002;16(6):736–41.

58. Cook VL, Blikslager AT. Use of systemically administered lidocaine in horses with gastrointestinal tract disease. J Am Vet Med Assoc 2008;232(8):1144–8.

59. Meyer GA, Lin HC, Hanson RR, et al. Effects of intravenous lidocaine overdose on cardiac electrical activity and blood pressure in the horse. Equine Vet J 2001; 33(5):434–7.

60. Murrell JC, White KL, Johnson CB, et al. Investigation of the EEG effects of intravenous lidocaine during halothane anaesthesia in ponies. Vet Anaesth Analg 2005;32(4):212–21.

61. Torfs S, Delesalle C, Dewulf J, et al. Risk factors for equine postoperative ileus and effectiveness of prophylactic lidocaine. J Vet Intern Med 2009;23(3):606–11.

62. Cohen ND, Lester GD, Sanchez LC, et al. Evaluation of risk factors associated with development of postoperative ileus in horses. J Am Vet Med Assoc 2004; 225(7):1070–8.

63. Cook VL, Jones Shults J, McDowell M, et al. Attenuation of ischaemic injury in the equine jejunum by administration of systemic lidocaine. Equine Vet J 2008; 40(4):353–7.

64. Malone E, Turner T, Wilson J. Intravenous lidocaine for the treatment of equine ileus. Paper presented at: 6th Equine Colic Research Symposium. Athens (GA), 1998.

65. Dickey EJ, McKenzie HC, Brown KA, et al. Serum concentrations of lidocaine and its metabolites after prolonged infusion in healthy horses. Equine Vet J 2008; 40(4):348–52.

66. Milligan M, Kukanich B, Beard W, et al. The disposition of lidocaine during a 12-hour intravenous infusion to postoperative horses. J Vet Pharmacol Ther 2006;29(6):495–9.

67. Feary DJ, Mama KR, Wagner AE, et al. Influence of general anesthesia on pharmacokinetics of intravenous lidocaine infusion in horses. Am J Vet Res 2005; 66(4):574–80.

68. Farstvedt EG, Hendrickson DA. Intraoperative pain responses following intraovarian versus mesovarian injection of lidocaine in mares undergoing laparoscopic ovariectomy. J Am Vet Med Assoc 2005;227(4):593–6.

69. Knobloch M, Portier CJ, Levionnois OL, et al. Antinociceptive effects, metabolism and disposition of ketamine in ponies under target-controlled drug infusion. Toxicol Appl Pharmacol 2006;216(3):373–86.

70. Peterbauer C, Larenza PM, Knobloch M, et al. Effects of a low dose infusion of racemic and S-ketamine on the nociceptive withdrawal reflex in standing ponies. Vet Anaesth Analg 2008;35(5):414–23.

71. Elfenbein JR, Sanchez LC, Robertson SA. The systemic effects of prolonged ketamine continuous rate infusion in clinically normal horses. Paper presented at The American College of Veterinary Internal Medicine Forum. Anaheim (CA), June 9–12, 2010.

72. Fass J, Bares R, Hermsdorf V, et al. Effects of intravenous ketamine on gastrointestinal motility in the dog. Intensive Care Med 1995;21(7):584–9.

73. Kawasaki T, Ogata M, Kawasaki C, et al. Ketamine suppresses proinflammatory cytokine production in human whole blood in vitro. Anesth Analg 1999;89(3):665–9.

74. DeClue AE, Cohn LA, Lechner ES, et al. Effects of subanesthetic doses of ketamine on hemodynamic and immunologic variables in dogs with experimentally induced endotoxemia. Am J Vet Res 2008;69(2):228–32.

75. Boatwright CE, Fubini SL, Grohn YT, et al. A comparison of N-butylscopolammonium bromide and butorphanol tartrate for analgesia using a balloon model of abdominal pain in ponies. Can J Vet Res 1996;60(1):65–8.

76. Roelvink ME, Goossens L, Kalsbeek HC, et al. Analgesic and spasmolytic effects of dipyrone, hyoscine-N-butylbromide and a combination of the two in ponies. Vet Rec 1991;129(17):378–80.

77. Luo T, Bertone JJ, Greene HM, et al. A comparison of N-butylscopolammonium and lidocaine for control of rectal pressure in horses. Vet Ther 2006;7(3):243–8.

78. Merritt AM, Xie H, Lester GD, et al. Evaluation of a method to experimentally induce colic in horses and the effects of acupuncture applied at the Guan-yuan-shu (similar to BL-21) acupoint. Am J Vet Res 2002;63(7):1006–11.

79. Thomasy SM, Slovis N, Maxwell LK, et al. Transdermal fentanyl combined with nonsteroidal anti-inflammatory drugs for analgesia in horses. J Vet Intern Med 2004;18(4):550–4.

80. Blackshaw LA, Brierley SM, Hughes PA. TRP channels: new targets for visceral pain. Gut 2009;59(1):126–35.

81. Burnstock G. Purinergic mechanosensory transduction and visceral pain. Mol Pain 2009;5:69.

82. Achem SR. New frontiers for the treatment of noncardiac chest pain: the adenosine receptors. Am J Gastroenterol 2007;102(5):939–41.

# Pain in Osteoarthritis

P. René van Weeren, DVM, PhD*, Janny C. de Grauw, DVM

**KEYWORDS**

- Osteoarthritis • Joint pain • Articular cartilage
- Pharmacologic management of joint pain

Osteoarthritis (OA), also known as osteoarthrosis or degenerative joint disease, is the most important chronic musculoskeletal disorder in both humans and horses. Although not a life-threatening disease, OA is considered one of the major concerns in human health care because of the vast number of people involved and the severe impact this literally crippling disease can have on quality of life. In the United States alone, total costs of OA were estimated at $89.1 billion in 2001[1] and a more recent article estimates that, compared with 2005, total hip replacements will have gone up by 673% in 2030 to a total of 3.5 million surgeries per year.[2] In France, direct costs of OA exceeded $2 billion in 2002 and accounted for 13 million physician visits. That year's figures represented a 156% increase in costs over 1993, which was for more than 90% because of an increase in the number of patients, rather than because of the increase of costs per patient.[3] The substantial direct and indirect costs of OA make this disease a major economic burden, in addition to a cause of loss of quality of life for hundreds of millions of people. In horses, articular disorders, most of which are related to osteoarthritic pain, account for the greatest single economic loss to the equine industry,[4] and likewise form a major animal welfare concern.

This article focuses on pain associated with OA. It first describes the basic biology of articular cartilage and other joint structures and the defining features of the osteoarthritic disease process. Subsequently, the possible origins of pain in OA are discussed before embarking on how to manage this clinical entity. The emphasis is on the pharmacologic management of joint pain, and attention is paid to systemic therapeutic strategies as well as to local (intra-articular [IA]) treatment modalities. Nonmedical ways of modulating joint pain are briefly mentioned, but not extensively discussed, as these are outside the scope of this article.

## BIOLOGY OF THE DIARTHRODIAL JOINT AND CHARACTERISTICS OF OA

The fluid-filled cavity of the diarthrodial joint is surrounded by a limited number of tissues. These always include articular cartilage and the synovial membrane, in some cases supplemented by IA structures such as ligaments and menisci. Of these

Department of Equine Sciences, Faculty of Veterinary Medicine, Utrecht University, Yalelaan 114, NL-3584 CM, Utrecht, The Netherlands
* Corresponding author.
E-mail address: R.vanWeeren@uu.nl

Vet Clin Equine 26 (2010) 619–642
doi:10.1016/j.cveq.2010.07.007
0749-0739/10/$ – see front matter © 2010 Elsevier Inc. All rights reserved.

tissues, articular cartilage has been studied most extensively, probably followed by subchondral bone, a tissue that is not normally in direct contact with the joint cavity but may become exposed to it in severe cases of OA or in other joint disorders like IA fractures or osteochondrosis. Notwithstanding the historical focus of research interest on articular cartilage and subchondral bone, it is increasingly being recognized that synovial joints should be regarded more comprehensively as complex organs in which all constituent tissues play an important role: IA homeostasis is key to maintaining joint health, and impaired homeostasis is central to the pathogenesis and progression of joint degeneration.[5,6]

## Biology of the Diarthrodial Joint

The main function of diarthrodial joints is to enable smooth articulation of 2 adjoining bone ends, at the same time providing both strength to accommodate the forces generated by the combined influences of gravity, locomotion, and inertia, and resilience necessary to attenuate the shocks generated by locomotion. All articular tissues participate in accomplishing this complex task that poses severe biomechanical challenges to some of them, as opposing requirements like the need for simultaneous resilience and strength are hard to reconcile.

The joint capsule is a stiff fibrous tissue that offers structural support. It is often functionally and anatomically reinforced by other supporting structures, such as collateral ligaments. The inner lining of the joint capsule, the synovial membrane, consists of an inner thin (1–3 cells thick) cellular layer, variably supported by an outer stromal layer consisting of adipose and fibrous tissue that is well innervated and vascularized and that becomes continuous with the outer fibrous joint capsule. Owing to the lack of a basement membrane, the gaps between adjacent synoviocytes, and the close proximity of subsynovial blood vessels, there is ample possibility of exchange of all components but macromolecules between plasma and synovial fluid, and the latter can hence be considered an ultrafiltrate of the former.[7] The synovial membrane is populated by 3 types of cells. Synovial type A cells are mainly phagocytic, B cells are active paracrine secretors and produce hyaluronic acid (HA), and C cells are believed to be intermediate between the two. The high degree of vascularization of the subsynovial tissue and the capacity of the synovial cells to produce a wide variety of inflammatory mediators and catabolic enzymes make the synovial membrane a key player in all forms of joint inflammation or arthritis.

The hyaline cartilage that covers the articular surfaces of bones is a highly specialized connective tissue with biomechanical characteristics that make it particularly suitable for load bearing and shock absorption.[8] A sparse population of chondrocytes (1%–2% of articular cartilage volume) is distributed throughout the extracellular matrix, which consists mainly of type II collagen, proteoglycans, glycoproteins, and water. The physical properties of the tissue depend on the structure and organization of the macromolecules in the extracellular matrix.[9,10] The collagen molecules are organized in a dense cross-linked fibrillar network that is packed with proteoglycans, which are strongly negatively charged as a result of their polyanionic glycosaminoglycan sidechains. This creates a large osmotic swelling pressure, drawing water into the tissue and expanding the collagen network. It is this balance within the extracellular matrix between the tension in the collagen network and the osmotic swelling pressure of the proteoglycans that gives articular cartilage its unique biomechanical characteristics, as it provides a combination of high compressive stiffness and resilience. These properties are critically dependent on both the integrity of the collagen network and the synthesis and retention of proteoglycans.[9,11,12]

Articular cartilage is connected to the underlying subchondral bone via the calcified cartilage layer. The subchondral bone consists of a so-called subchondral plate of dense cortical bone that is supported by trabecular bone with a more open structure. The thickness of the subchondral bone plate may vary and can be heavily influenced by pathology. Distal tarsal subchondral bone plate thickness has been measured at 2 to 4 mm in normal horses[13] and is in the same order of magnitude in other joints. The subchondral bone provides structural support for the overlying cartilage; its mechanical properties are therefore vital to the accommodation of forces of locomotion by the articular cartilage.

The joint cavity is filled with synovial fluid (SF), which as discussed can be considered an ultrafiltrate of blood plasma, with molecules smaller than 10 KDa existing in full equilibrium between plasma and SF.[14] Synovial fluid is highly viscous, mainly because of its high concentration of HA. Synovial fluid is a key component in joint homeostasis, as it acts both as a lubricant to allow nearly frictionless joint motion and as the medium for transport of nutrients and waste products to and from the avascular articular cartilage. From a research point of view, it is also uniquely suited to monitor IA events, as all changes evoked by a disturbance of joint homeostasis, such as influx of cells or locally produced inflammatory mediators and cytokines but also by-products of tissue turnover, which all have the potential to be used as biomarkers of disease, can be detected in the SF.[15]

## Osteoarthritis

Recently, 3 of the world's most prominent OA researchers agreed on the following definition of OA: *"Osteoarthritis can be described as the failed repair of damage that has been caused by excessive mechanical stress (defined as force/unit area) on joint tissues."*[16] This implies that although multiple factors may lead to OA, mechanical impact (either as a major single event or as repetitive microtrauma) is central to all of these, and that the sequence of events that ensues represents the intrinsic repair process, which may either fail or be successful in restoring joint function.

The focus on biomechanical influences as the sole primary etiological factor in OA is not uncontested. In the horse, synovitis is also regarded as an important primary, or at least concomitant, event.[17] Irrespective of whether there are only single or multiple primary factors, there is general consensus that after this primary event a vicious cycle may ensue that comprises both inflammatory and degradative components. There is no doubt that inflammation in OA is much less prominent than in rheumatoid arthritis (RA), and OA has even long been considered a noninflammatory degenerative disorder. However, in the genomic era of molecular biology, this view can no longer be maintained[18] and it is now widely recognized that synovial inflammation is an important component of OA, contributing to the dysregulation of chondrocyte catabolic and anabolic activities (**Fig. 1**).[19] In OA, bouts of more intense inflammatory activity typically alternate with (often long) quiescent spells in which joint abnormalities are minimal. This slow and insidious progression of the disease is reflected by the intermittent occurrence of clinical symptoms, with "flare-ups" and overt lameness often alternating with periods in which the joint may be largely asymptomatic.[20] Although OA can be managed relatively well for prolonged periods if loading can be adapted to the (reduced) carrying capacity of the joint, often this is not the case and instead the joint enters a vicious cycle of inflammation, structural damage, further loss of resistance to loading, aggravated inflammatory response, and so forth. In this respect, it is important to realize that articular cartilage is not able to fully repair itself because of the extremely long turnover time of collagen type II (half-life of human collagen type II has been calculated at 117 years[21]). Instead, cartilage damage will be

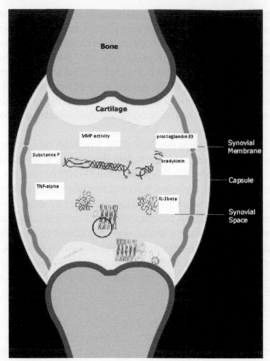

**Fig. 1.** Simplified, schematic view of a joint with active synovitis. The fluid-filled synovial cavity contains a plethora of mediators and activated catabolic enzymes released by the synovial membrane as well as by chondrocytes, which will in turn affect the cleavage as well as synthesis of articular cartilage matrix components like collagen type II and proteoglycans.

repaired by fibrocartilage that is mainly composed of collagen type I and that has inferior biomechanical qualities compared with the original tissue.

The cumulative damage will eventually lead to softening, fibrillation, ulceration, and loss of articular cartilage (**Fig. 2**); hypertrophy and fibrosis of the synovial membrane and joint capsule; sclerosis and eburnation of subchondral bone; and formation of

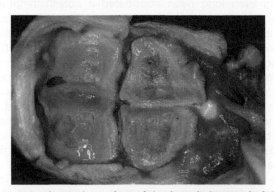

**Fig. 2.** View of the proximal articular surface of the first phalanx and of the articular side of the sesamoid bones from a metacarpophalangeal joint that was heavily affected by late-stage OA.

osteophytes and/or subchondral cysts.[22] Both at this end stage and at each interme-diate stage of the disease process, there are many potential sources of joint pain.

## PAIN IN OA

Joint pain (often intermittent) is one of the hallmarks of OA and the major cause of lameness associated with the disease. It has been described as "the most prominent but least well-studied feature of OA."[23]

### The Origin of Pain

For the perception of pain, 2 general conditions need to be met: first, a pain stimulus must be generated, and second this stimulus must be detected, transduced, and transmitted by the nervous system to the brain where pain perception can take place. Two general types of pain stimuli in synovial joints can be distinguished: mechanical stimuli, generated by (severe) mechanical changes in the environment of the joint (eg, by direct trauma), and chemical stimuli resulting from tissue inflammation. These stimuli are detected and forwarded by different types of receptors, mechanorecep-tors, and nociceptors, the distribution and relative abundance of which differ in various joint tissues. The signal is then carried by A$\delta$ or C-nerve fibers in peripheral nerves to the dorsal horn of the spinal cord, where neuromodulators and neurotransmitters are located within synapses between primary and secondary neurons. The latter decus-sate within the spinal cord and travel to the brain where the signal is further processed, modulated, and finally perceived.[24]

### Innervation of Articular Tissues

Articular cartilage is unique in that it is both aneural and avascular (at least in mature individuals). As a result, damage limited to the cartilage layer will not immediately be detected, and this may explain how cartilage erosion as seen in OA can silently prog-ress for a long time before becoming clinically manifest. Of the other articular tissues, both subchondral bone and the joint capsule are innervated, the latter quite densely. This is also the case for IA ligaments and menisci. In articular tissues, 4 types of afferent receptors can be discerned.[25] Type 1 receptors are low-threshold mechano-receptors, consisting of thinly encapsulated end organs of medium size (80–100 µm) connected to medium-sized myelinated nerve fibers. They can be found in the joint capsule, but not in the synovial membrane, and serve mainly a proprioceptive func-tion. Type 2 receptors are large encapsulated end organs (280–300 µm), connected to 9- to 12-µm myelinated nerve fibers. They are low-threshold mechanoreceptors and can be found typically at the junction of the fibrous joint capsule and the subsy-novial adipose tissue, hence in closer proximity to the joint cavity. These receptors are rapidly adapting and are activated only when the joint is in motion, acting as dynamic proprioceptive sensors. Type 3 receptors are relatively large (150 × 600 µm), thinly encapsulated end organs located near the bony insertions of IA and peri-artic-ular ligaments. They have a high threshold and are inactive in static conditions and during limited passive movement. These receptors are activated when joint motion reaches its physiologic limits; they have both mechanoreceptive and nociceptive potential and can be seen as safety mechanisms. They are connected to very rapidly conducting myelinated fibers. Type 4 receptors, also known as polymodal nocicep-tors, are not really anatomically discernible as receptors, but rather consist of free nerve endings of afferent nonmyelinated C-fibers or small myelinated A$\delta$ fibers. They are abundant in the entire joint capsule and can even be found in limited numbers within the synovial membrane. Also, the periosteum directly adjacent to the joint margins has a dense supply of these receptors. Type 4 receptors are high-threshold nociceptors that respond to thermal and chemical, but also mechanical, stimuli, whereby chemical stimuli (like those evoked by inflammatory mediators) may augment the responsiveness to mechanical stimuli, hence sensitizing the joint to these and causing hyperalgesia as well as allodynia.

Pain transmission through afferent fibers is not the simple one-way procedure it may appear to be. Peripheral sensory neurons function as afferent conductors, but they also exert important efferent functions mediated by neuropeptides.[26] Neuropeptides are small molecules that are synthesized in the dorsal root and autonomic ganglion neurons and from there are transported via the axon to peripheral nerve terminals. They are potent bioactive substances that can induce the release of other mediators, such as cytokines, prostaglandins, and nitric oxide (NO). Their active range is usually limited, both in space and time, owing to their chemically labile character. In healthy or regenerating tissue, they may have growth factorlike functions[27] and thus they do not only play a role during inflammation but also in the maintenance of joint homeostasis. Well-known neuropeptides include substance P (SP), calcitonin gene–related peptide (CGRP), vasoactive intestinal polypeptide (VIP), neuropeptide Y (NPY), and somatostatin (SOM).[26] Neuropeptides play an important role in the complex mechanisms that modulate and mitigate nociceptive input; for instance, VIP is thought to be instrumental in the augmentation of the responsiveness to mechanical stimuli in case of joint inflammation.[28]

### Pathophysiological Sources of Pain in OA

Numerous processes in the course of OA can contribute to the joint pain experienced by affected subjects, and very rarely can the precise tissue origin of pain be identified in the individual patient (**Fig. 3**). The previously described sensory innervation patterns of the subchondral bone, marginal periosteum, synovial membrane, and joint capsule will contribute to a variable extent to OA pain and loss of function, depending on individual disease stage and activity. In addition, alterations of central nervous system pathways associated with chronic pain states (central sensitization or "wind-up")

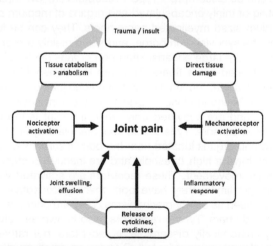

**Fig. 3.** Simplified schematic diagram of the vicious cycle of osteochondral damage and cartilage degeneration in OA, showing key processes that may contribute to joint pain associated with the disease.

have also been identified in human patients with OA and may partially explain the difficulty in long-term management of OA pain.[29] Within the joint tissues, subchondral bone exposure, remodeling, and/or marrow edema (causing a rise in intraosseous pressure), as well as marginal periosteal activation associated with osteophyte formation, have been implicated as sources of pain in more advanced stages of OA.[25] Synovitis is an important factor that contributes to pain in OA both through joint effusion, swelling, and/or fibrosis that in turn will activate mechanoreceptors in the joint capsule, and through direct chemical stimulation of nociceptors.

## Pathways of Inflammatory Pain

Whereas the stimulation of mechanoreceptors by mechanical influences is relatively straightforward, nociception will in most cases be stimulated or enhanced by inflammation. In this context, the interrelationship between the 2 receptor types needs to be pointed out: not only can mechanoreceptors become sensitized by chemical stimuli released during inflammatory processes, as alluded to previously, but mechanical stimulation itself may, through tissue damage, elicit an inflammatory response with release of pro-nociceptive mediators.

Pain is 1 of the 5 classic characteristics of inflammation (rubor, tumor, dolor, calor, and functio laesa), as already formulated in Antiquity by Celsus (30BC–38AD). In inflammation, pain originates from the chemical stimulation of nerve afferents by a variety of endogenous mediators. It is commonly accepted that interleukin-1 (IL-1) and tumor necrosis factor alpha (TNF-$\alpha$) are the 2 major cytokine players in the pathogenesis of OA.[30] IL-1 and TNF-$\alpha$ increase the synthesis of prostaglandin $E_2$ (PGE$_2$) by stimulating cyclooxygenase (COX)-2, microsomal PGE synthase-1 (MPES-1), and soluble phospholipase $A_2$ (SPLA$_2$), and they upregulate the production of nitric oxide via inducible nitric oxide synthetase (iNOS).[23] IL-1$\beta$ is known to induce the production of other proinflammatory cytokines also, including IL-6, -17, and -18 (for a review, see Goldring and Goldring[31]). Relatively little work has been devoted to the exact identification of pain-related mediators in joint disease, which supports the earlier quoted statement that pain is one of the principal but least researched symptoms of OA.[23] Prostaglandins have always been incriminated as the major pain mediators in arthritis,[32] but this key role is not as clear-cut and unambiguous as it may seem. In a dog study, significant positive correlations were established between PGE$_2$ levels in SF and subjective lameness score,[33] but in another dog study comparing normal and osteoarthritic tissues, a significant increase in COX-2 protein was found in OA specimens without an increase in PGE$_2$ concentration.[34] In a study using human synovial tissue and comparing early and established OA, COX-2 expression was higher in early OA, but cytokine-induced PGE$_2$ production in culture was similar.[35] In a horse study where PGE$_2$ levels in SF were compared in lame horses that did or did not respond to IA analgesia, no significant difference was found. Interestingly, however, when comparing the SF PGE$_2$ levels of these lame horses (blocking to a low 4-point or 6-point perineural nerve block) to those of sound horses, the lame horses had significantly higher and more variable PGE$_2$ levels than the sound controls.[36] There are indications that the other branch of the arachidonic acid cascade, the pathway that leads via 5-lipoxygenase (LOX) to the formation of leukotrienes, may play a role in articular nociception too. In the previously mentioned dog study,[34] there was a trend ($P = .069$) toward upregulation of LOX in OA-affected animals. Further, leukotriene $B_4$ (LTB$_4$) has been shown to be implicated in hyperalgesia in joints of mice.[37] In the horse, LTB$_4$ levels have been shown to be increased in animals suffering from osteochondrosis (OC) and may be involved in the extensive joint distension that is seen in many of these cases.[38] However, lameness in these patients is uncommon and thus far no link between $LTB_4$ and joint pain in the horse has been established.

Various neuropeptides have been identified as direct pain mediators in joint disease in humans. These include neuropeptide Y, serotonin, and calcitonin gene–related peptide.[39,40] In the horse, substance P has been suggested to play a role in the signaling and maintenance of pain associated with OA,[41] but could not be related to radiographic OA status of a joint.[42] However, substance P was the only mediator from a panel of possible mediators that could be directly linked to outcome of IA analgesia in the study by De Grauw and colleagues.[36] Kinins, with bradykinin as the main representative,[43,44] the major inflammatory cytokines themselves, and chemokines, a rather novel family of cytokines that now has been linked to the induction and maintenance of chronic pain,[45] have all been implicated in the generation of joint pain and are involved in the regulation of sensory neuron function (for an overview see Miller and colleagues[46]). None of these pain mediators have yet been investigated in the horse, with the exception of bradykinin, the concentration of which was not related to the outcome of IA analgesia,[36] but did show a strong correlation with lameness and joint hyperalgesia in chemically induced synovitis.[47]

## MANAGEMENT OF JOINT PAIN

Pain is the most salient clinical feature of OA and has the biggest impact on both welfare and performance. Pain management is therefore of great importance when managing osteoarthritis; however, it should be realized that treatment aimed at pain reduction does not necessarily treat the underlying primary disease process and may even interfere negatively with it. In fact, it has been suggested that long-term use of nonsteroidal anti-inflammatory drugs might enhance the pathologic process of cartilage degeneration by removing the regulatory role of $PGE_2$ on IL-1 synthesis.[48] On the other hand, treatment aimed primarily at pain relief may, through anti-inflammatory actions, also positively affect the articular cartilage by means of inhibition of release of catabolic factors.[49]

Chronic pain attributable to OA is mostly managed pharmacologically, but other ways of modulating joint pain are available and may prove efficacious. The following section first discusses systemic medical treatment of OA pain, followed by IA or other topical therapies, to conclude with a paragraph on nonpharmacologic modulation of joint pain.

### Systemic Treatment of Joint Pain

The nonsteroidal anti-inflammatory drugs (NSAIDs) are by far the most important class of compounds in this category. However, several other systemically administered OA drugs also provide some extent of analgesia, although this is secondary to their influence on the primary process and not the principal *rationale* for their use.

### Nonsteroidal anti-inflammatory drugs

NSAIDs inhibit the enzyme cyclooxygenase (COX) in the arachidonic acid cascade, thus inhibiting prostaglandin production. Most of the older NSAIDs indiscriminately inhibit both COX-1 and -2 iso-enzymes, and therefore also affect constitutive prostaglandin production by COX-1 that exerts physiologic functions among which is protection of mucosal barriers in the gastrointestinal tract. Newer generation NSAIDs have been developed that are more selective COX-2 inhibitors and these have demonstrated a superior gastrointestinal safety profile in humans, while providing comparable analgesic and anti-inflammatory potency.[50] Preferential and selective COX-2 inhibitors have also become available for the treatment of OA in the horse, but traditional nonselective NSAIDs are still routinely used, with phenylbutazone maintaining its prominent place over the past decades. **Table 1** summarizes dosages and ways of administration for the most commonly used NSAIDs, which will be dealt with in somewhat more detail in the following paragraphs.

Phenylbutazone (PBZ), or "bute" as it is sometimes semi-affectively called, is the most widely used drug in equine orthopedic practice and is often cited as the most cost-effective treatment for OA pain.[51] Its use is not entirely uncontested, though, as the drug may have severe adverse health effects on humans. Butazones have been associated with a (slightly) increased risk of aplastic anemia in humans[52] and potential genotoxic and carcinogenic effects were identified in mice and rat studies[53]; for this reason, the drug has been withheld from official registration for equine use in some countries. Recently, concern was expressed about the possible public health effect of PBZ in horse meat exported from the United States. In the United States, horse meat is not regularly sold for human consumption, but many slaughter horses are exported, and eventually enter the food chain.[54] PBZ is mostly used orally in a dose of 2.2 mg/kg twice a day (or tapered to once a day) after an initial loading dose of 4.4 mg/kg twice a day for 2 consecutive days. Intravenous formulations are also available, but carry some risk of perivenous irritation.[51] Most equine clinicians will agree that PBZ is very effective in treating articular pain, and this is indeed supported by literature, but comparative research on clinical efficacy versus other NSAIDs in horses is surprisingly limited.[55–58] The information on the effects of PBZ on cartilage or chondrocytes (ie, on the primary disease process), is even scarcer and stems mainly from in vitro studies that have produced conflicting results. Beluche and colleagues[59] reported detrimental inhibition of proteoglycan synthesis in articular cartilage of horses that were administered PBZ in vivo, whereas Frean and colleagues

**Table 1**
Overview of the most commonly used NSAIDs with their route of administration and dosage

| Name of Drug | Route of Application | Dosage | Remarks |
|---|---|---|---|
| Phenylbutazone | Oral | 2.2 mg/kg BID (Initial loading dose often 4.4 mg/kg for 2 days and for long-term use standard dose tapered to SID) | In some countries not permitted because of perceived risks for human health |
| Flunixin | Oral or IV | 1.1 mg/kg SID | IM application possible, but has been associated with myonecrosis |
| Carprofen | IV or oral | 0.7 mg/kg (IV) SID 1.4 mg/kg (oral) SID | |
| Ketaprofen | IV or IM | 2.2 mg/kg SID | In oral form not bioavailable |
| Vedaprofen | Oral | Initial dose 2 mg/kg BID, maintenance 1 mg/kg BID | |
| Meloxicam | Oral | 0.6 mg/kg SID | A positive effect on cartilage metabolism has been demonstrated in vivo[49] |
| Naproxen | Oral or IV | 10 mg/kg BID or SID | |

Abbreviations: BID, twice a day; IM, intramuscular; IV, intravenous; SID, once a day.

and Jolly and colleagues failed to demonstrate any such effect after in vitro exposure of cartilage to PBZ.[60,61] Fradettte and colleagues[62] showed that administration of PBZ increased osteocalcin levels in synovial fluid in healthy equine joints, but found no effects on biomarkers of both collagen and proteoglycan metabolism. PBZ has a narrower safety margin than most other equine NSAIDs and may have severe toxic side effects when recommended dosages are exceeded and/or in susceptible animals (which include geriatric horses, ponies, foals, and those with vascular, renal, or hepatic compromise[63]). These adverse effects include gastrointestinal ulceration, renal papillary necrosis, and thrombosis and are potentially lethal.

Flunixin has found its widest application in equine practice in the treatment of abdominal pain. It is, however, also effective for the alleviation of lameness[64] and was shown to be equally efficacious to PBZ in horses with navicular disease[58] and to provide longer postoperative analgesia.[57] Flunixin suppresses induced $PGE_2$ production by synovial membrane in vitro without detrimental effects on function or viability of the tissue,[65] but has been shown to increase IL-6 production by synoviocytes, albeit at very high doses.[48] Other possible effects of the drug on joint homeostasis have not been investigated. Flunixin is generally administered at a dose of 1.1 mg/kg once a day orally or intravenously (IV). Toxicity is low, with adverse effects only becoming apparent at 5 times the recommended daily dose.[66]

Carprofen was shown to be a relatively potent analgesic in horses, with duration of postoperative analgesia intermediate between that of flunixin and PBZ.[57] It is administered at a dose of 0.7 mg/kg IV or 1.4 mg/kg orally in countries where the oral dosage form carries market authorization for horses. Several in vitro studies have focused on the potential influence of the drug on joint homeostasis and indicated possible positive effects. Carprofen, which exists as 2 enantiomers, attenuated lipopolysaccharide (LPS)-induced IL-6 increase in cultured synoviocytes and the S enantiomer did the same in chondrocytes.[67] Also, (S-)carprofen stimulated proteoglycan synthesis in chondrocytes[68] and in cartilage explants.[69] Carprofen is considered a safe NSAID but has a relatively narrow therapeutic index, with adverse effects developing at twice the recommended dose.[70] Because of its potential beneficial effects on articular tissues, it has been suggested that carprofen could become a future NSAID of choice in OA,[51] but thus far the drug has not really challenged the position of PBZ and data on tissue effects in vivo are lacking.

Ketoprofen has been shown to accumulate in inflamed tissues, which has been suggested to result in improved efficacy in inflamed joints[71]; given that most NSAIDs are weak acids, accumulation in an inflamed environment should however not be unique to ketoprofen. In a direct comparison with PBZ in induced synovitis, the drug was found to be inferior to PBZ in treating acute joint inflammation,[56] although it proved equally effective at alleviating hoof pain.[72] The recommended dosage of ketoprofen is 2.2 mg/kg IV once a day. Ketoprofen is a relatively safe NSAID[73] but the main disadvantage of the drug precluding its routine use in chronic joint disease is that it is not orally bioavailable, restricting routes of administration to either intramuscular (IM) or IV.

This restriction does not apply to the related drug vedaprofen that has been registered for oral use (initial dosage 2 mg/kg twice a day, maintenance 1 mg/kg twice a day) in several countries. Vedaprofen seems to have more affinity for COX-1 than COX-2.[74] Nothing is known about its effects on the primary process of OA or about its efficacy against musculoskeletal pain in general. On clinical impression it has been suggested that the analgesic efficacy of vedaprofen for orthopedic pain compares unfavorably with that of PBZ, which may be because of its relatively short-lived reduction of $PGE_2$,[74] but no well-designed comparative clinical efficacy studies have been performed. In countries where the use of PBZ is either illegal or restricted, however, meloxicam rather than vedaprofen seems to have become the preferred oral NSAID for orthopedic diseases.

Meloxicam (orally dosed at 0.6 mg/kg once a day) was shown to be a potent anti-inflammatory and analgesic drug in an equine arthritis model.[75] Meloxicam was also shown to be the most selective COX-2 inhibitor of 4 examined NSAIDs (with PBZ, flunixin, and carprofen) when tested in vitro at the level of 50% inhibition (IC50), although at 80% inhibition, COX-2 selectivity was relatively less, whereas that of other NSAIDs increased.[76] Meloxicam is the only NSAID for which data exist regarding the in vivo effects of treatment on cartilage metabolism over the course of acute synovitis. In an LPS-induced arthritis model, De Grauw and colleagues[49] demonstrated a significant clinical effect on lameness and a local anti-inflammatory effect in the joint, as evidenced by suppression of $PGE_2$, bradykinin, and substance P release in the synovial fluid of the affected joints. Interestingly, matrix metalloproteinase (MMP) activity in synovial fluid was also lower than in placebo-treated joints, as were markers of proteoglycan breakdown and collagen II turnover. This indicated that meloxicam was able to mitigate the catabolic effects of acute joint inflammation on articular cartilage, although it remains to be established whether this also translates into chondroprotection in the longer term.

Naproxen does not seem to find wide application for use in equine musculoskeletal pain given the virtual absence of the drug in samples taken from track fatalities in a recent study, which was in contrast to PBZ and, to a lesser extent, flunixin.[77] Efficacy for treating equine OA has not been compared with other more commonly used drugs; therefore, no reliable data are known.[51] However, naproxen did prove more potent than PBZ in an equine myositis model.[78] Naproxen is administered orally or IV at a dosage of 10 mg/kg twice or once a day and has a wide safety margin.

***Other systemic treatments***

Horses suffering from OA or other chronic joint disorders are frequently orally treated with so-called "neutraceuticals," which are supposed to have a disease-modifying effect and in most cases contain, among other ingredients, mixtures of chondroitin sulfate and glucosamine. There has been (and still is) much controversy about the potential usefulness and mechanisms of action of these products in horses (for reviews see Trumble,[79] Goodrich and Nixon,[51] and Richardson and Loinaz[80]). Although some of the proposed modes of action include some level of anti-inflammatory activity, implying an indirect analgesic effect, these drugs are not primarily given to alleviate pain and will not be discussed further here.

Tiludronate is a bis-phosphonate that has been reported to be effective in cases of navicular disease or bone spavin characterized by osteolytic lesions.[81] Although tiludronate is not a primary analgesic agent, it was found to be effective against pain caused by osteoarthritic lesions of the thoracolumbar vertebral column.[82] There are no reports on its effects on OA in the appendicular skeleton.

Other systemic treatments for OA in horses include IM polysulfated glycosaminoglycans (PSGAG) and IV or oral sodium hyaluronate (HA). Various modes of action of each of these drugs have been identified in vitro, but precisely which of these contribute(s) most to clinical effects remains to be established. Intramuscular PSGAG was shown to reduce lameness (and hence pain) as well as effusion in an equine carpitis model,[83] but in 2 other in vivo studies using a carpal chip–induced OA model, no clinical (analgesic) benefit and no disease-modifying effect on any of the joint tissues were detected.[84,85]

Hyaluronan (HA; sodium hyaluronate) is available for systemic use in an IV formulation and in some countries also as an oral gel. The in vivo mode of action of intravenous HA on joint pain is thought to be mainly anti-inflammatory, although the way this effect comes about remains uncertain given the very rapid clearance of exogenous HA from the systemic circulation (terminal half-life after IV administration in horses of 43 minutes[86]). Interestingly, HA has been shown to have a direct analgesic effect through interaction with peripheral nerve endings in joints,[87] which could contribute to observed analgesic effects in horses.[88]

## LOCAL TREATMENT OF JOINT PAIN

Topical therapies for joint pain in the vast majority of cases comprise IA injection of corticosteroids (for an overview of most commonly used drugs and dosages see **Table 2**). The principal aims of corticosteroid use are attenuation of inflammation and pain relief (ie, mitigation of symptoms). The corticosteroids are discussed to some extent in the following section. In addition, there are a few other intra-articularly applied pharmaceuticals that principally target the primary process of OA, but may have some effect on pain perception and these are also mentioned briefly.

### Corticosteroids

Intra-articular corticosteroids were first used in human medicine in the early 1950s.[89] Application in veterinary practice soon followed suit.[90] Corticosteroids inhibit the nuclear factor (NF)-$\kappa$B signaling pathway, which plays an important role in the sequence of events leading to inflammatory mediator production, thereby acting as a potent upstream inhibitor of inflammation.[91,92] They are known to regulate gene expression levels of not only inflammatory but also matrix genes (eg, collagen type II and aggrecan gene expression) and hence can also affect cartilage turnover and repair.[93]

Corticosteroids inhibit inflammatory mediator production by inhibiting phospholipase $A_2$ through the production of anti-phospholipase proteins called lipocortins.[94] Because of their mode of action upstream in the arachidonic acid cascade, corticosteroids not only inhibit COX-1/2 derived mediators (including prostaglandins, thromboxanes, and lipoxins), but also the LOX-derived mediators like leukotrienes.

It should be realized that corticosteroids are primarily potent anti-inflammatory agents, exerting their analgesic action indirectly via the suppression of inflammation.

**Table 2**
**Overview of the most commonly used corticosteroids for intra-articular use**

| Name of Drug | Duration of Action | Dosage | Remarks |
|---|---|---|---|
| Methylprednisolone acetate | Long | 40–100 mg | The lower end of the dosage range is recommended for an optimal effect while avoiding damage at a longer term |
| Bethamethasone acetate | Medium to long | 3–18 mg | |
| Triamcinolone acetonide | Medium | 6–18 mg | Most commonly used |

In case of a combination of a corticosteroid and hyaluronic acid (HA), the former is commonly used at its normal dosage and HA often at approximately 20 mg/joint (but there are relatively large differences in molecular weight and purity among commercially available HA preparations and recommendations by the manufacturer may differ).

They are not specific analgesics. This explains the differences in analgesic efficacy in various joint disorders. Corticosteroids have been found to be most effective in those conditions where inflammation is the most important hallmark of the joint disorder, such as RA and juvenile idiopathic arthritis in humans.[95] In conditions like OA, where inflammation is less prominent and tissue degradation is at the forefront, they provide less effective pain relief. In humans, corticosteroid use in knee OA produced temporary pain relief for 3 weeks only; in RA this was much longer.[96]

Although first hailed as a more or less magic class of drugs in joint disease, corticosteroid use became controversial after reports on steroid-induced deterioration of articular tissues, which soon became known as "steroid arthropathy."[97,98] The issue has led to decades of debate about the suitability and even the ethical acceptability of IA corticosteroid use in horses, but seems to have settled down in recent years as a result of dedicated research and the publication of more long-term clinical data. In human medicine, IA use of corticosteroids is common practice for many conditions, including RA, juvenile idiopathic arthritis, and OA.[95] Multiple injections of 40 mg of triamcinolone into the knee joint at 3-month intervals for a period of 2 years did not lead to loss of joint space over time[99]; however, frequent repetition of IA injections with corticosteroids (up to 20 injections with half-week intervals) may lead to deleterious effects.[100] In horses, studies that showed negative matrix effects of corticosteroids have generally tended to use relatively high, repeated doses, and/or looked at effects in healthy joints. In a joint with preexistent synovitis, inflammatory gene expression is upregulated and catabolic enzyme activity increased, and the positive inhibitory effects of corticosteroids on these processes exceed the potential negative effects on cartilage matrix.[101,102] There now seems to be common agreement that, if used judiciously with respect to frequency and interval and not excessively dosed, the beneficial effects of IA corticosteroids in joint disease outweigh the disadvantages and possible risks.[51]

Other potential risks of corticosteroid use include an increased risk of joint infection and masking of signs thereof because of the immunosuppressive action of corticosteroids, and occurrence of so-called "flare," a transient but occasionally severe aseptic synovitis. The perceived risk of joint infection is low. A rate of 1:25,000 has been reported in humans.[103] Although the risk is low, the potential consequences of joint infection in the horse may be devastating and strict asepsis is imperative when performing the arthrocentesis. The routine use of antibiotics as practiced by many can be questioned, but is understandable when conditions are less than optimal. Joint flare after IA injection is seen in approximately 2% of cases in human medicine.[104] In the horse, the condition is known too. It is self-limiting, but may require treatment with NSAIDs.

There are several types of corticosteroids that are used in equine practice. They differ mainly in duration of action. Most commonly used are methylprednisolone acetate, betamethasone, and triamcinolone, which are discussed briefly in the following paragraphs.

Methylprednisolone acetate (MPA) is a long-acting corticosteroid with a recommended dose of 40 to 100 mg per joint. However, it is advised to aim for the lower end of this dose range. Doses between 10 and 40 mg have been shown to have a clear anti-inflammatory effect while preserving the normal joint environment.[105,106]

Betamethasone acetate is a medium- to long-acting corticosteroid. It has been used in equine medicine for more than 40 years.[107] The advised dose is 3 to 18 mg per joint. The drug did not have deleterious effects 7 weeks after application in both exercised and unexercised horses in an osteochondral chip model.[108] However, in vitro work showed suppression of proteoglycan synthesis at low to medium doses.[60]

Triamcinolone acetonide is probably the most widely used corticosteroid in equine orthopedics. It has a medium duration of action and was shown to have potent analgesic action in an LPS-induced lameness model in the horse.[109] In vitro studies have indicated that triamcinolone may potentially effectively suppress inflammation without negative effects on the transcription of extracellular matrix genes[110]; work by Frisbie and colleagues[111] even suggested minimization of OA development in an osteochondral chip model. However, as with all corticosteroids, the potential for unintentional alteration of cartilage metabolism is also present with triamcinolone, as evidenced by changes in SF biomarkers in healthy horses after 3 consecutive IA injections with 2-week intervals.[112]

## Opioids

Opioids, of which morphine is most widely used for medical purposes, are analgesic drugs par excellence. The IA use of morphine was introduced for postoperative analgesia after arthroscopic knee surgery in human medicine in the early 1990s.[113] Morphine produces analgesia in joints by the interaction with opioid receptors in the synovial membrane, which are upregulated in inflammation. The efficacy of the treatment is not uncontested. An initial meta-analysis of results from multiple clinical trials showed that intra-articularly administered morphine had a definite but small analgesic effect,[114] but a more recent one did not corroborate this.[115] In veterinary medicine, the technique has been adopted quite quickly in small animal practice,[116] but only recently has work been published in the horse. Santos and colleagues[117] compared the effect of IA morphine in horses with experimentally induced synovitis with the local anesthetic ropivacaine and found the analgesic effect of morphine to have a slower onset, but also to be stronger and longer lasting (up to 24 hours). The effects of IA morphine in an LPS-induced synovitis model were also studied recently by Lindegaard and colleagues[118,119] and Van Loon and colleagues[47]; the latter showed a significant effect of IA morphine on lameness, joint effusion, behavioral expression of pain, and on SF inflammatory mediators ($PGE_2$ and bradykinin). Interestingly, morphine had no effect on biomarkers of cartilage metabolism (De Grauw and colleagues, unpublished results, 2009) or on substance P release. Although IA morphine has been suggested as an alternative treatment for chronic joint pain in humans,[120,121] it is unlikely that the drug will be used in the horse for this purpose because of its relatively short duration of action as well as regulatory issues associated with opiate usage.

## Hyaluronic Acid

Hyaluronic acid (HA), also called hyaluronan, is a large unsulphated glycosaminoglycan that consists of repeating units of D-gluronic acid and N-acetylglucosamine. It has been used extensively as IA treatment in horses (for a review, see Caron[122]) initially mainly as visco-supplementation, but later more on the basis of its anti-inflammatory capacities that seem to be more crucial to clinical efficacy.[51] Although HA is supposed to positively affect the primary disease process and its principal use is not to provide analgesia, as is the case with corticosteroids or NSAIDs, HA reportedly also has some analgesic effect itself.[123] In humans there are various reports on the analgesic effects of HA in OA but publication bias and flaws in experimental design may have overestimated the beneficial effects in many studies. A meta-analysis showed only a relatively small positive effect of HA application compared with placebo.[124] In the horse, there are various studies reporting reduction of lameness following IA HA treatment, but many of these suffer from flaws in the experimental design, such as lack of description of randomization and blinding, and absence of a control group or use of an inappropriate control group, which may have affected the trustworthiness of the results.[80] A well-controlled study comparing the effects of IA polysulphated glycosaminoglycans and IA HA in an osteochondral chip model showed positive effects of HA at the tissue level, but failed to substantiate any clinical effect.[84]

The combination of IA corticosteroids and HA is popular in equine practice, as it permits the reduction of the dose of corticosteroids and, at least intuitively, may counteract the possible deleterious effects of these drugs on the cartilage either through such dose reduction and/or through a possible "chondroprotective" action of HA.[122] Unfortunately, no controlled trials have been reported to date that compare the clinical (analgesic) efficacy and cartilage matrix effects of IA HA, IA steroids, and IA steroid plus HA. Although it can indeed be assumed that the combination will have a substantial analgesic effect, in vitro studies so far have not provided support for the premise that HA might counteract potentially negative steroid effects on the articular cartilage.[125,126]

### Other Local Treatments

Topical administration of NSAIDs to specific joints has been investigated in horses, but has not found widespread application in practice thus far, probably because of the convenience of oral administration in practical circumstances. Iontophoric administration of ketoprofen to the middle carpal joint of sound horses has been tried, but was found to have far insufficient delivery efficiency.[127] A study investigating topical application of the NSAID diclofenac in a liposomal cream formulation in an equine-induced OA model was more successful, showing a significant reduction of lameness scores versus untreated controls that was comparable with that produced by PBZ.[55] Interestingly though, diclofenac was detected in the joint fluid only at concentrations far below that needed for effective COX-inhibition, and indeed did not reduce synovial fluid $PGE_2$ concentration compared with untreated controls, whereas PBZ did. This again highlights the less than simple direct relationship between clinical pain or lameness and SF prostaglandin concentration. Whether the lesser radial carpal bone sclerosis and overall gross cartilage erosion with topical diclofenac versus PBZ was somehow also related to the lack of reduction of SF $PGE_2$ concentration or was rather because of a COX-independent effect of the cream remained unclear.

Gene therapy has been used in the horse in an experimental setting.[128,129] It proved feasible to elevate expression of the IL-1 receptor antagonist for a prolonged period, thus exerting an anti-inflammatory effect that may indirectly affect pain perception.[128] Although promising and scientifically highly interesting, it cannot be expected that gene therapy will find wide application for alleviation of joint pain in the horse in the foreseeable future.

## NONPHARMACEUTICAL WAYS TO MODULATE CHRONIC JOINT PAIN

There are various nonpharmacological ways to influence pain from osteoarthritic joints (for an extensive overview, see Malone[130]). The most radical way is surgical arthrodesis of the affected joint, which eliminates joint motion but consequently also joint pain. For certain joints, particularly the proximal interphalangeal joints and the smaller tarsal joints, this is a viable therapeutic option in the horse, as it does not preclude athletic performance. Performed in other joints such as the metacarpophalangeal, metatarsophalangeal, or carpal joints, arthrodesis usually is a salvage procedure for valuable breeding stock. Most arthrodeses are performed using osteosynthetic techniques,[131,132] but other techniques such as chemical arthrodesis through IA injection of ethyl alcohol[133] have also been described.

A wide variety of complementary therapeutic modalities are available that are of potential utility in the treatment of chronic OA pain in horses. These include, but are not limited to, physiotherapy, acupuncture, extracorporeal shock wave treatment (ESWT), magnetic field therapy, transcutaneous electric nerve stimulation (TENS), therapeutic ultrasound, and laser therapy.[130] Of these, few have stood (or even have been subjected to) the test of rigorous scientific scrutiny, either in horses or in humans, and much of the "evidence" regarding these therapies is anecdotal at best. Interferential and patterned muscle stimulation has been claimed to be effective in the treatment of pain associated with knee OA in humans,[134] but the overall conclusion with regard to the efficacy of TENS for pain relief in OA is inconclusive, as published trials are small and of questionable quality.[135] In horses, ESWT has been suggested by some to be a viable option for pain relief from OA,[136] but recently it was shown to have no clinical or disease-modifying beneficial effect in a carpal chip model of induced OA,[137] and caution seems warranted as another recent study in rats demonstrated degeneration of articular cartilage caused by ESWT treatment.[138] For most other modalities, no studies that can stand the test of scientific rigor have been performed in horses.

## SUMMARY

Pain is the most important clinical hallmark of OA and OA pain management is an important item for the equine practitioner whose caseload on average consists of 67% orthopedic cases, most of them attributable to joint disorders. It is important to repeat here that pain is a symptom generated by the underlying disease process. Pain relief alone may have a favorable (short- to midterm) clinical effect, but could have adverse effects on the underlying disease process and hence on long-term outcome if overall management of the athletic horse is not altered (ie, exercise regimes adjusted accordingly) and/or if analgesia is not combined with other strategies that target the underlying degenerative process. Therefore, any pain treatment that is instituted in patients suffering from OA should be critically evaluated in this context. Progress in pain management in OA will likely come from 2 sources. First, it will stem from research on the disease process itself. The global research effort on human as well as animal OA is tremendous, and rapid progress is being made on both fundamental issues such as the detailed elucidation of pathogenetic mechanisms, and in areas with great therapeutic potential like the exciting field of tissue engineering.[139] Second, progress can be expected in our knowledge of systemic and local nociceptive pathways and pharmacologic modulation thereof. Both sources of progress are related. Knowledge of the molecular events in the pathogenesis of OA will lead to the identification of novel targets for pain therapy, which may include key receptors, ion channels, and neurotrophins.[140]

Progress can be expected to be most rapid in human medicine, given the huge research effort and research funding in this field compared with veterinary medicine. However, basic joint biology and pathogenetic mechanisms of common joint disorders such as OA have proven to be highly conserved among mammalian species and there is no doubt that pain control in the equine orthopedic patient will directly benefit from the research performed on behalf of its human counterpart.

## REFERENCES

1. Leigh JP, Seavey W, Leistikow B. Estimating the costs of job related arthritis. J Rheumatol 2001;28:1647–54.
2. Bitton R. The economic burden of osteoarthritis. Am J Manag Care 2009; 15(Suppl 8):S230–5.

3. Le Pen J, Reygrobellet C, Gérentes I. Financial costs of osteoarthritis in France. The "COART" France study. Joint Bone Spine 2005;72:567–70.
4. Frisbie DD. Synovial joint biology and pathology. In: Auer JA, Stick JA, editors. Equine surgery. 3rd edition. St. Louis (MO): Saunders; 2006. p. 1037–55.
5. Samuels J, Krasnokutsky S, Abramson SB. Osteoarthritis. A tale of three tissues. Bull NYU Hosp Jt Dis 2008;66:244–50.
6. Saris DB, Dhert WJ, Verbout AJ. Joint homeostasis. The discrepancy between old and fresh defects in cartilage repair. J Bone Joint Surg Br 2003;85:1067–76.
7. Todhunter RJ. General principles of joint pathobiology. In: McIlwraith CW, Trotter GW, editors. Joint disease in the horse. Philadelphia: Saunders; 1996. p. 1–28.
8. Palmer JL, Bertone AL. Joint biomechanics in the pathogenesis of traumatic arthritis. In: McIlwraith CW, Trotter GW, editors. Joint disease in the horse. Philadelphia: WB Saunders; 1996. p. 104–19.
9. Kempson GE. The mechanical properties of articular cartilage. In: Sokoloff L, editor. The joints and synovial fluid, vol. 2. New York: Academic Press; 1980. p. 177–238.
10. Jurvelin J, Säämänen AM, Arokoski J, et al. Biomechanical properties of canine knee articular cartilage as related to matrix proteoglycans and collagen. Eng Med 1988;17:147–62.
11. Eyre DR, Wu JJ. Collagen structure and cartilage matrix integrity. J Rheumatol Suppl 1995;43:82–5.
12. Van Weeren PR, Brama PA. Physiology and pathology of the equine joint. Pferdeheilk 2001;17:307–18.
13. Branch MV, Murray RC, Dyson SJ, et al. Is there a characteristic distal tarsal subchondral bone plate thickness pattern in horses with no history of hindlimb lameness? Equine Vet J 2005;37:450–5.
14. Knox P, Levick JR, McDonald JN. Synovial fluid. Its mass, macromolecular content, and pressure in major limbs of the rabbit. Q J Exp Physiol 1988;73:33–6.
15. Van Weeren PR, Firth EC. Future tools for early diagnosis and monitoring of musculoskeletal injury: biomarkers and CT. Vet Clin North Am Equine Pract 2008;24:153–75.
16. Brandt KD, Dieppe P, Radin E. Etiopathogenesis of osteoarthritis. Med Clin North Am 2009;93:1–24.
17. McIlwraith CW. General pathobiology of the joint and response to injury. In: McIlwraith CW, Trotter GW, editors. Joint disease in the horse. Philadelphia: WB Saunders; 1996. p. 40–70.
18. Attur MG, Dave M, Akamatsu M, et al. Osteoarthritis or osteoarthrosis: the definition of inflammation becomes a semantic issue in the genomic era of molecular medicine. Osteoarthritis Cartilage 2002;10:1–4.
19. Loeser RF. Molecular mechanisms of cartilage destruction: mechanics, inflammatory mediators, and aging collide. Arthritis Rheum 2006;54:1357–60.
20. Trotter GW, McIlwraith CW. Clinical features and diagnosis of equine joint disease. In: McIlwraith CW, Trotter GW, editors. Joint disease in the horse. Philadelphia: WB Saunders; 1996. p. 120–45.
21. Verzijl N, DeGroot J, Thorpe SR, et al. Effect of collagen turnover on the accumulation of advanced glycation end products. J Biol Chem 2000;50:39027–31.
22. Kuettner K, Goldberg VM. Introduction. In: Kuettner K, Goldberg VM, editors. Osteoarthritic disorders. Rosemont (IL): American Association of Orthopedic Surgeons; 1995. p. xxi–xxv.

23. Goldring MB, Goldring SR. Osteoarthritis. J Cell Physiol 2007;213:626–34.
24. Raffa RB. Mechanism of action of analgesics used to treat osteoarthritis pain. Rheum Dis Clin North Am 2003;29:733–45.
25. Caron JP. Neurogenic factors in joint pain and disease pathogenesis. In: McIlwraith CW, Trotter GW, editors. Joint disease in the horse. Philadelphia: WB Saunders; 1996. p. 71–80.
26. Niissalo S, Hukkanen M, Imai S, et al. Neuropeptides in experimental and degenerative arthritis. Ann N Y Acad Sci 2002;966:384–99.
27. Haegerstrand A, Dalsgaard CJ, Jonzon B, et al. Calcitonin gene-related peptide stimulates proliferation of human endothelial cells. Proc Natl Acad Sci U S A 1990;87:1299–303.
28. Schuelert N, McDougall JJ. Electrophysiological evidence that the vasoactive intestinal peptide receptor antagonist VIP6-28 reduces nociception in an animal model of osteoarthritis. Osteoarthritis Cartilage 2006;14:1155–62.
29. Gwilym SE, Keltner JR, Warnaby CE, et al. Psychophysical and functional imaging evidence supporting the presence of central sensitization in a cohort of osteoarthritis patients. Arthritis Rheum. 2009;61(9):1226–34.
30. Calich AL, Domiciano DS, Fuller R. Osteoarthritis: can anti-cytokine therapy play a role in treatment? Clin Rheumatol 2010;29:451–5.
31. Goldring SR, Goldring MB. The role of cytokines in cartilage matrix degradation in osteoarthritis. Clin Orthop Relat Res 2004;427(Suppl):S27–36.
32. Pettipher ER. Pathogenesis and treatment of chronic arthritis. Sci Prog 1989;73:521–34.
33. Trumble TN, Billinghurst RC, McIlwraith CW. Correlation of prostaglandin E2 concentrations in synovial fluid with ground reaction forces and clinical variables for pain or inflammation in dogs with osteoarthritis induced by transection of the cruciate ligament. Am J Vet Res 2004;65:1269–75.
34. Lascelles BD, King S, Roe S, et al. Expression and activity of COX-1 and 2 and 5-LOX in joint tissues from dogs with naturally occurring coxofemoral joint osteoarthritis. J Orthop Res 2009;27:1204–8.
35. Benito MJ, Veale DJ, FitzGerald O, et al. Synovial tissue inflammation in early and late osteoarthritis. Ann Rheum Dis 2005;64:1263–7.
36. De Grauw JC, van de Lest CH, van Weeren R, et al. Arthrogenic lameness of the fetlock: synovial fluid markers of inflammation and cartilage turnover in relation to clinical joint pain. Equine Vet J 2006;38:305–11.
37. Guerrero AT, Verri WA, Cunha TM, et al. Involvement of LTB4 in zymosan-induced joint nociception in mice: participation of neutrophils and PGE2. J Leukoc Biol 2008;83:122–30.
38. De Grauw JC, Brama PA, Wiemer P, et al. Cartilage-derived biomarkers and lipid mediators of inflammation in horses with osteochondritis dissecans of the distal intermediate ridge of the tibia. Am J Vet Res 2006;67:1156–62.
39. Suzuki T, Segami N, Nishimura M, et al. Bradykinin expression in synovial tissues and synovial fluids obtained from patients with internal derangement of the temporomandibular joint. Cranio 2003;21:265–70.
40. Bouloux GF. Temporomandibular joint pain and synovial fluid analysis: a review of the literature. J Oral Maxillofac Surg 2009;67:2497–504.
41. Fortier LA, Nixon AJ. Distributional changes in substance P nociceptive fiber patterns in naturally osteoarthritic articulations. J Rheumatol 1997;24:524–30.
42. Kirker-Head CA, Chandna VK, Agarwal RK, et al. Concentrations of substance P and prostaglandin E2 in synovial fluid of normal and abnormal joints of horses. Am J Vet Res 2000;61:714–8.

43. Dray A. Kinins and their receptors in hyperalgesia. Can J Physiol Pharmacol 1997;75:704–12.
44. Meini S, Maggi CA. Knee osteoarthritis: a role for bradykinin? Inflamm Res 2008; 57:351–61.
45. Charo IF, Ransohoff RM. The many roles of chemokines and chemokine receptors in inflammation. N Engl J Med 2006;354:610–21.
46. Miller RJ, Hosung J, Bhangoo SK, et al. Cytokine and chemokine regulation of sensory neuron function. Handb Exp Pharmacol 2009;194:417–49.
47. Van Loon JP, de Grauw JC, van Dierendonck M, et al. Intra-articular opioid analgesia is effective in reducing joint pain and inflammation in an equine LPS induced synovitis model. Equine Vet J 2010;42(5):412–9.
48. Landoni MF, Foot R, Frean S, et al. Effects of flunixin, tolfenamic acid, R(-) and S (+) ketoprofen on the response of equine synoviocytes to lipopolysaccharide stimulation. Equine Vet J 1996;28:468–75.
49. De Grauw JC, van de Lest CH, Brama PA, et al. *In vivo* effects of meloxicam on inflammatory mediators, MMP activity and cartilage biomarkers in equine joints with acute synovitis. Equine Vet J 2009;41:693–9.
50. Chen YF, Jobanputra P, Barton P, et al. Cyclooxygenase-2 selective non-steroidal anti-inflammatory drugs (etodolac, meloxicam, celecoxib, rofecoxib, etoricoxib, vadecoxib and lumiracaxib) for osteoarthritis and rheumatoid arthritis: a systematic review and economic evaluation. Health Technol Assess 2008;12. 1–278.
51. Goodrich LR, Nixon AJ. Medical treatment of osteoarthritis in the horse— a review. Vet J 2006;171:51–69.
52. Risks of agranulocytosis and aplastic anemia. A first report of their relation to drug use with special reference to analgesics. The International Agranulocytosis and Aplastic Anemia Study. JAMA 1986;256:1749–57.
53. National Toxicology Program. NTP Toxicology and Carcinogenesis Studies of Phenylbutazone (CAS No. 50-33-9) in F344/N Rats and B6C3F1 Mice (Gavage Studies). Natl Toxicol Program Tech Rep Ser 1990;367:1–205.
54. Dodman N, Blondeau N, Marini AM. Association of phenylbutazone usage with horses bought for slaughter: a public health risk. Food Chem Toxicol 2010;48(5): 1270–4.
55. Frisbie DD, McIlwraith CW, Kawcak CE, et al. Evaluation of topically administered liposomal cream for treatment of horses with experimentally induced arthritis. Am J Vet Res 2009;70:210–5.
56. Owens JG, Kamerling SG, Stanton SR, et al. Effects of pretreatment with ketoprofen and phenylbutazone on experimentally induced synovitis in the horse. Am J Vet Res 1996;57:866–74.
57. Johnson CB, Taylor PM, Young SS, et al. Postoperative analgesia using phenylbutazone, flunixin or carprofen in horses. Vet Rec 1993;133:336–8.
58. Erkert RS, MacAllister CG, Payton ME, et al. Use of force plate analysis to compare the analgesic effects of intravenous administration of phenylbutazone and flunixin meglumine in horses with navicular syndrome. Am J Vet Res. 2005; 66(2):284–8.
59. Beluche LA, Bertone AL, Anderson DE, et al. Effects of oral administration of phenylbutazone to horses on *in vitro* articular cartilage metabolism. Am J Vet Res 2001;62:1916–21.
60. Frean SP, Cambridge H, Lees P. Effects of anti-arthritic drugs on proteoglycan synthesis by equine cartilage. J Vet Pharmacol Ther 2002;25: 289–98.

61. Jolly WT, Whittem T, Jolly AC, et al. The dose-related effects of phenylbutazone and a methylprednisolone acetate formulation (Depo-Medrol) on cultured explants of equine carpal articular cartilage. J Vet Pharmacol Ther 1995;18: 429–37.

62. Fradette ME, Céleste C, Beauchamp RH, et al. Effects of continuous oral administration of phenylbutazone on biomarkers of cartilage and bone metabolism in horses. Am J Vet Res 2007;68:128–33.

63. Owens JG, Clark TP. Analgesia. Vet Clin North Am Equine Pract 1999;15(3): 705–23.

64. Houdeshell JW, Hennessy PW. A new non-steroidal, anti-inflammatory analgesic for horses. J Equine Med Surg 1977;1:57–63.

65. Moses VS, Hardy J, Bertone AL, et al. Effects of anti-inflammatory drugs on lipopolysaccharide-challenged and -unchallenged equine synovial explants. Am J Vet Res 2001;62:54–60.

66. Trillo MA, Soto G, Gunson DE. Flunixin toxicity in a pony. Equine Pract 1984;6: 21–9.

67. Armstrong S, Lees P. Effects of carprofen (R and S enantiomers and racemate) on the production of IL-1, IL-6 and TNF-alpha by equine chondrocytes and synoviocytes. J Vet Pharmacol Ther 2002;25:145–53.

68. Frean SP, Abraham LA, Lees P. In vitro stimulation of equine articular cartilage proteoglycan synthesis by hyaluronan and carprofen. Res Vet Sci 1999;67: 183–90.

69. Armstrong S, Lees P. Effects of R and S enantiomers and a racemic mixture of carprofen on the production and release of proteoglycan and prostaglandin E2 from equine chondrocytes and cartilage explants. Am J Vet Res 1999;60: 98–104.

70. May SA, Lees P. Nonsteroidal anti-inflammatory drugs. In: McIlwraith CW, Trotter GW, editors. Joint disease in the horse. Philadelphia: WB Saunders; 1996. p. 223–37.

71. Owens JG, Kamerling SG, Barker SA. Pharmacokinetics of ketaprofen in healthy horses and horses with acute synovitis. J Vet Pharmacol Ther 1995;18:187–95.

72. Owens JG, Kamerling SG, Stanton SR, et al. Effects of ketoprofen and phenylbutazone on chronic hoof pain and lameness in the horse. Equine Vet J 1995;27: 296–300.

73. MacAllister CG, Morgan SJ, Borne AT, et al. Comparison of adverse effects of phenylbutazone, flunixin meglumine, and ketoprofen in horses. J Am Vet Med Assoc 1993;202(1):71–7.

74. Lees P, May SA, Hoeijmakers M, et al. A pharmacodynamic and pharmacokinetic study with vedaprofen in an equine model of acute nonimmune inflammation. J Vet Pharmacol Ther 1999;22:96–106.

75. Toutain PL, Cester CC. Pharmacokinetic-pharmacodynamic relationships and dose response to meloxicam in horses with induced arthritis in the right carpal joint. Am J Vet Res 2004;65:1533–41.

76. Beretta C, Caravaglia G, Cavalli M. COX-1 and COX-2 inhibition in horse blood by phenylbutazone, flunixin, carprofen and meloxicam: an in vitro analysis. Pharmacol Res 2005;52:302–6.

77. Dirikolu L, Woods E, Boyles J, et al. Nonsteroidal anti-inflammatory agents and musculoskeletal injuries in thoroughbred racehorses in Kentucky. J Vet Pharmacol Ther 2009;32:271–9.

78. Jones EW, Hamm D. Comparative efficacy of PBZ and naproxen in induced equine myositis. J Equine Med Surg 1978;2:341–7.

79. Trumble TN. The use of neutraceuticals for osteoarthritis in horses. Vet Clin North Am Equine Pract 2005;21:575–97.

80. Richardson DW, Loinaz R. An evidence-based approach to selected joint therapies in the horse. Vet Clin North Am Equine Pract 2007;23:443–60.

81. Denoix JM, Thibaud D, Riccio B. Tiludronate as a new therapeutic agent in the treatment of navicular disease: a double-blind placebo-controlled clinical trial. Equine Vet J 2003;35:407–13.

82. Coudry V, Thibaud D, Riccio B, et al. Efficacy of tiludronate in the treatment of horses with signs of pain associated with osteoarthritic lesions of the thoraco-lumbar vertebral column. Am J Vet Res 2007;68:329–37.

83. White GW, Stites T, Jones W, et al. Efficacy of intramuscular chondroitin sulfate and compounded acetyl-d-glucosamine in a positive controlled study of equine carpitis. Proc Am Assoc Equine Pract 2004;50:264–9.

84. Frisbie DD, Kawcak CE, McIlwraith CW, et al. Evaluation of the effect of extracorporeal shock wave treatment on experimentally induced osteoarthritis in middle carpal joints of horses. Am J Vet Res 2009;70:449–54.

85. Trotter GW, Yovich JV, McIlwarith CW, et al. Effects of intramuscular polysulfated glycosaminoglycans on chemical and physical defects in equine articular cartilage. Can J Vet Res 1989;53:224–30.

86. Popot MA, Bonnaire Y, Guéchot J, et al. Hyaluronan in horses: physiological production rate, plasma and synovial fluid concentration in control conditions and following sodium hyaluronate administration. Equine Vet J 2004;36:482–7.

87. Peña Ede L, Sala S, Rovira JC, et al. Elastoviscous substances with analgesic effects in joint pain reduce stretch-activated ion channel activity in vitro. Pain 2002;99:501–8.

88. Kawcak CE, Frisbie DD, Trotter GW, et al. Effects of intravenous administration of sodium hyaluronate on carpal joints in exercising horses after arthroscopic surgery and osteochondral fragmentation. Am J Vet Res 1997;58:1132–40.

89. Hollander JL, Brown EM, Jessar RA, et al. Hydrocortisone and cortisone injected into arthritic joints; comparative effects of and use of hydrocortisone as a local antiarthritic agent. J Am Med Assoc 1951;147:1629–35.

90. Van Pelt RW. Clinical and synovial fluid response to intrasynovial injection of 6alpha-methylprednisolone acetate into horses and cattle. J Am Vet Med Assoc 1963;143:738–48.

91. Shalom-Barak T, Quach J, Lotz M. Interleukin-17-induced gene expression in articular chondrocytes is associated with activation of mitogen-activated protein kinase and NF-kappaB. J Biol Chem 1998;273:467–73.

92. Garvican ER, Vaughan-Thomas A, Redmond C, et al. MMP-mediated collagen breakdown induced by activated protein C in equine cartilage is reduced by corticosteroids. J Orthop Res 2010;28:370–8.

93. Kydd AS, Reno CR, Tsoa HW, et al. Early inflammatory arthritis in the rabbit: the influence of intraarticular and systemic corticosteroids on mRNA levels in connective tissues of the knee. J Rheumatol 2007;34:130–9.

94. Di Rosa RJ, Flower F, Hirata L, et al. Nomenclature announcement. Anti-phospholipase proteins. Prostaglandins 1984;28:441–2.

95. Habib GS, Saliba W, Nashashibi M. Local effects of intra-articular corticosteroids. Clin Rheumatol 2010;29:347–56.

96. Bellamy N, Campbell J, Robinson V, et al. Intraarticular corticosteroid for treatment of osteoarthritis of the knee. Cochrane Database Syst Rev 2002;2:CD005328.

97. Chandler GN, Wright V. Deleterious effect of intra-articular hydrocortisone. Lancet 1958;7048:661–3.
98. Salter RB, Gross A, Hamilton Hall J. Hydrocortisone arthropathy—an experimental investigation. Can Med Assoc J 1967;97:374–7.
99. Raynauld JP, Buckland-Wright C, Ward R, et al. Safety and efficacy of long-term intraarticular steroid injections in osteoarthritis of the knee: a randomised, double-blind, placebo-controlled trial. Arthritis Rheum 2003;48:370–7.
100. Parikh JR, Houpt JB, Jacobs S, et al. Charcot's arthropathy of the shoulder following intraarticular corticosteroid injections. J Rheumatol 1993;20:885–7.
101. Todhunter RJ, Fubini SL, Vernier-Singer M, et al. Acute synovitis and intra-articular methylprednisolone acetate in ponies. Osteoarthritis Cartilage 1998;6: 94–105.
102. MacLeod JN, Fubini SL, Gu DN, et al. Effect of synovitis and corticosteroids on transcription of cartilage matrix proteins. Am J Vet Res 1998;59:1021–6.
103. Pal B, Morris J. Perceived risks of joint infection following intra-articular corticosteroid injections: a survey of rheumatologists. Clin Rheumatol 1999;18:264–5.
104. Hollander JL. Intrasynovial corticosteroid therapy in arthritis. Md State Med J 1970;19:62–6.
105. Farquhar T, Todhunter RJ, Fubini SL, et al. Effect of methylprednisolone and mechanical loading on canine articular cartilage in explant culture. Osteoarthritis Cartilage 1996;4:55–62.
106. Todhunter RJ, Fubini SL, Wootton JA, et al. Effect of methylprednisolone acetate on proteoglycan and collagen metabolism of articular cartilage explants. J Rheumatol 1996;23:1207–13.
107. Houdeshell JW. Field trials of a new long-acting corticosteroid in the treatment of equine athropathies. Vet Med Small Anim Clin 1969;64:782–4.
108. Foland JW, McIlwraith CW, Trotter GW, et al. Effect of betamethasone and exercise on equine carpal joints with osteochondral fragments. Vet Surg 1994;23:369–76.
109. Kay AT, Bolt DM, Ishihara A, et al. Anti-inflammatory and analgesic effects of intra-articular injection of triamcinolone acetonide, mepivacaine hydrochloride, or both on lipopolysaccharide-induced lameness in horses. Am J Vet Res 2008;69:15646–54.
110. Richardson DW, Dodge GR. Dose-dependent effects of corticosteroids on the expression of matrix-related genes in normal and cytokine-treated articular chondrocytes. Inflamm Res 2003;52:39–49.
111. Frisbie DD, Kawcak CE, Trotter GW, et al. Effects of triamcinolone acetonide on an in vivo equine osteochondral fragment exercise model. Equine Vet J 1997;29: 349–59.
112. Céleste C, Ionescu M, Poole RA, et al. Repeated intraarticular injections of triamcinolone acetonide alter cartilage matrix metabolism measured by biomarkers in synovial fluid. J Orthop Res 2005;23:602–10.
113. Stein C, Comisel K, Haimerl E, et al. Analgesic effect of intraarticular morphine after arthroscopic knee surgery. N Engl J Med 1991;325:1123–6.
114. Gupta A, Bodin L, Holmström B, et al. A systematic review of the peripheral analgesic effects of intraarticular morphine. Anesth Analg 2001;93:761–70.
115. Rosseland LA. No evidence for analgesic effect of intra-articular morphine after knee arthroscopy: a qualitative systematic review. Reg Anesth Pain Med 2005; 30:83–98.
116. Pascoe PJ. Opioid analgesics. Vet Clin North Am Small Anim Pract 2000;30: 757–72.

117. Santos LC, de Moraes AN, Saito ME. Effects of intraarticular ropivacaine and morphine on lipopolysaccharide-induced synovitis in horses. Vet Anaesth Analg 2009;36:280–6.
118. Lindegaard C, Gleerup KB, Thomsen MH, et al. Anti-inflammatory effects of intra-articular administration of morphine in horses with experimentally induced synovitis. Am J Vet Res 2010;71:69–75.
119. Lindegaard C, Thomsen MH, Larsen S, et al. Analgesic efficacy of intra-articular morphine in experimentally induced radiocarpal synovitis in horses. Vet Anaesth Analg 2010;37:171–85.
120. Likar R, Schäfer M, Paulak F, et al. Intraarticular morphine analgesia in chronic pain patients with osteoarthritis. Anesth Analg 1997;84:1313–7.
121. Fine PG, Mahajan G, McPherson ML. Long-acting opioids and short-acting opioids: appropriate use in chronic pain management. Pain Med 2009;10(Suppl 2):S79–88.
122. Caron JP. Intra-articular injections for joint disease in horses. Vet Clin North Am Equine Pract 2005;21:559–73.
123. Moskowitz RW. Hyaluronic acid supplementation. Curr Rheumatol Rep 2000;2:466–71.
124. Lo GH, LaValley M, McAlindon T, et al. Intra-articular hyaluronic acid in treatment of knee osteoarthritis: a meta-analysis. JAMA 2003;290:3115–21.
125. Yates AC, Stewart AA, Byron CR, et al. Effects of sodium hyaluronate and methylprednisolone acetate on proteoglycan metabolism in equine articular chondrocytes treated with interleukin-1. Am J Vet Res 2006;67:1980–6.
126. Doyle AJ, Stewart AA, Constable PD, et al. Effects of sodium hyaloronate and methylprednisolone acetate on proteoglycan synthesis in equine articular cartilage explants. Am J Vet Res 2005;66:48–53.
127. Eastman T, Panus PC, Honnas CM, et al. Cathodic iontophoresis of ketoprofen over the equine middle carpal joint. Equine Vet J 2001;33:614–6.
128. Frisbie DD, Ghivizzani SC, Robbins PD, et al. Treatment of experimental equine osteoarthritis by in vivo delivery of the equine interleukin-1 receptor antagonist gene. Gene Ther 2002;9:12–20.
129. Goodrich LR, Brower-Toland BD, Warnick L, et al. Direct adenovirus-mediated IGF-1 gene transduction of synovium induces persisting synovial fluid IGF-1 ligand elevations. Gene Ther 2006;13:1253–62.
130. Malone ED. Managing chronic arthritis. Vet Clin North Am Equine Pract 2002;18:411–37.
131. Auer JA. Arthrodesis techniques. In: Equine surgery, editors. Auer JA, Stick JA. 3rd edition. St. Louis (MO): Saunders; 2006. p. 1073–86.
132. Jones P, Delco M, Beard W, et al. A limited surgical approach for pastern arthrodesis in horses with severe osteoarthritis. Vet Comp Orthop Traumatol 2009;22:303–8.
133. Shoemaker RW, Allen AL, Richardson CE, et al. Use of intra-articular administration of ethyl alcohol for arthrodesis of the tarsometatarsal joint in healthy horses. Am J Vet Res 2006;67:850–7.
134. Burch FX, Tarro JN, Greenberg JJ, et al. Evaluating the benefits of patterned stimulation in the treatment of osteoarthritis of the knee: a multi-center, randomized single-blind, controlled study with an independent masked evaluator. Osteoarthritis Cartilage 2008;16:865–72.
135. Rutjes AW, Nüesch E, Sterchi R, et al. Transcutaneous electrostimulation for osteoarthritis of the knee. Cochrane Database Syst Rev 2009;4:CD002823.
136. Revenaugh MS. Extracorporeal shock wave therapy for treatment of osteoarthritis in the horse: clinical applications. Vet Clin North Am Equine Pract 2005;21:609–25.

137. Frisbie DD, Kawcak CE, McIlwraith CW. Evaluation of the effect of extracorporeal shock wave treatment on experimentally induced osteoarthritis in middle carpal joints of horses. Am J Vet Res 2009;70:449–54.

138. Mayer-Wagner S, Ernst J, Maier M, et al. The effect of high-energy extracorporeal shock waves on hyaline cartilage of adult rats in vivo. J Orthop Res 2010; 28(8):1050–6.

139. Ahmed TA, Hincke MT. Strategies for articular cartilage lesion repair and functional restoration. Tissue Eng Part B Rev 2010;16(3):305–29.

140. Dray A, Read SJ. Future targets to control osteoarthritis pain. Arthritis Res Ther 2007;9:212.

# Laminitic Pain: Parallels with Pain States in Humans and Other Species

Simon N. Collins, PhD[a,b,c,]*, Christopher Pollitt, BVSc, PhD[a],
Claire E. Wylie, BVM&S, MRCVS, MSc[d],
Kaspar Matiasek, DVM, DrMedVet, DrMedVetHabil, FTA-Neuropath, MRCVS[c,e,]*

> **KEYWORDS**
>
> - Laminitis • Neuropathic pain • Inflammatory pain • Nociception
> - Dorsal root ganglia

Laminitis is a serious disease of the foot that results in debilitation, development of pronounced digital pain, and great suffering in the afflicted animal. The disease poses a threat to all horses, and is widely considered as being one of the most important diseases of horses and a global equine welfare problem.[1–3] Epidemiologic estimates from around the world variously suggest a population prevalence ranging between 7% and 14%.[4–8] It is estimated that 15% of horses in the United States are afflicted with laminitis over the course of their lifetime, and 75% of these horses develop severe or chronic lameness and debilitation that necessitates euthanasia.

Laminitis results in pathologic changes to the foot that cause severe discomfort, leading to abnormal foot placement and limb loading. These events can, if treatment is unsuccessful, lead ultimately to permanent anatomic changes within the foot, locomotor dysfunction, and reduced athletic performance, with continual or recurrent

[a] School of Veterinary Science, The University of Queensland, Gatton Campus, Gatton, Queensland 4343, Australia
[b] Orthopaedic Research Group, Centre for Equine Studies, Animal Health Trust, Lanwades Park, Kentford, Newmarket, Suffolk, UK
[c] Neuromuscular Research Group, Animal Health Trust, Lanwades Park, Kentford, Newmarket, Suffolk, UK
[d] Epidemiology Research Group, Centre for Preventive Medicine, Animal Health Trust, Lanwades Park, Kentford, Newmarket, Suffolk, UK
[e] Neuropathology Laboratory, Animal Health Trust, Lanwades Park, Kentford, Newmarket, Suffolk, UK
* Corresponding author. Simon N. Collins, School of Veterinary Science, The University of Queensland, Gatton Campus, Gatton, Queensland 4343, Australia; Kaspar Matiasek, Neuromuscular Research Group, Animal Health Trust, Lanwades Park, Kentford, Newmarket, Suffolk, UK.
*E-mail addresses:* simon.collins@aht.org.uk; kaspar.matiasek@aht.org.uk

Vet Clin Equine 26 (2010) 643–671
doi:10.1016/j.cveq.2010.08.001
0749-0739/10/$ – see front matter © 2010 Elsevier Inc. All rights reserved.

bouts of severe foot pain. Rather than failure of remedial foot treatments per se, it is the inability to manage the unrelenting and severe pain associated with the disease that is the single most common cause of euthanasia in laminitic horses. Indeed all too often foot treatment is curtailed before it can take full effect, due to the owner's inability to tolerate the persistent and refractory pain exhibited by the afflicted animal. If suffering was not so overt then improved treatment outcomes could arguably result.

Effective pain management is therefore of primary clinical importance.[9,10] However, despite these facts the precise pathophysiological processes that result in laminitic pain are poorly defined, and hence the delivery of effective palliative care is clinically challenging. Two recent, and highly recommended reviews[11,12] have highlighted the pathobiologic complexity of pain within the laminitic horse. These reviews have also commented on knowledge of the mechanistic basis of pain in the laminitic horse being limited, and that research is at an early stage in "unlocking Pandora's box" to gain understanding of the critical events that occur in this devastating and debilitating disease, This understanding remains a key research priority in the quest to "conquer" the threat posed by laminitis.[2]

Knowledge and understanding of pain states in other animal species may further aid the elucidation of equine laminitic pain mechanisms, guide the search for treatable causes of this multifactorial problem, and thereby help achieve enhanced therapeutic and palliative care. However, parallels drawn from pain states in other animals must consider species differences in both anatomy and physiology, and the specific nature of the laminitic disease process.

## DISEASE DEVELOPMENT AND PROGRESSION

Comprehensive knowledge of the pathologic events that occur within the laminitic foot, and their functional consequences, is essential in developing an understanding of the mechanistic basis of laminitic pain and in formulating appropriate pain management strategies. These events have been extensively reviewed elsewhere[13-20] and should be fully appreciated by all involved in the management of the laminitic horse.

In summary, laminitis triggers a complex series of pathophysiological events that lead to the development of digital pain. The onset of clinical signs of pain marks progression from the developmental or prodromal stage to the acute phase of the disease (**Table 1**).[21,22] Subsequently, the affected animal may either recover fully to enter a subacute phase, or conversely progresses into the chronic phase of the disease. It is important to appreciate that the subacute laminitic animal remains at potential risk of entering into the chronic phase of the condition until such time (up to 9 months) as normal hoof horn production has fully regenerated the hoof capsule of the affected foot.

Most notably, laminitis pathophysiology causes anatomic change within the interdigitating epidermal and dermal lamellae that forms an integral part of the suspensory apparatus of the distal phalanx (SADP), threatening its structural and functional integrity. The SADP (referred to elsewhere as the hoof-bone attachment apparatus[17,18]) unites the distal phalanx (DP) and the hoof wall via the lamellar dermis, and suspends the appendicular skeleton within the hoof capsule. The SADP is of major biomechanical importance because it enables these structures to act as a single structural and functional entity.[16,18,23-25] The SADP facilitates pain-free force transference between ground and skeleton during weight bearing, with the hoof wall, rather than the sole or digital pad, acting as the principal weight-bearing structure. This anatomic arrangement is unique to the ungulate foot, and in the horse it represents the principal mechanism by which weight-bearing forces are accommodated and resisted.[16,18,23] During weight bearing, the hoof capsule deforms in a regular and repeatable manner, and the DP moves relative to the hoof wall to generate internal forces that counter the loading forces associated with weight bearing. These events are accommodated painlessly by the dermal tissues. This unguligrade mode of weight bearing differs fundamentally from that which occurs in either the digigrade or plantigrade foot.[16,23]

Lamellar pathology initiated during the prodromal phase of the disease[26] progressively degrades the structural integrity of the SADP, and may reduce the ultimate strength by 90% within 48 hours of the onset of acute-phase laminitis.[27] This process leads to increased levels of DP movement within the hoof capsule in response to loading, causing elevated soft tissue strain and associated tissue damage within the affected foot. Ultimately the degree of lamellar pathology may exceed the mechanical limits of the SADP, leading to SADP failure. Failure of the SADP results in permanent dislocation of the DP, and irreversibly changes the normal anatomic interrelationships between hoof capsule, dermis, and DP (and the other osseous and nonosseous components of the foot) (**Fig. 1**). This dislocation event, which others describe as "structural failure" and "digital collapse," marks the onset of chronic-phase laminitis.[18,21,22,28] Dislocation of the DP further compromises normal foot function and leads to additional digital pain. Affected animals may present clinically as either chronic remissive laminitics (CRL), which are responsive to conventional methods of palliative care, or conversely as refractory exacerbative laminitics (REL),[29] which remain nonresponsive to these palliative methods.

Although wound-healing responses occur to restore the structural integrity of the damaged SADP, the mechanical properties of the regenerated lamellar structure are adversely affected.[30] In particular, research has shown that the rigidity of the regenerated SADP in the affected horse is significantly reduced and the failure strength of the SADP can be reduced by up to 58%.[30] Collectively, these changes leave the affected horse susceptible to recrudescent traumatic SADP injury, the development of secondary pathologies, and concurrent exacerbations and remissions of digital pain.

## SENSORY INNERVATION OF THE HORSE FOOT

Understanding of the local sensory innervation and the pathologic microenvironment is crucial in elucidating the pathobiology of laminitic pain. The distal forelimb and hindlimb are innervated by sensory nerves emanating from C7-C8 and L6-S1-S2, respectively, with innervation of the foot achieved by ramifications arising from the medial and lateral digital nerve, and the dorsal branch of the palmar/plantar nerve.[31–37]

Although the fine detail of the sensory innervation pattern is not completely defined, sensory inputs to the afferent nerves of the peripheral nervous system (PNS) are ultimately conveyed to the central nervous system (CNS) via the dorsal root. These sensory inputs include proprioceptive (posture movement and spatial orientation), nociceptive (noxious stimulation), and enteroceptive/viscerosensory (internal homeostatic state) input.

Lamellated Paccinian-like and Ruffini corpuscles are focally located within the palmar aspect of the dermis of the frog and heel bulbs.[31,33] These pressure-sensitive proprioceptors convey information by fast-conducting myelinated type Aα-fibers, and provide proprioceptive sensory information relating to foot placement and the hoof-ground interaction. With Merkel cell-neurite complexes in the coronary epithelium, there is another type of pressure receptors, responsible for discriminatory tactile senses at the dorsal and lateral aspects of the foot (**Fig. 2**). The precise role of these suspected high-resolution receptors in this area remains unclear.

**Table 1**
Summary of disease progression detailing pathophysiological events that can occur within the affected animal and the associated pain mechanisms that may be evoked

| Disease Phase | Duration | Clinical Signs | Structural/Functional Integrity of the SADP | Key Anatomic, Pathologic and Pathomechanical Events | Potential Pain Mechanism |
|---|---|---|---|---|---|
| Prodromal | 24–72 h | No clinical signs of pain | | Onset of lamellar degradation and basement membrane lysis in response to either vascular, inflammatory, enzymatic, endocrinopathic, or mechanical disease processes | Inflammatory pain, Nociceptive pain |
| Acute | 48–72 h Affected animal may recover ands enter a subacute phase or alternatively enters the chronic disease phase | Onset of clinical signs of pain, Stance and gait irregularities, Adoption of classic laminitic stance | | Lamellar dysadhesion and SADP compromise, Vascular dysfunction, Vasoconstriction, vasodilation, Vascular coagulopathy, Inflammation, Ischemia/reperfusion, Compartment injury, Free radical production, Metabolic dysfunction | |
| Subacute | 9–12 mo Subacute animals may recovery or progress into the chronic disease | Foot soreness, Reduced athletic performance | SADP compromise, Focal lamellar damage, Compromised lamellar interface yet maintains significant digital stability, Hoof dermis and DP retains its function integrity | Tissue modeling and wound healing processes, Potential for ongoing mechanical trauma | Nociceptive pain, Peripheral sensitization |

| | | | | |
|---|---|---|---|---|
| Chronic | Reduced athletic performance | SADP failure and digital collapse | Degenerative changes to the anatomy of the foot | Inflammatory pain |
| Permanent | Lameness and permanent locomotor impairment | Anatomic dislocation of the DP within the hoof capsule | Soft tissue trauma | Peripheral sensitization |
| | Recurrent bouts of severe digital pain | CRL animals display digital stability in response to therapeutic farriery | compartment injury and edema formation | Thermal and mechanical hypergesia |
| | Chronic recrudescent lameness and associated pain | REL display digital instability despite therapeutic farriery | Lamellar stretching and separation | Central sensitization |
| | Animals may present as either CRL responsive to traditional methods of palliative care or conversely, REL, nonresponsive to these methods of palliative care | | Hemorrhage exudate and "seroma" formation | Sodium channel accumulation, redistribution, and altered expression |
| | Recurrent bouts of acute-phase laminitis or recrudescent pain | | Compression of coronary and solear dermis | Changes in vanilloid receptor expression |
| | | | Papillary reorientation, coronary band separation, and shear lesion formation | α-Receptor expression |
| | | | Wound healing and soft tissue remodeling | Sympathetic sprouting |
| | | | Disruption to normal pattern of hoof horn | Increased transmission |
| | | | Development of secondary foot pathologies | Reduced inhibition |
| | | | Lamellar wedge formation | |
| | | | Bone modeling and lysis | |
| | | | Solear prolapse and abscessation | |
| | | | "Hidden dangers" arising from inward growing hoof horn | |

Abbreviations: CRL, chronic remissive laminitis; REL, refractory exacerbative laminitis; SADP, suspensory apparatus of the distal phalanx.

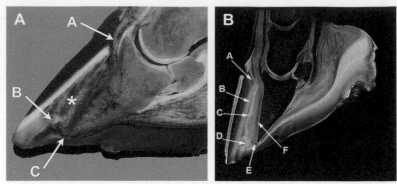

**Fig. 1.** (*A*) Sagittal section of a foot with severe chronic laminitis showing presence of a large lamellar wedge (*asterisk*). The attachment between the distal phalanx (DP) and the dorsal hoof wall (the suspensory apparatus of the distal phalanx) has failed and hoof and bone are now widely separated. The anatomic dislocation of the unsupported DP within the hoof capsule has affected the normal alignment of the dermal papillae, resulting in distorted inward growth of the proximal hoof wall and leading to compression of the coronary dermis (A). The material apparent between the inner aspect of the hoof wall and the DP is abnormal, and consists of dysplastic epidermal tissue that forms a weak, pathologic structure called the lamellar wedge (B). This results in increased soft tissue strain levels (tension and shear) during weight bearing There is evidence of extensive exudation and hemorrhage within the lamellar wedge. Anatomic dislocation of the DP has caused the sole to become convex instead of concave (dropped sole), and is causing compression and vascular trauma within the solear dermis in the region of the distal margin of the DP (C). (*B*) High-resolution sagittal 3D fat-saturated T1 SPGR magnetic resonance (MR) image of a chronic laminitic foot showing a range of pathologies associated with the failure of the suspensory apparatus of the distal phalanx, and the subsequent dislocation of the distal phalanx within the affected hoof. A: distortion of the proximal hoof wall, with stretching of the coronary dermis, and soft tissue compression resulting from inward growing hoof horn. B: linear hypointense MR feature at the dorsal margin of the lamellar interface, indicating traumatic lamellar separation, with associated hemorrhage and exudate formation. C: lamellar wedge formation (high MR signal intensity within the lamellar interface indicating extensive epidermal dysplasia and soft tissue modeling. Note that the dysplastic epidermal tissues expands distally and encroaches inwards (D). E: hypointense MR signal showing vascular trauma associated with compression of the solear dermis in the region of the distal border of the distal phalanx. F: Hypointense MR signal indicating vascular trauma within the sublamellar dermis resulting from elevated soft tissue strain levels (shear and tension) during weight bearing.

Transmission of nociceptive signals is achieved by a network of slow-conducting myelinated type Aβ fibers, thinly myelinated type Aδ fibers, and unmyelinated type C nerve fibers. These noxious signals are registered by free nerve endings, which are distributed throughout the coronary, lamellar, and solear dermis of the foot. As polymodal receptors, these nerve endings convert harmful mechanical, chemical, and thermal stimuli into sensory impulses. The density and distribution of these nerve fibers is poorly defined; however, both peptidergic[32–34] and adrenergic fibers[38] have been identified within the dermal tissues of the foot.

Based on their investigations of the ramification pattern within the lamellar and sublamellar dermis, it is the authors' view to divide the dermis of the dorsum of the foot into 3 morphologically distinct zones of innervation (**Fig. 3**).

Zone 1 contains large multifascicular nerves (**Fig. 4**) that run parallel to the parietal surface of the DP. Short branches of these nerves (**Fig. 5**), and longer ones from proximally located and lateral rami, run as neurovascular bundles within Zone 2 and extend

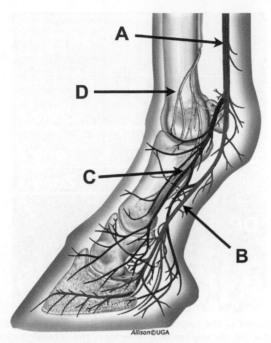

Allison©UGA

**Fig. 2.** Sensory nerves of the distal limb and digit. A, palmar nerve and B, palmar digital nerve (*red*); C, dorsal branch of the palmar digital nerve (*blue*); D, palmar metacarpal nerve (*yellow*). (*Courtesy of* Andrew Parks, VetMB, MS, MRCVS, University of Georgia, Athens, GA.)

toward the primary lamellae, where single nerve fibers and small clusters emanate close to the dermoepidermal junction at the base of the primary epithelial lamellae (**Fig. 6**A).

From there they run along the axis of the primary dermal lamellae, associated with the small blood vessels, and release small endings in the secondary dermal lamellae (Zone 3). Other studies[31,33] have shown that an extensive innervation pattern also exists within the papilliated perioplic, coronary, and solear dermis, with nerve fibers extending centrally toward the apex of each dermal papilla. In horses and other species, free endings are present within the basal and suprabasal epithelial layers of the skin. Occasionally, small unmyelinated nerve fibers/endings can be seen within the suprabasal layers of the secondary epidermal lamellae (**Fig. 6**B).

In addition to the somatic senses, sympathetic nerve fibers maintain vascular tone within the dermal tissues of the foot (**Fig. 7**), regulate the action of a complex system of arteriovenous anastomoses, and modulate the chemical milieu within the dermis.[38] Their afferent signals similarly employ unmyelinated fibers.[34,35] The efferent viscero-motor signals of these reflex arches are delivered to the vascular smooth muscles via small myelinated fibers that synapse to the postganglionic neurons, which are located within large to medium-sized dermal nerve fascicles (**Fig. 8**).

Knowledge of the sensory innervation pattern of the DP is extremely limited. Deep branches of the medial and lateral digital nerve enter the solear foraminae of the DP, accompanying the digital artery.[36] Nerve fibers are also known to enter the DP close to the insertion of the deep digital flexor tendon,[36,39] and the medullary spaces between the bone trabecula are richly populated with nerve fibers.[40]

Collectively, the neural inputs contribute to the sensory digital nerve, and to a varying extent appear to be directly involved in pathologic pain associated with laminitis.

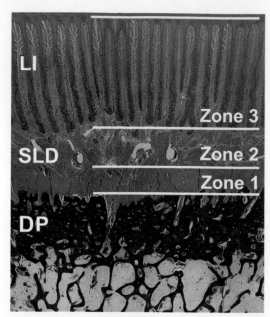

**Fig. 3.** Transverse section of the suspensory apparatus of the distal phalanx, which unites the hoof wall to the DP via the lamellar interface: the interdigitation of dermal and epidermal lamellae (LI) and the sublamellar dermis (SLD), and the proposed 3-zone innervation pattern proposed by the authors. Zone 1 deep within the SLD is innervated predominantly by large multifascicular nerves emanating from the dorsal branch of the palmar nerve. Short branches of these nerves, and longer ones from proximally located and lateral rami, run as neurovascular bundles within Zone 2 and extend toward the primary dermal lamellae, where single nerve fibers and small clusters emanate close to the dermoepidermal junction at the base of the primary dermal lamellae. From there they run along the axis of the primary dermal lamellae, associated with the small blood vessels, and release small endings in the secondary dermal lamellae, and the suprabasal cells of the secondary epidermal lamellae (Zone 3). Hematoxylin-eosin stain; subgross image.

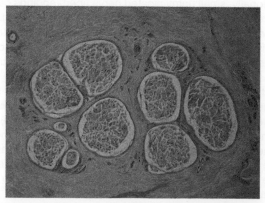

**Fig. 4.** Transverse section of a large multifascicular nerve located within Zone 1 of the sublamellar dermis (hematoxylin-eosin stain, original magnification ×375).

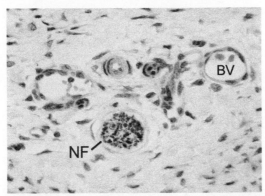

**Fig. 5.** Small nerve fascicle (NF) in close association with blood vessels (BV) of Zone 2. Note the immunopositivity for the neuropeptide and transmitter substance P (*brown*) (hematoxylin-eosin stain, original magnification ×375).

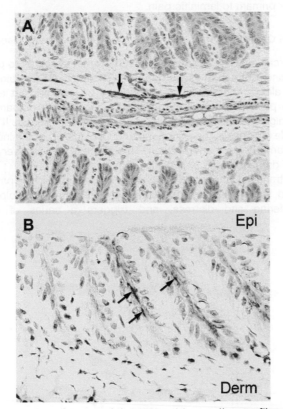

**Fig. 6.** Sensory innervation of Zone 3. (*A*) CGRP-positive small nerve fiber (*arrows*) crossing toward the apex of the primary dermal lamella. (*B*) Further CGRP-positive single fibers (*arrows*) are occasionally observed in the suprabasal layers of the secondary epidermal lamellae if met in plane of section. Epi, epidermis; Derm, dermis (hematoxylin couterstain; original magnification ×375 for A, ×750 for B).

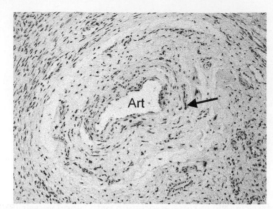

**Fig. 7.** CGRP-positive (*brown*) sympathetic fibers (*arrow*) addressing a large dermal artery (Art) (hematoxylin counterstain, original magnification ×187).

Conversely, discriminatory tactile senses (skin sensitivity to mechanical stimuli) are restricted to aspects of the distal limb proximal to the foot, and hence are unlikely to contribute per primam to laminitic pain.

## PAIN STATES: AN OVERVIEW

The ability to perceive pain is an adaptive mechanism and serves to protect the individual from imminent or actual tissue damage. This physiologic pain offers biologic advantage and allows coordinated responses to be evoked that act to minimize damage. Hence pain is normally only elicited when intense or damaging noxious stimuli activate high-threshold nociceptive primary sensory nerves. If tissue damage occurs, reversible changes in the peripheral and CNS follow, which induce hypersensitivity in the inflamed or damaged region. This process aids recovery by minimizing contact with the damaged area until healing has occurred.

In contrast to transient and adaptive physiologic pain, persistent pathologic pain is maladaptive and serves no biologic advantage. Persistent pathologic pain leads directly to suffering and distress, and triggers a series of catabolic and

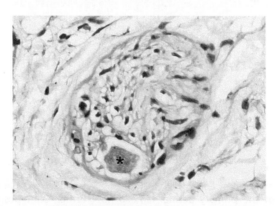

**Fig. 8.** Medium-sized nerve fascicle of Zone 2 harboring a postganglionic autonomic nerve cell (*asterisk*). Periodic acid-Schiff stain; mild artificial changes due to repeated freezing/thawing cycles (original magnification ×375).

immunocompromising neuroendocrine consequences.[41,42] Pathologic pain results from either continuous employment (firing) of nociceptors or damage to the nervous system at the level of the peripheral nerve, the dorsal root ganglia and dorsal horn, and/or the CNS. This latter type of pathologic pain is referred to as neuropathic pain.[43,44]

The relationship that exists between etiology, mechanism, and clinical signs in neuropathic pain is complex and varied, with the clinical signs often persisting after full resolution of the initiating disease. Indeed, it is important to remember that no particular pain mechanism is inevitable as a consequence of a specific disease, and a single pain mechanism can elicit different clinical signs in different animals. Most strikingly, the same clinical signs can arise as a consequence of different pain mechanisms. Hence the identification of the causal mechanisms that give rise to neuropathic pain in a particular disease is essential if optimized treatment strategies are to be developed.[45]

## CAUSES OF PAIN WITHIN THE LAMINITIC FOOT

Although laminitis has traditionally been viewed as an inflammatory disease of the lamellae (which historically gave rise to the term laminitis), the disease has been shown to be far more complex than a simple inflammatory process. It is therefore important, in ensuring that effective and optimized treatment is given to the afflicted animal, that the clinician is fully conversant with the disease pathogenesis and is aware of all potential pathophysiological events that can induce digital pain.

Although the precise mechanistic cause of laminitic pain remains unclear, it is likely to be multifactorial in nature and related to the primary disease process, biomechanical factors, reactive secondary pathology, and also to changes in the pain perception pathways.[11,12] Thus laminitic pain is most likely composed of nociceptive, inflammatory, and neuropathic components, with the contributions of each varying at different phases of the disease (see **Table 1**).

It is generally accepted that inflammatory mediators are of central importance in the development of digital pain in a laminitic horse. The acute phase of the disease is characterized by the onset of clinical signs of digital pain, resulting in stance and gait alterations. There are differing views regarding the specific pathophysiological processes that trigger digital pain. Central to this discussion is an ongoing debate as to whether disease progression is associated with vasoconstrictive or vasodilatory events within the lamellar tissues of the foot. For detailed discussion of these matters, the reader is directed elsewhere to excellent reviews of the subject.[27,46–48]

Proponents of a vasoconstrictive etiology suggest that digital pain arises as a consequence of a process involving an ischemic crisis, epidermal necrosis, reperfusion injury, and oxidative stress.[27] Conversely, proponents of a vasodilatory etiology state that pain arises as a consequence of basement membrane degradation, associated epidermal cell damage and insidious but inexorable SADP failure. It is generally agreed, however, that both of these mechanistic pathways induce an inflammatory cascade within the foot, which leads directly to the development of a classic inflammatory pain state.[49,50]

Because digital pain appears to precede inflammatory infiltrates in the early stage of the acute phase, the actual trigger might be exposure of the nerve endings to ischemia, pH and electrolyte shifts, pressure, release of arachidonic degradation products, cytokines and chemokines, and upregulation of matrix metalloproteinases (**Fig. 9**). Moreover, sympathetic nerve fibers of the affected region may release adenosine triphosphate (ATP) and thereby stimulate purinergic (ATP-receptive) nociceptors, in response to the inflammation as has been demonstrated in other species.[51]

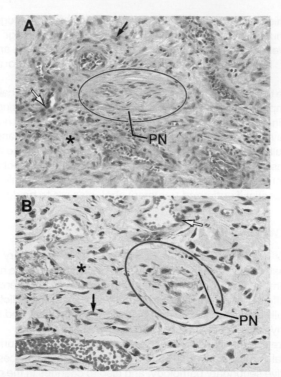

**Fig. 9.** Two sections of small nerve fascicles taken from the laminitic dermis in 2 different horses affected by chronic exacerbative laminitis (CEL). (*A*) The remarkably spared nerve fascicle and its perineural (PN) sheath (*encircled by red line*) passes an area with activated fibroblasts (*black arrow*), pericellular collagen deposition (*asterisk*), and vascular proliferates with endothelial hypertrophy (*white arrow*). Plasma cell aggregates are seen throughout (hematoxylin-eosin stain, original magnification x375). (*B*) In contrast to the former, the encircled nerve fascicle in this area presents with perineural edema and dyscompaction (PN) surrounding an endoneurium, which shows loss of nerve tissue and fibroplasia (compare with *A*). The stroma also contains activated fibroblasts (*black arrow*) and blood vessels (*white arrow*). Compared with *A*, there is less (eosinophilic) collagen deposition but interstitial edema (*asterisk*) (hematoxylin-eosin stain, original magnification ×750).

This inflammatory response is believed to induce dermal edema, and because the dermal tissues are constrained within the confines of the hoof capsule, compartment injury may develop. The increasing dermal pressure gradient is likely to influence homeostasis of the fascicular nerve fibers contained within the dermis. Animal experiments have shown that interstitial pressures of approximately 20 mm Hg significantly reduce the epineurial venular flow and thereby the endoneurial blood perfusion,[52] whereas compartment pressures of more than 30 mm Hg impair axoplasmic transport[52] and the maintenance of myelin sheath integrity is affected at pressures exceeding 50 mm Hg.[53] In an inflamed environment, as in acute laminitis, exposed nerve fibers become increasingly mechanosensitive and transform pressure gradients arising within the hoof capsule and above (eg, during palpation of proximal and middle phalanges) into painful sensory A- and C-fiber impulses.[54] Hence this hyperexcitability evokes pain without nociceptor employment.

As in other tissues, increased dermal compartment pressures affect the blood circulation via compression of the veins and venules and to a lesser extent the arteries.

Venous engorgement and subsequent hypertension of the bone marrow triggers both persistent pain and bone modeling in clinical and experimental settings.[55–58] Experimental work on goats revealed that a twofold increase of the normal baseline intraosseous pressure induces limb pain by as yet unclear mechanisms.[59–61] Hence, pressures of 35 mm Hg in the caprine tibia,[59,61] 45 mm Hg in the equine third metatarsal bone,[60] and 50 mm Hg in the equine navicular bone are associated with resting limb pain.[62] The latter also seems to be responsible for referred palmar foot pain.[62] Due to the foot's encapsulated anatomy, the intraosseous pressure in the DP of horses with and without laminitis has rarely been recorded. However, histologic assessment of the DP of chronic laminitic feet, euthanized because of unrelenting foot pain, often reveals extensive bone modeling and endosteal edema (**Fig. 10**) (Collins and colleagues, unpublished results, 2009).

The inflammatory processes and vascular dysfunction are further compounded by increased DP movement during weight bearing as lamellar pathology develops over time. Excessive movement of the DP within the hoof capsule of the laminitic foot and/ or dislocation of the DP following SADP failure is likely to cause elevated levels of shear and tensile deformation within the lamellar and sublamellar dermis, leading to both vascular occlusion and vascular and neural trauma within these tissues. Similarly, this will also lead to increased loading of the solear dermis inducing vascular compromise, and nerve compression and/or nerve crush injuries. Soft tissue deformation can directly stimulate nociceptors and damage the perivascular nerve fascicles, triggering neuropathic mechanisms. Similar to their hyperexcitability for pressure, nerves crossing inflamed areas become sensitive to stretching. In experimental settings, a 3% nerve segment elongation leads directly to ectopic impulse generation in A and C fibers.[54] The distal displacement of the DP within the laminitic hoof capsule during weight bearing is expected to exceed this critical value of nerve fiber elongation, and may likewise trigger ectopic pain. While nociceptive pain caused by increased DP displacement during loading will, in part, be determined by the severity of the lamellar degradation, its effect will be more pronounced in those laminitic horses that present with a greater body weight. Standardbred horses developed more severe lamellar degradation than ponies despite laminitis being induced by the same pronged hyperinsulinemic induction model.[63] Similarly, it is intuitively to be expected that obese laminitic cases will exhibit a heightened pain response to weight bearing compared with their less obese counterparts because DP displacement will be greater in the heavier animal, thereby generating a larger mechanoceptive stimulus.

Traditionally, digital pain in the chronic laminitic horse has been thought to arise from responses to secondary foot pathologies, including abscessation and reactive bone modeling and lysis, resulting from SADP failure, DP dislocation, and abnormal biomechanical foot function. Perpetuation of local inflammation does indeed chronically expose nerves to a chemical environment that stimulates those nerve endings equipped with vanilloid receptors, and also those nerve endings that are sensitive to protons and products of purine metabolism.[51] In addition, leukocytes may release mediators with algogenic activities (eg, bradykinins, cytokines, prostaglandins, and growth factors) that lower the excitation threshold of the afferent neurons. This threshold lowering induces peripheral sensitization, which causes innocuous local stimuli to be perceived as pain.[51]

Both these primary and secondary effects on the pain pathways fit nicely into the paradigm of laminitis being an inflammatory disorder of the dermis. However, pain and hypersensitivity are also present in horses that receive early anti-inflammatory treatments. Thus perpetuation of pain in these horses must result from sources other

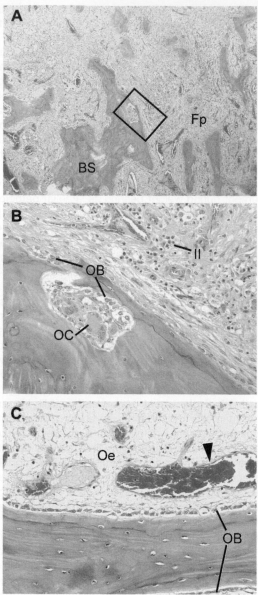

**Fig. 10.** Soft tissue and bone remodeling associated with SADP failure. (*A*) The low-power field image features multiple DP bone spicules (BS) separated by soft dermal tissue undergoing extensive, disorganized fibroplasia (Fp) (hematoxylin-eosin stain, original magnification ×375). (*B*) Closer view on the enframed area of *A*. Ongoing bone remodeling is indicated by clusters of osteoclasts (OC) intermingling with an extensive osteoblastic activity (OB). The fibrous stroma shows diffuse mononuclear inflammatory infiltrates (II) (hematoxylin-eosin stain, original magnification ×187). (*C*) The endosteal compartment of the DP likewise presents with an osteoblastic lining (OB). In most CEL cases there is an endosteal edema (Oe) associated with congestion of the venous blood vessels (*arrowhead*) (hematoxylin-eosin stain, original magnification ×375).

than nociception and inflammation. The key to understanding the devastating and nonsteroidal anti-inflammatory drug (NSAID)-resistant pain in REL horses lies in: (1) the physical damage of the digital nerves[64] and (2) the hypersensitivity of regenerating axons that sprout into the areas of active soft tissue remodeling, that is, the lamellar wedge.[16]

Only recently has the association between laminitic pain and physical injury of the digital sensory nerves been conclusively established.[64] This study found severe damage to both unmyelinated and myelinated sensory nerve fibers, and increased expression of the activation marker ATF3 (a specific marker for nerve cell damage) in the corresponding dorsal root ganglion cells of some laminitic horses.[64]

Potential sources of peripheral nerve damage within the confines of the hoof capsule have been outlined. SADP failure and DP dislocation collectively lead to dermal hemorrhage, seroma formation, submural edema, ischemia and reperfusion, and compartment injury. In addition, excessive DP movement, DP dislocation and sol-ear weight bearing causes further tissue damage and vascular occlusion within the solear dermis. This damage is especially pronounced around the distal margin of the DP, where crush-type injury occurs as the dermal tissues (and presumably the peripheral nerves contained within) are compressed between bone and sole horn. Furthermore, the "hidden dangers" associated with DP dislocation, that is, compression of the coronary, solear, and distal lamellar dermis by inward growing hoof horn (resulting from solear and coronary papillar reorientation),[16,17] are likely to cause further compression of peripheral nerve fibers. Chronic compression and entrapment has been shown in other species to interfere with the endoneurial perfusion and directly damage both axons and myelin sheath.[65] It is this axonal injury that induces neuropathic pain. Unlike nociceptive pain, neuropathic pain is resistant to NSAIDs, and unlike inflammatory pain it is also nonresponsive to opioid treatment.[66]

While ectopic impulse generation may be the first problem in subtotally damaged fibers, the disruption of afferent signaling leads to neuroplastic changes in the outer laminae of the dorsal horn of the spinal cord, whereas nociceptive fibers are supposed to synapse to the second-order neuron. This synapse is under tonic inhibition by regulatory fibers from the upper pain control centers. Deafferentation by loss of previously established synaptic connections from the dorsal root ganglia (DRG) leaves the neuron "craving" for new functional connections and synaptic impulses. Hence it becomes responsive to subthreshold signals from the sensory nerves and, secondly, starts shedding factors, which attract other afferent nerve fibers to establish new connections. In this manner, functional nociceptive afferent fibers may increase their number of activated neurons and thereby their receptive field disproportionately. Moreover, mechanoceptive terminals from the neighboring inner lamina may form new synapses and thereby falsely project their innocuously evoked signals onto the pain pathways. The synaptic remodeling is long lasting once the synaptic transmission has been achieved and the anatomic changes are not easily controlled pharmacologically.[67,68]

After peripheral nerve damage by the aforementioned mechanisms, the axons attempt to reinnervate the dermis and epidermis by axonal sprouting. The immature sprouts are hyperexcitable, and are prone to spontaneous firing similar to painful neuromas.[69] With C fibers, the ensheathing Remak cells occasionally cluster groups of axons into one pocket, which allows for jumping of impulses on neighboring fibers. That way thermoceptive fibers may cross-depolarize nociceptive fibers and induce pain. Peripheral nerve damage can also incite a concurrent sprouting of sympathetic nerve fibers into both the diseased dermis and the DRG tissue, in which the reactive and degenerating nerve cells are embedded.[70] The subsequent activity of the fibers has been associated with sympathetically maintained pain,[71] in which the discomfort is accompanied by attendant autonomic dysregulation leading to additional vasodilation and edema.[72] Taken together, in chronic laminitis the ongoing nociceptive stimulation is accompanied by threshold lowering at different areas of the pain pathways (hyperalgesia), a general hypersensitivity of sensory fibers (hyperesthesia), nociceptive signaling by innocuous stimuli (allodynia), and spontaneous excitation of damaged and regenerating nerves, including those that project onto the central pain pathways.

As suggested by Jones and colleagues,[66] the DRG mirrors nicely the damage of the digital nerves in chronic laminitis (**Fig. 11**). In long-standing cases with REL, histologic slides show the dropout of lethally damaged sensory neurons. The true impact on the nerve cells, however, becomes far more obvious in preparations stained by the cell death marker Fluorojade (**Fig. 12**). It is noteworthy, however, that it is the surviving neurons that are responsible for the persistent pain. Directly damaged nerve cells may express the activation marker ATF3,[64] nonspecifically indicating peripheral axonal damage and regeneration.[73]

Other phenomena seen in association with peripheral nerve damage in other species may indicate the presence of hitherto unreported responses within the laminitic horse, and can better direct interpretative questioning of empirical data. For example, does the upregulation of neuroactive peptides calcitonin-gene related peptide (CGRP) and substance P in large type A neurons (reported by Jones and

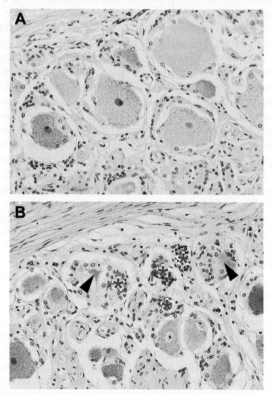

**Fig. 11.** Dorsal root ganglion C8 of a normal horse (*A*) and an animal affected by ipsilateral front limb CEL (*B*). Note the abundance of degenerating ganglion cells (*arrowheads*) and their replacement by reactive satellite cells, so-called Nageotte bodies (*asterisks*) (hematoxylin-eosin stain, original magnification ×375).

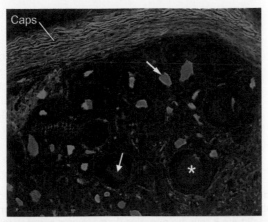

**Fig. 12.** Staining of C8 ganglia in CEL cases with the marker Fluorojade C reveals a selective uptake of the fluorochrome by degenerating nerve cells (*yellow arrow*) if compared with fluoronegative large type A (*asterisk*) and small type B cells (*white arrow*). Nonspecific staining is observed in nonneural fibrocollagenous elements of the ganglion capsule (Caps). (original magnification ×187).

colleagues[64]) indicate a phenotypic shift that would result in the projection of previously innocuous signals onto the pain pathways (**Fig. 13**)?

Another candidate for gaining further understanding of the mechanistic causes of laminitic pain, and in identifying a target molecule for advanced palliative treatment is the calcium channel subunit $\alpha 2\delta$. This ionophore protein is involved in signal transmission between first- and second-order sensory neurons in the dorsal horn of the spinal cord. In rodent pain models, $\alpha 2\delta$ expression is increased (independent of stimuli) in states of hyperalgesia and allodynia.[74] Analogously, the authors have found this ionophore protein to be expressed strongly in DRG neurons of REL-affected horses (Matiasek and Collins, unpublished results, 2009–2010) (**Fig. 14**). This finding suggests that refractory exacerbative pain in a laminitic horse could possibly be targeted better by alternative, nonanalgesic drugs. Although there are no previous evidence-based research data to confirm this assertion, anticonvulsant drugs have proved effective in

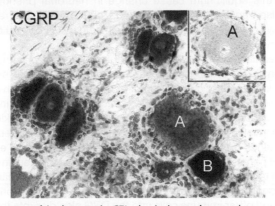

**Fig. 13.** Chronic neuropathic changes in CEL also induces abnormal expression of the neuropeptide CGRP (*brown color complex*) in large type A neurons if compared with nonaffected animals and noninvolved cervical DRGs (*inset*) (hematoxylin couterstain, original magnification ×375).

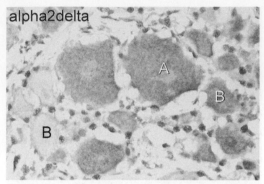

**Fig. 14.** Long-standing laminitis cases reveal a strong (*brown*) immunopositivity for the calcium channel subunit $\alpha2\delta$ in a majority of both type A and B neurons within the DRG of C8. Only a few small type B cells are negative (hematoxylin counterstain, original magnification ×375).

treating chronic pain states both in the horse and in other animal species.[74] In addition, empirical observations suggest that the anticonvulsant drug gabapentin demonstrates noticeable clinical analgesic effects in chronic laminitic horses.

## NEUROPATHIC COMPONENTS IN LAMINITIC PAIN?

Chronic neuropathic pain is a complex syndrome that results directly from injury to the PNS due to trauma, compression, inflammation, neurotoxins, and metabolic disease. Peripheral nerve injury results in anatomic, physiologic, and neurochemical modification to the sensory neurons, which causes spontaneous aw well as abnormal responses to both painful (noxious) and nonpainful (nonnoxious) stimuli. The range of changes depends on several factors including (1) lesion type (axotomy or compression), (2) location, and (3) distance from the neuronal cell body (located in the DRG). Normal neuronal function is dependent on an activity-maintained equilibrium between the neuron, its supporting nonneural cells, and the immediate microenvironment. Disturbances to this equilibrium cause change in neuronal phenotype, sensitivity, excitability, impulse transmission, growth status, and survival. The reader is directed to excellent reviews on the subject of neuropathic pain by Gilron and colleages,[70] Klusáková and Dubový,[75] and Woolf and Mannion.[76]

As discussed earlier, inflammatory mediators can sensitize nociceptor terminals causing hypersensitized responses to thermal and mechanical stimuli. Likewise, inflammation within a nerve or ganglia can directly affect neuronal chemistry function, as well as survival. Recent studies in other species suggest that inflammatory and proinflammatory cytokines (including interleukin-1 and -6), chemokines, and neurotropic factors are involved in the initiation of neuropathic pain states, and that cytokines and chemokines are able to directly influence afferent nerve excitation. These findings may be of particular relevance in laminitis because interleukin-1$\beta$ and -6 levels have been shown to increase significantly following epidermal cell damage and basement membrane degradation, at an early stage of disease progression.[27,77,78] Invasion of macrophages and other immune cells into the DRG also disrupts the normal activation equilibrium of the neuron, and causes heightened excitability in DRG neurons. Associated neuronal cell death induces reactive changes in the surrounding neurons, further amplifying the effects of any disturbance to the equilibrium state.

Direct peripheral nerve injury can also disturb the equilibrium state, and likewise, insults that cause changes in activity or sensory input to the CNS also have long-term effects on neuronal phenotype and function. Phenotypic changes occur within the perikarya following disease/injury; these include chromatolysis, eccentric displacement of the nucleus, and shrinkage. These pathognomonic degenerative changes are known to mirror dysfunction.[79] Nerve lesions also induce changes in the glial cells surrounding the DRG neurons, such as satellite cells and Schwann cells. Schwann cells serve not only to insulate the axon through myelin production but also regulate sensory neuron function by controlling expression and distribution of ionophores, and growth factor synthesis.[80] Schwann cell responses in other species result in changes in sodium and calcium channel expression. Investigations in the authors' laboratories have similarly demonstrated phenotypic changes within the DRG of C7 of chronic exacerbative laminitis (CEL) horses (see **Figs. 11** and **13**).

In addition to these changes, the distal stump of the damaged nerve undergoes Wallerian degeneration, leading to cytokine and chemokine production, in response to immune cell infiltration. A breakdown of the blood-nerve barrier results in their transportation to both damaged and intact neurons in the immediate vicinity of the lesion, and systemically to the DRG. Wallerian degeneration is thought to be a major component in the development of neuropathic pain. Neuroma formation occurs at the distal end of the proximal stump of the transected nerve, and is associated with spontaneous ectopic neural activity (in both the neuroma and the DRG), as a consequence of artificial impulse transmission between injured and noninjured neurons. The functional consequences of nerve compression resulting from crush-type injury are less well defined than transection injury. However, the functional responses are considered to be determined by injury site and severity.[65,75] For example, the distal part of the peripheral nerve is more susceptible to crush injury than more proximal sites, due to its simple fascicular structure and small amount of protective connective tissue.[75] This factor may be of direct relevance regarding laminitic pain, given that it is the distal part of the peripheral nerve that is exposed to the pathophysiological and biomechanical events associated with disease progression. Nerve compression is known to result in epineurial and endoneurial edema, as well as in nerve strangulation, triggering a series of events that culminates in persistent pain, and may be of significance especially in the solear dermis following DP dislocation, where tissues are focally compressed between the distal margin of the DP and the sole horn.

Initial changes following PNS injury lead to decreased threshold sensitivity of the peripheral nociceptors and thereby to enhancement of painful impulses to the CNS. Additional painful impulses are generated by spontaneous ectopic activity from damaged neurons, and also from cross-excitation of undamaged neurons. Degeneration of neuronal cell bodies within the DRG, and the subsequent central deafferentation, initiates terminal sprouting of large myelinated type A axons within the dorsal horn. These sprouting extensions invade that part of the dorsal horn which normally contains nociceptive neurons activated by high-intensity pain stimuli. Injury to the PNS can also result in wide-scale changes in gene expression including a switch in protein phenotype (including the neuropeptide substance P), which leads to changes in neuron excitability.

## TREATMENT PERSPECTIVES

Pain control is the single most important task in clinical management of laminitic horses. The multifactorial pathogenesis of laminitic pain poses a challenging task to the clinician, who aims to elucidate and tackle the actual triggers of discomfort and suffering. Throughout all phases of laminitis, nociceptive, inflammatory, and neuropathic mechanisms are interwoven (see **Table 1**). An understanding of the aforementioned—and still incompletely defined—cascades of local damage and their pathophysiological and anatomic consequences is essential to develop effective palliative treatments. Given the complexity of the situation, it is the authors' view that a multimodal therapeutic approach is needed (**Table 2**).

At early stages, when pain directly results from inflammatory and nociceptive stimuli associated with SADP failure, conventional analgesia by use of NSAIDs tackles both the inflammation and pain. Hence, pain relief is presumed to be achievable by blockage of cyclooxygenase (COX) activity in association with foot management and farriery that achieves digital stability and protects the SADP from further damage. Even though this concept seems well grounded, NSAIDs employ COX-independent mechanisms and do not necessarily diminish inflammation in the foot. Moreover, the selective role of COX isoforms 1 and 2 in laminitic pain requires further elucidation. At the present stage, the pan-COX inhibitor phenylbutazone and the COX-1 preferential ketoprofen appear to be most effective in reducing foot pain.[12,81]

With progression of the disease, other pain mechanisms are likely to gain importance. Thus, in chronic laminitis even high doses of NSAIDs may still not lead to pain relief within 3 days of administration.[81,82] The clinician also needs to consider the potential adverse side effects of long-term exposure to NSAIDs, which include right dorsal colitis, gastric ulceration, and renal tubular necrosis. Hence long-term use cannot be justified unless immediate relief is achieved.[83] It is also important to consider that NSAIDs can also potentiate matrix metalloproteinases[82] and could therefore actually be contraindicated. These adverse effects may be fewer with application of COX-2 selective drugs. However, NSAIDs tackling both COX-1 and COX-2 have been shown to be far more effective analgesics in laminitic horses.[12]

As an adjunct to conventional analgesics that are frequently used, dimethylsulfoxide (DMSO) is used as an anti-inflammatory drug and hydroxyl radical scavenger to counteract the effects of ischemia/reperfusion injury.

The ongoing research on inflammatory pain in rodents has elucidated some other candidate pathways to be targeted by non–anti-inflammatory drugs. Spontaneous firing and peripheral sensitization of nerve fibers in inflamed compartments in many species, for example, can be effectively antagonized by opioids that bind to δ-, μ-, and κ-receptors.[51] Their expression on primary afferent neurons increases in response to opiate production by leukocytes infiltrating tissues during inflammation.[84] However, in the horse clinical experience with modern opiates is limited. Most of the traditional μ- and κ-receptor agonists cause significant gastrointestinal, hemodynamic, and/or behavioral side effects that may or may not be controlled by use of additional drugs such as α2-agonists.[12] No data currently exist on the possibility of opioid-induced hyperalgesia in horses, which is a feared complication of long-term application of μ-agonists in other mammals.[85]

Of note, both inflammation and soft tissue trauma lead to local production of neurotrophic factors, which serves to guarantee the survival of disconnected nerve cells and to promote axonal sprouting. In particular, nerve growth factor (NGF) appears to be extensively upregulated with chronic inflammation, inducing expression of the nociceptor molecule TRPV-1 (transient receptor potential cation channel, subfamily V, member 1) within the exposed sensory nerves.[86] This vanilloid-like receptor, after being integrated into the membrane of the distal (intralesional) nerve ending, is very responsive to thermal stimuli as occurs during inflammation. This receptor upregulation therefore contributes to a "vicious circle" during which inflammatory hyperalgesia develops.[86] TRPV-1 expressing neurons can be lethally stimulated by local injection of the agonist resiniferatoxin at the nerve endings. Resiniferatoxin experimentally leads

**Table 2**
Summary of hypothesized mechanisms involved with inflammatory, nociceptive, and neuropathic components of laminitic pain

| Pain Mechanism | Topography | Mechanism | Treatment |
|---|---|---|---|
| Inflammatory pain | Area infiltrated by leukocytes | • pH decrease<br>• Proinflammatory cytokines<br>• Neuroactive peptides<br>• Chronic stimulation (gating)<br>• Release of ATP | • NSAIDs<br>• Opiates<br>• Specific vanilloid receptor antagonists |
| Nociceptive pain | The foot | • SADP compromise and increased soft tissue deformation during loading<br>• SADP failure and soft tissue trauma<br>• Seroma formation<br>• Lamellar wedge formation<br>• "Hidden dangers" following lamellar wedge formation<br>• Bone lysis and endosteal edema | • Supportive farriery to stabilize the foot<br>• Therapeutic foot trimming<br>• Remedial farriery including coronary band fenestration and peel and distal hoof wall resection<br>• Controlled weight loss in obese cases |
| Neuropathic pain: peripheral sensitization | Nerve endings | • Increased nociceptors density<br>• Decreased excitation threshold | • Vanilloid receptor antagonists<br>• Sodium channel blockers |
| Neuropathic pain: central sensitization | Synapse to second-order neuron | • Presynaptic increase of calcium channels<br>• Threshold lowering at postsynaptic membrane (increased sensitivity, decreased inhibitory tone) | • Presynaptic inhibition of neurotransmitter release (eg, gabapentinoids)<br>• Postsynaptic interference with glutamate (eg, ketamine) |
| Neuropathic pain: sodium channel accumulation, redistribution, and altered expression | Upregulation at site of nerve damage | Ectopic and spontaneous excitations (spontaneous pain) | Anticonvulsants and sodium blockers (eg, lidocaine) |
| Neuropathic pain: changes in vanilloid receptor expression | Production site: dorsal root ganglion<br>Insertion: nociceptive nerve endings | NGF-induced expression | Specific antagonists or lethal agonists |
| Neuropathic pain: α-receptor expression sympathetic sprouting | • Areas with extensive tissue pathology<br>• Dorsal root ganglia | Excitation of thermoceptive fibers | α-Antagonists |

*Abbreviations:* ATP, adenosine triphosphate; DRG, dorsal root ganglion; NGF, nerve growth factor; NSAID, nonsteroidal anti-inflammatory drug.

to a selective decay of C and Aδ pain fibers without afflicting changes to proprioceptive or motor axons.[87,88] This approach has been successful in dogs suffering from osteoarthritis and osteosarcoma,[89] and has recently been recommended for pain control in horses.[90] These investigators have established a quantitative test to measure TRPV-1 in the equine DRG. This technique provides veterinarians with the opportunity to assess TRPV-1 expression levels in laminitic horses and will help confirm whether resiniferatoxin treatment would, in principle, be appropriate in the treatment of chronic laminitic pain. Although there is at present no molecular data on the TRPV expression in the authors' cases, preliminary morphometry studies performed in their laboratories have revealed an increase in DRG neuron size in laminitic horses, indicating a neurotrophic effect (Matiasek and Collins, unpublished results, 2009). Hence, it may be speculated that NGF (or other growth factors) plays a role in laminitic pain as well, and that TRPV-1 induction is therefore probable. Hence the judicious use of therapeutic hypothermia (distal limb cryotherapy) may not only be of value in preventing disease development and/or in ameliorating its severity during the acute phase of the disease,[23,91–94] but may also assist in breaking the "vicious circle" of inflammatory hyperalgesia, and thus help prevent the development of chronic exacerbative neuropathic pain.

It is important to remember that pain-inducing pathology within the dermis and the DP cannot be reversed easily, hence it is imperative that therapeutic foot treatments should be instigated at the earliest opportunity to: (1) stabilize the foot, (2) prevent DP dislocation, and (3) reduce the risk posed by lamellar wedge formation. For detailed discussion of appropriate preventative and therapeutic farriery and foot management, the reader is directed elsewhere for expert discourse on treatment options at various stages during disease progression.[15,95–101]

Retrograde digital venography provides the clinician with the means of identifying areas of tissue compression, venous deficit, and potential hypoxia, and identifying the presence of "hidden dangers" within the affected foot. This technique can also serve as a means of assessing the effectiveness of foot treatments in restoring normal digital circulation and relief of focal tissue compression. Readers are directed to recent reviews on this subject by Rucker,[102,103] and Pollitt and colleagues.[104]

Specifically in respect of the "hidden dangers" associated with lamellar wedge formation, which are only now being fully recognized, timely resection of the proximal and distal dorsal hoof wall is required to allow reorientation of the dermal papillae of the sole and realignment of the coronary dermis.[105] This intervention facilitates restoration of the normal pattern of hoof horn production. In addition, treatment shoes and sole inserts should support the palmar/plantar aspect of the foot and spare (relieve) any sole pressure beneath the dorsal margin of the dislocated DP that would elevate strain levels within the solear dermis. Shoe breakover should align with the dorsodistal margin of the DP to minimize strain levels within the lamellar dermis, thereby protecting the weakened SADP.

It is also important to instigate a controlled program of weight loss in those laminitic horses that present with an obese body condition, to further reduce the amount of DP displacement during loading and to minimize soft tissue strain levels and its associated mechanoceptive stimulus. To achieve this, a careful balance between dietary manipulation and exercise is needed that fully takes into account the compromised nature of the SADP and the timeline of the disease.

Given the complex multifactorial nature of the pain generating mechanisms associated with laminitis, an alternative and potentially optimized treatment approach would be to "target pain" at a common location along the sensory nerve pathway that was not dependent on the actual pain-generating stimuli. In this regard, all afferent signals have to induce an action potential in the second-order sensory neuron of the dorsal horn to enter the central pain pathways toward the somesthetic cortex. Transmission onto these neurons depends notably on presynaptic voltage-gated calcium channels. In experimental models of neuropathic pain, both hyperalgesia and allodynia have been shown to be triggered by an increased expression of the calcium channel subunit $\alpha2\delta$ protein.[74] This protein subunit appears to facilitate the transmitter release of substance P and CGRP,[106] and glutamate. Their action is considered to be independent of the actual stimulus type that induced the action potential within the afferent nerve fiber. This seemingly ubiquitous ionophore can be selectively inhibited by so-called gabapentinoids, namely gabapentin and pregabalin.[106,107] It is believed that these drugs interfere with ionophore trafficking and functional integration into the presynaptic membrane.[107,108] Hence by inhibiting these ionophores, gabapentinoids potentially represent a very potent analgesic capable of managing multifactorial pain states. There are isolated empirical accounts of successful pain management in laminitic horses; however, clinical trials have not yet been undertaken. To preclinically screen for scientific evidence sufficient to warrant future gabapentinoid testing in laminitic horses, the authors have conducted preliminary immunohistochemical investigations to confirm the presence of the target $\alpha2\delta$ subunit in DRGs of laminitic horses. These investigations have revealed significant expression of the subunit in CEL horses. Unfortunately, however, gabapentin has been shown to have a potent sedative effect in the horse and low oral bioavailability.[109] Further studies are needed on the pharmacokinetics of gabapentin and pregabalin (which exerts less sedative effects) to firmly establish appropriate and safe dosage rates in the horse before palliative efficacy for the treatment of laminitic pain can be fully assessed.

Similarly specific drug therapies aimed at blocking the excitatory glutamate receptors on the postsynaptic membrane of the second-order neuron would achieve pain relief irrespective of the evoking stimuli. Impulse transmission blockage can be achieved by the N-methyl-D-aspartate receptor antagonist ketamine. Like the gabapentinoids, ketamine has an antiallodynic and antihyperalgesic activity that has been proven in other species.[110,111] Ketamine also exhibits synergism with conventional analgesics, and as an adjunct can help prevent adverse side effects encountered with conventional analgesics. However,, in the horse subanesthetic ketamine substitution on its own does not lead consistently to pain control, even when administered by long-term infusion.[112]

## SUMMARY

Despite the severe and debilitating effect of pain associated with laminitis, relatively little is known as to the precise pathophysiological process leading to its development and progression, and the respective role played by inflammatory and neuropathic pain mechanisms. Gaining better understanding of these processes through evidence-based research remains an essential first step to enable the development of effective palliative care for the afflicted horse. Successful development of effective pain management strategies will create the desired "window of opportunity" to allow foot treatments time to take their therapeutic effect, and thereby give the horse a better opportunity for recuperation, disease remission, and return to paddock soundness or even athletic performance.

## ACKNOWLEDGMENTS

The authors specifically want to thank Ray Wright, Animal Heath Trust, Newmarket, UK, for his expertise in histologic preparations.

## REFERENCES

1. Moore RM. Welcome to the 2nd American Association of Equine Practitioners Foundation, equine laminitis research workshop. J Equine Vet Sci 2010;30:73.
2. Moore RM. Vision 20/20—conquer laminitis by 2020. J Equine Vet Sci 2010;30: 74–6.
3. Moore RM. Barbaro injury highlights need for laminitis research funding. 2006. Available at: http://www.aaep.org/press_room.php?term=2006&id=242. Accessed July 20, 2010.
4. Wylie CE, Collins SN, Durham AE, et al. An epidemiological study of laminitis in the new millenium. In: Proceedings of the 12th Symposium of the International Society for Veterinary Epidemiology and Economics. Durban (South Africa), 2009. p. 559.
5. Hinckley KA. Endocrine and haemodynamic investigations of normal and laminitic horses [PhD Thesis]. Sheffield (UK): University of Sheffield; 1996.
6. Hinckley KA, Henderson IW. The epidemiology of equine laminitis. In: Proceedings of the British Equine Veterinary Association Congress. Warwick (UK), 2009. p. 62–3.
7. Kane AJ, Traub-Dargatz JL, Losinger WC, et al. The occurrence and causes of lameness and laminitis in the U.S. horse population. In: Proceedings of the American Association of Equine Practitioners Annual Congress. 2009. p. 277–82.
8. Anon. Lameness & laminitis in U.S. horses. Fort Collins (CO): USDA:APHIS:VS, CEAH, National Animal Health Monitoring System, # N318.0400; 2000.
9. Rendle D. Equine laminitis 1. Management in the acute stage. In Pract 2006;28: 434–43.
10. Rendle D. Equine laminitis 2. Management and prognosis in the chronic stage. In Pract 2006;28:526–36.
11. Yaksh TL. The pain state arising from the laminitic horse: insights into future analgesic therapies. J Equine Vet Sci 2010;30:79–82.
12. Driessen B, Bauquier SH, Zarucco L. Pain (neuropathic) management of chronic laminitis. Vet Clin North Am Equine Pract 2010;26(2):315–37.
13. Johnson PJ, Messer NT, Ganjam VK. Cushing's syndromes, insulin resistance and endocrinopathic laminitis. Equine Vet J 2004;36:194–8.
14. Pollitt CC, Daradka M. Hoof wall wound repair. Equine Vet J 2004;36:210–5.
15. Pollitt CC. Equine laminitis; current concepts. Canberra (Australia): Rural Industries Research and Development Council; 2008.
16. Collins SN, van Eps AW, Pollitt CC, et al. The lamellar wedge. Vet Clin North Am Equine Pract 2010;26:179–95.
17. Pollitt CC, Collins SN. Chronic laminitis. In: Ross M, Dyson S, editors. Diagnosis and management of lameness in the horse. St Louis (MO): Saunders; 2010.
18. Hood DM. The mechanisms and consequences of structural failure of the foot. Vet Clin North Am Equine Pract 1999;15:437–61.
19. Morgan SJ, Grosenbaugh DA, Hood DM. The pathophysiology of chronic laminitis. Pain and anatomic pathology. Vet Clin North Am Equine Pract 1999;15: 395–417.
20. Geor R, Frank N. Metabolic syndrome-from human organ disease to laminar failure in equids. Vet Immunol Immunopathol 2009;129:151–4.
21. Hood DM, Stevens KA. Pathophysiology of equine laminitis. Compend Contin Edu Pract Vet 1981;3(Suppl):454–60.
22. Hood DM. Laminitis in the horse. Vet Clin North Am Equine Pract 1999;15: 287–94.

23. van Eps AW, Collins SN, Pollitt CC. Supporting limb laminitis. Vet Clin North Am Equine Pract 2010;26(2):287–302.
24. Pellmann R. Struktur und Funktion des Hufbeintraegers beim Pferd. Berlin: Free University of Berlin; 1995 [in German].
25. Budras KD, Bragulla H, Pellmann R, et al. Das Hufbein mit Perios und Insertionszone des Hufbeintraegers. Wien Tieraerztl Monatsschr 1997;84:241–7 [in German].
26. Visser MB, Pollitt CC. The timeline of acute phase laminitis. Equine Vet J, in press.
27. Hood DM. The pathophysiology of developmental and acute laminitis. Vet Clin North Am Equine Pract 1999;15:321–43.
28. Parks AH, Mair TS. Laminitis: a call for unified terminology. Equine Vet Educ 2009;21:102–6.
29. Linford RL. Laminitis (founder). In: Smith BP, editor. Large animal internal medicine. 2nd edition. St Louis (MO): Mosby; 1996. p. 1300–9.
30. Burt NW, Baker SJ, Wagner IP, et al. Digital instability as a potential prognostic indicator in horses with chronic laminitis. In: Hood DM, Wagner IP, Jacobson AC, editors. Proceedings of the Hoof Project. College Station (TX): Private Publishers Texas A & M; 1997. p. 105–15.
31. Krawarik F. Ueber Nerven in der Klauen- und Huflederhaut unserer Haussaeugetiere. Zeitschr f Anat u Entwicklungsgesch 1938;108:211–44 [in German].
32. Bowker RM, Brewer AM, Vex KB, et al. Sensory receptors in the equine foot. Am J Vet Res 1993;54:1840–4.
33. Bowker RM, Linder KE, Sonea IM. Sensory nerve fibres and receptors in equine distal forelimbs and their potential role in locomotion. Equine Vet J 1995;18 (Suppl):141–6.
34. Buda O, Budras KD. Segment specific nerve supply of the equine hoof. Pferdeheilkunde 2005;21:280–4.
35. Bowker RM. Innervation of the equine foot: its importance to the horse and to the clinician. In: Floya A, Mansmann R, editors. Equine podiatry. St Louis (MO): Saunders; 2007. p. 74–89.
36. Sack WO. Nerve distribution in the metacarpus and front digit of the horse. J Am Vet Med Assoc 1975;167:298–305.
37. Parks A. Form and function of the equine digit. Vet Clin North Am Equine Pract 2003;19:285–307.
38. Molyneux GS, Haller CJ, Mogg K, et al. The structure, innervation and location of arteriovenous anastomoses in the equine foot. Equine Vet J 1994;26: 305–12.
39. Bowker RM, Rockershouser SJ, Linder K, et al. A silver-impregnation and immunocytochemical study of innervation of the distal sesamoid bone and its suspensory ligaments in the horse. Equine Vet J 1994;26:212–9.
40. Engiles JB. Pathology of the distal phalanx in equine laminitis: more than just skin deep. Vet Clin North Am Equine Pract 2010;26:155–65.
41. Khoromi S, Muniyappa R, Nackers L, et al. Effects of chronic osteoarthritis pain on neuroendocrine function in men. J Clin Endocrinol Metab 2006;91: 4313–8.
42. Clauw DJ, Chrousos GP. Chronic pain and fatigue syndromes: overlapping clinical and neuroendocrine features and potential pathogenic mechanisms. Neuroimmunomodulation 1997;4:134–53.
43. Zimmermann M. Pathobiology of neuropathic pain. Eur J Pharmacol 2001;429: 23–37.

44. Treede RD, Jensen TS, Campbell JN, et al. Neuropathic pain: redefinition and a grading system for clinical and research purposes. Neurology 2008;70: 1630–5.

45. Scholz J, Woolfe CJ. Can we conquer pain? Nat Neurosci 2002;5:1062–7.

46. Moore RM, Eades SC, Stokes AM. Evidence for vascular and enzymatic events in the pathophysiology of acute laminitis: which pathway is responsible for initiation of this process in horses? Equine Vet J 2004;36:204–9.

47. Eades SC. Overview of current laminitis research. Vet Clin North Am Equine Pract 2010;26:51–63.

48. Pollitt CC. Update on the pathophysiology of laminitis. In: Proceedings of the 10th Geneva Congress of Equine Medicine and Surgery. Geneva (Switzerland), 2009. p. 12–5.

49. Van Eps AW, Leise B, Watts M, et al. Digital hypothermia inhibits early laminar inflammatory signaling in the oligofructose laminitis model. In: Proceedings of ACVIM Forum. Anaheim (CA), 2010.

50. Belknap JK, Giguere S, Pettigrew A, et al. Lamellar pro-inflammatory cytokine expression patterns in laminitis at the developmental stage and at the onset of lameness: innate vs. adaptive immune response. Equine Vet J 2007;39:42–7.

51. Kidd BL, Urban LA. Mechanisms of inflammatory pain. Br J Anaesth 2001;87: 3–11.

52. Rydevik B, Lundborg G, Bagge U. Effects of graded compression on intraneural blood blow. An in vivo study on rabbit tibial nerve. J Hand Surg Am 1981;6:3–12.

53. Dahlin LB, McLean WG. Effects of graded experimental compression on slow and fast axonal transport in rabbit vagus nerve. J Neurol Sci 1986;72:19–30.

54. Dilley A, Lynn B, Pang SJ. Pressure and stretch mechanosensitivity of peripheral nerve fibres following local inflammation of the nerve trunk. Pain 2005;117:462–72.

55. Arnoldi CC. Intraosseous hypertension. A possible cause of low back pain? Clin Orthop Relat Res 1976;115:30–4.

56. Arnoldi CC, Lemperg K, Linderholm H. Intraosseous hypertension and pain in the knee. J Bone Joint Surg Br 1975;57:360–3.

57. Arnoldi CC, Linderholm H, Mussbichler H. Venous engorgement and intraosseous hypertension in osteoarthritis of the hip. J Bone Joint Surg Br 1972;54: 409–21.

58. Morisset S, Hawkins JF, Kooreman K. High intraosseous pressure as a cause of lameness in a horse with a degloving injury of the metatarsus. J Am Vet Med Assoc 1999;215:1478–80.

59. Welch RD, Johnston CE 2nd, Waldron MJ, et al. Intraosseous infusion of prostaglandin E2 in the caprine tibia. J Orthop Res 1993;11:110–21.

60. Welch RD, Johnston CE 2nd, Waldron MJ, et al. Bone changes associated with intraosseous hypertension in the caprine tibia. J Bone Joint Surg Am 1993;75:53–60.

61. Welch RD, Waldron MJ, Hulse DA, et al. Intraosseous infusion using the osteoport implant in the caprine tibia. J Orthop Res 1992;10:789–99.

62. Pleasant RS, Baker GJ, Foreman JH, et al. Intraosseous pressure and pathologic changes in horses with navicular disease. Am J Vet Res 1993;54:7–12.

63. De Laat MA, McGowan CM, Sillence MN, et al. Equine laminitis: Induced by 48 h hyperinsulinaemia in Standardbred horses. Equine Vet J 2010;42:129–35.

64. Jones E, Vinuela-Fernandez I, Eager RA, et al. Neuropathic changes in equine laminitis pain. Pain 2007;132:321–31.

65. Rempel D, Dahlin L, Lundborg G. Pathophysiology of nerve compression syndromes: response of peripheral nerves to loading. J Bone Joint Surg Am 1999;81:1600–10.

66. Dellemijn P. Are opioids effective in relieving neuropathic pain? Pain 1999;80: 453–62.
67. Miletic G, Dumitrascu CI, Honstad CE, et al. Loose ligation of the rat sciatic nerve elicits early accumulation of Shank1 protein in the post-synaptic density of spinal dorsal horn neurons. Pain 2010;149:152–9.
68. Wall PD. Neuropathic pain and injured nerve: central mechanisms. Br Med Bull 1991;47:631–43.
69. Truini A, Cruccu G. Pathophysiological mechanisms of neuropathic pain. Neurol Sci 2006;27(Suppl 2):S179–82.
70. Gilron I, Watson CP, Cahill CM, et al. Neuropathic pain: a practical guide for the clinician. CMAJ 2006;175:265–75.
71. Koltzenburg M, McMahon SB. The enigmatic role of the sympathetic nervous system in chronic pain. Trends Pharmacol Sci 1991;12:399–402.
72. Baron R, Levine JD, Fields HL. Causalgia and reflex sympathetic dystrophy: does the sympathetic nervous system contribute to the generation of pain? Muscle Nerve 1999;22:678–95.
73. Reid AJ, Welin D, Wiberg M, et al. Peripherin and ATF3 genes are differentially regulated in regenerating and non-regenerating primary sensory neurons. Brain Res 2010;1310:1–7.
74. Li CY, Zhang XL, Matthews EA, et al. Calcium channel alpha2delta1 subunit mediates spinal hyperexcitability in pain modulation. Pain 2006;125:20–34.
75. Klusakova I, Dubovy P. Experimental models of peripheral neuropathic pain based on traumatic nerve injuries—an anatomical perspective. Ann Anat 2009;191:248–59.
76. Woolf CJ, Mannion RJ. Neuropathic pain: aetiology, symptoms, mechanisms, and management. Lancet 1999;353:1959–64.
77. Loftus JP, Black SJ, Pettigrew A, et al. Early laminar events involving endothelial activation in horses with black walnut- induced laminitis. Am J Vet Res 2007;68: 1205–11.
78. Fontaine GL, Belknap JK, Allen D, et al. Expression of interleukin-1beta in the digital laminae of horses in the prodromal stage of experimentally induced laminitis. Am J Vet Res 2001;62:714–20.
79. Burnett MG, Zager EL. Pathophysiology of peripheral nerve injury: a brief review. Neurosurg Focus 2004;16:E1.
80. De Felipe C, Hunt SP. The differential control of c-jun expression in regenerating sensory neurons and their associated glial cells. J Neurosci 1994;14:2911–23.
81. Sumano Lopez H, Hoyos Sepulveda ML, Brumbaugh GW. Pharmacologic and alternative therapies for the horse with chronic laminitis. Vet Clin North Am Equine Pract 1999;15:345–62.
82. Moyer W, Schumacher J. Are drugs effective treatment for horses with acute laminitis? In: 54th Annual Convention of the American Association of Equine Practitioners. San Diego (CA), 2008. p. 334–40.
83. Moses VS, Bertone AL. Nonsteroidal anti-inflammatory drugs. Vet Clin North Am Equine Pract 2002;18:21–37, v.
84. Stein C. Peripheral mechanisms of opioid analgesia. Anesth Analg 1993;76: 182–91.
85. Angst MS, Clark JD. Opioid-induced hyperalgesia: a qualitative systematic review. Anesthesiology 2006;104:570–87.
86. Anand U, Otto WR, Casula MA, et al. The effect of neurotrophic factors on morphology, TRPV1 expression and capsaicin responses of cultured human DRG sensory neurons. Neurosci Lett 2006;399:51–6.

87. Neubert JK, Mannes AJ, Karai LJ, et al. Perineural resiniferatoxin selectively inhibits inflammatory hyperalgesia. Mol Pain 2008;4:3.
88. Neubert JK, Karai L, Jun JH, et al. Peripherally induced resiniferatoxin analgesia. Pain 2003;104:219–28.
89. Brown DC, Iadarola MJ, Perkowski SZ, et al. Physiologic and antinociceptive effects of intrathecal resiniferatoxin in a canine bone cancer model. Anesthesiology 2005;103:1052–9.
90. da Cunha AF, Stokes AM, Chirgwin S, et al. Quantitative expression of the TRPV-1 gene in central and peripheral nervous tissue in horses. Int J Appl Res Vet Med 2008;6:15–23.
91. van Eps AW, Pollitt CC. Equine laminitis: cryotherapy reduces the severity of the acute lesion. Equine Vet J 2004;36:255–60.
92. van Eps AW, Pollitt CC. Equine laminitis model: cryotherapy reduces the severity of lesions evaluated seven days after induction with oligofructose. Equine Vet J 2009;41:741–6.
93. van Eps AW, Walters LJ, Baldwin GI, et al. Distal limb cryotherapy for the prevention of acute laminitis. Clin Tech Equine Pract 2004;3:64–70.
94. van Eps AW. Therapeutic hypothermia (cryotherapy) to prevent and treat acute laminitis. Vet Clin North Am Equine Pract 2010;26:125–33.
95. Goetz TE. Anatomic, hoof, and shoeing considerations for the treatment of laminitis in horses. J Am Vet Med Assoc 1987;190:1323.
96. Parks AH, Balch OK, Collier MA. Treatment of acute laminitis. Supportive therapy. Vet Clin North Am Equine Pract 1999;15:363–74.
97. Eustace RA, Caldwell MN. The construction of the heart bar shoe and the technique of dorsal wall resection. Equine Vet J 1989;21:367–9.
98. Peremans K, Verschooten F, De Moor A, et al. Laminitis in the pony: conservative treatment vs dorsal hoof wall resection. Equine Vet J 1991;23:243–6.
99. Steward ML. The use of the wooden shoe (Steward Clog) in treating laminitis. Vet Clin North Am Equine Pract 2010;26:207–14.
100. Curtis S, Ferguson DW, Luikart R, et al. Trimming and shoeing the chronically affected horse. Vet Clin North Am Equine Pract 1999;15:463–80.
101. Parks A, O'Grady SE. Chronic laminitis: current treatment strategies. Vet Clin North Am Equine Pract 2003;19:393–416.
102. Rucker A. Equine venography and its clinical application in North America. Vet Clin North Am Equine Pract 2010;26:167–77.
103. Rucker A. Chronic laminitis: strategic hoof wall resection. Vet Clin North Am Equine Pract 2010;26:197–205.
104. Pollitt CC, Baldwin H, Collins SN. Digital venography. In: Ross M, Dyson S, editors. Diagnosis and management of lameness in the horse. St Louis (MO): Saunders; 2010.
105. Eustace RA, Emery SL. Partial coronary epidermectomy (coronary peel), dorsodistal wall fenestration and deep digital flexor tenotomy to treat severe acute founder in a Connemara pony. Equine Vet Educ 2009;21:91–9.
106. Fehrenbacher JC, Taylor CP, Vasko MR. Pregabalin and gabapentin reduce release of substance P and CGRP from rat spinal tissues only after inflammation or activation of protein kinase C. Pain 2003;105:133–41.
107. Bauer CS, Nieto-Rostro M, Rahman W, et al. The increased trafficking of the calcium channel subunit alpha2delta-1 to presynaptic terminals in neuropathic pain is inhibited by the alpha2delta ligand pregabalin. J Neurosci 2009;29:4076–88.

108. Mich PM, Horne WA. Alternative splicing of the Ca2+ channel beta4 subunit confers specificity for gabapentin inhibition of Cav2.1 trafficking. Mol Pharmacol 2008;74:904–12.
109. Terry R, McDonnell S, van Eps AW, et al. Pharmacokinetic profile and behavioral effects of gabapentin in the horse. J Vet Pharm Ther, in press.
110. Qian J, Brown SD, Carlton SM. Systemic ketamine attenuates nociceptive behaviors in a rat model of peripheral neuropathy. Brain Res 1996;715:51–62.
111. Amr YM. Multi-day low dose ketamine infusion as adjuvant to oral gabapentin in spinal cord injury related chronic pain: a prospective, randomized, double blind trial. Pain Physician 2010;13:245–9.
112. Matthews NS, Fielding CI, Swineboard E. How to use a ketamine constant rate infusion in horses for analgesia. In: 50th Annual Convention of the American Association of Equine Practitioners. Denver (CO), 2004: p. 1431.

# Index

*Note:* Page numbers of article titles are in **boldface** type.

## A

$\alpha_2$-Adrenergic drugs, in visceral pain management, 607–609
Adrenergic receptors, pharmacology of, 515–517
$\alpha_2$-Agonist(s)
    analgesic actions of, 517–525
    in pain management, 478, **515–532**
        antagonists of, 525–526
        clinical relevance of, 526
    intraoperative use of, 523–525
    opioids and, 497–498
    pharmacokinetics of, 517
    routes of administration of, 517–522
        epidural, 521–522
        intercostal, 522
        intra-articular, 522
        intravenous regional, 522
        systemic, 517–521
Analgesia/analgesics
    intra-articular, opioids, 507–508
    ketamine and, 571–573
    opioid, **493–514.** See also *Opioid analgesia/analgesics.*
    spinal, **551–564.** See also *Spinal analgesia.*
    stress-induced, 481–482
    transdermal fentanyl analgesia, 508
Anesthesia/anesthetics
    inhalational, opioid analgesia/analgesics and, 499–501
    lidocaine, effects of, 539–540
    local, as pain therapy, 475–476, **533–549**
        systemic use of, historical perspective on, 533–534
    spinal, **551–564.** See also *Spinal anesthetics.*
    total intravenous, opioid analgesia/analgesics and, 498
Anti-inflammatory drugs, nonsteroidal, in pain management, 477
    joint pain, in osteoarthritis, 626–629
    visceral pain, 609
Antinociception, lidocaine-induced, mechanisms of, 535–539. See also *Lidocaine-induced antinociception.*
Antispasmodic(s), in visceral pain management, 612
Articular tissues, innervation of, osteoarthritis and, 623–624

## B

Betamethasone acetate, in joint pain management in osteoarthritis, 631
Butorphanol, in visceral pain management, 609–610

Vet Clin Equine 26 (2010) 673–679
doi:10.1016/S0749-0739(10)00100-8
0749-0739/10/$ – see front matter © 2010 Elsevier Inc. All rights reserved.

vetequine.theclinics.com

# Moving?

## Make sure your subscription moves with you!

To notify us of your new address, find your **Clinics Account Number** (located on your mailing label above your name), and contact customer service at:

**Email: journalscustomerservice-usa@elsevier.com**

**800-654-2452** (subscribers in the U.S. & Canada)
**314-447-8871** (subscribers outside of the U.S. & Canada)

**Fax number: 314-447-8029**

**Elsevier Health Sciences Division
Subscription Customer Service
3251 Riverport Lane
Maryland Heights, MO 63043**

*To ensure uninterrupted delivery of your subscription, please notify us at least 4 weeks in advance of move.

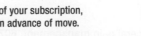

Printed and bound by CPI Group (UK) Ltd, Croydon, CR0 4YY

03/10/2024

01040458-0002